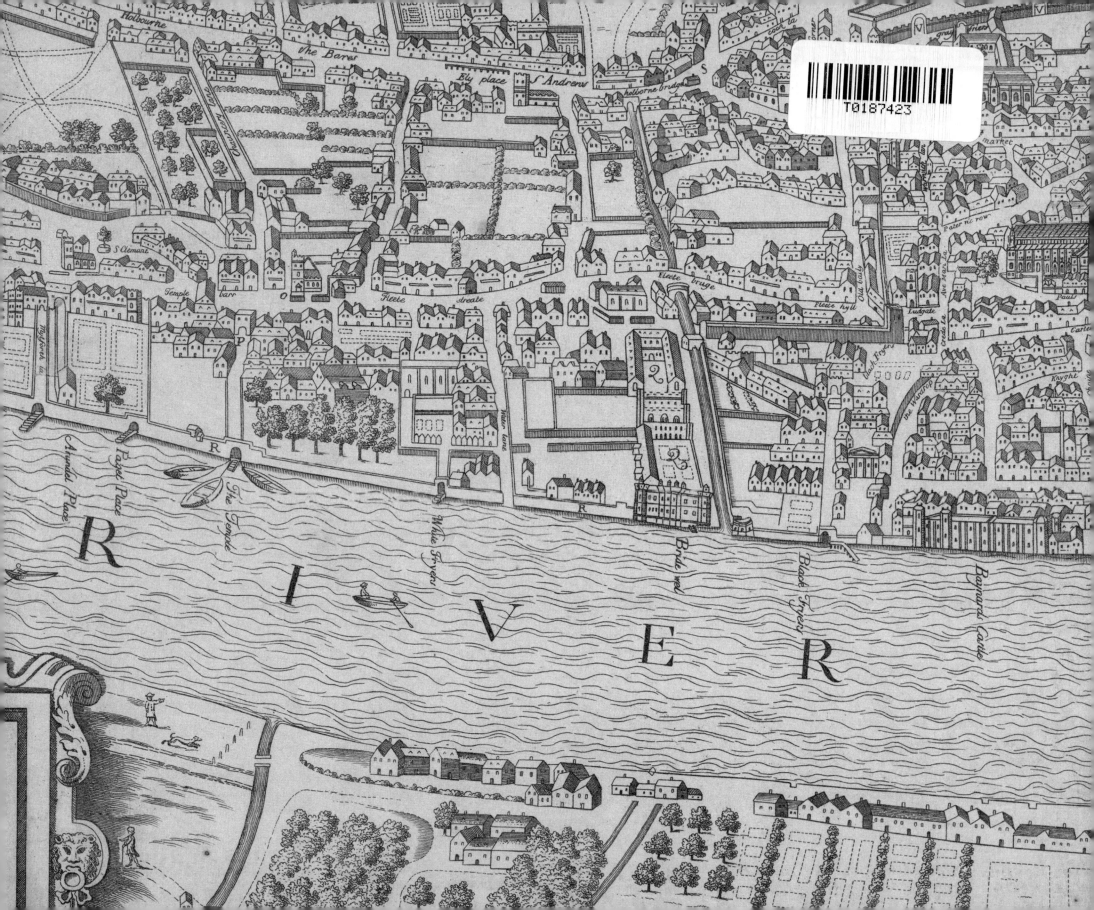

Holbourne
the Bares
Ely place   S.Andrew
helborne bridge
cook la
grey friers
market
S.Clemont
Pater no row
Temple   barr
Fleete   streate
Fleete bruge
Fleete hyll
Old baily
Pauls
Ludgate
Credo la   Ave Mar la
Carter
Black friers
the Wardrop
Knyght
Hofford la
Water lane
R
R
Arundel Place
Paget Place
The Temple
White Fryers
Bride wel
Black fryers
Baynards Castle

R I V E R

500 YEARS OF THE ROYAL COLLEGE OF PHYSICIANS

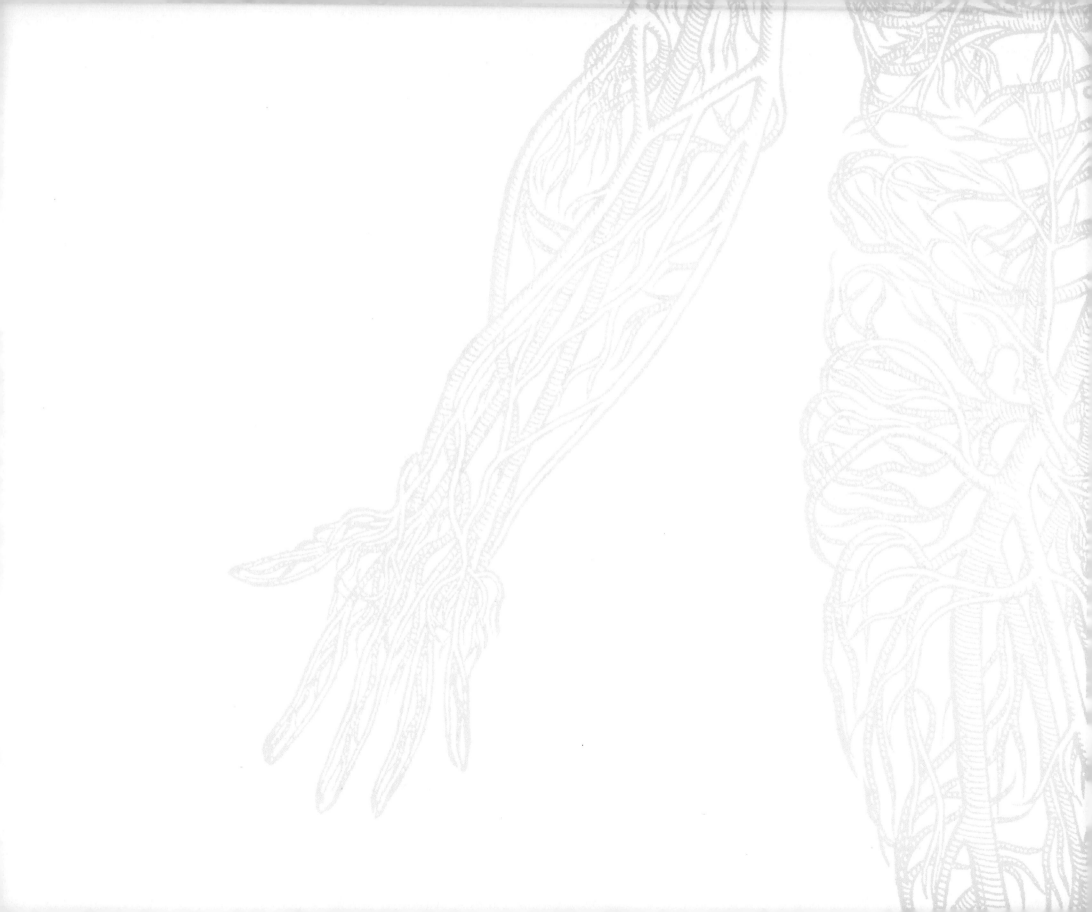

500 YEARS OF THE ROYAL COLLEGE OF PHYSICIANS

Edited by Linda Luxon *&* Simon Shorvon
with Julie Beckwith

Third Millenium Publishing

Contributors

J. Beckwith   H. Oakeley

S. Bowman   S. Shorvon

H. Hodgson   R. Thompson

L. Luxon

First published in Great Britain in 2018 by Third Millennium Publishing (an imprint of Profile Books Ltd)

Third Millennium Publishing Ltd
3 Holford Yard
Bevin Way
London WC1X 9HD
United Kingdom
www.tmbooks.com

ISBN: 978 1 781259 11 5

Project manager: Susan Millership
Design: John Dowling

Reprographics by BORN London.
Printed and bound in Italy
by L.E.G.O. SpA.

 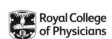

Royal College of Physicians

1518
2018
500 years of medicine

Contents

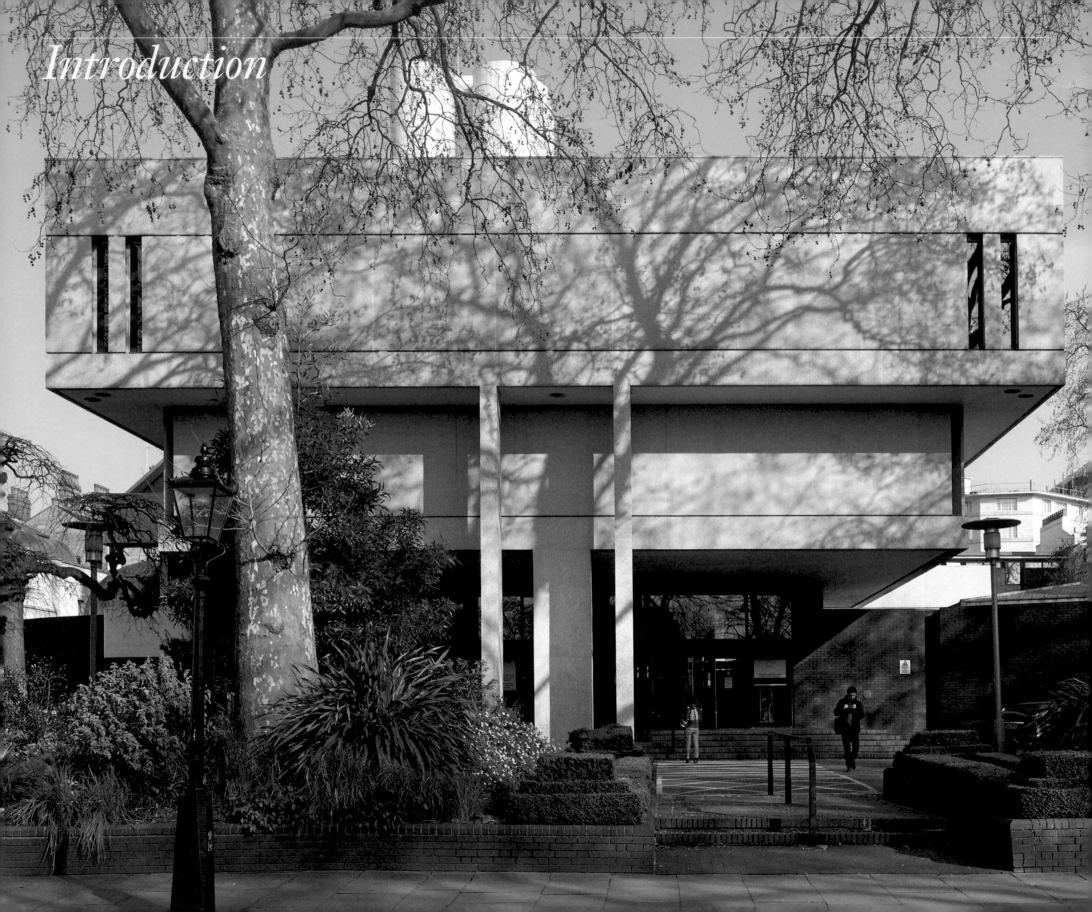

The year 2018 marks 500 years of the Royal College of Physicians – the oldest medical institution in England. Over this time, in different ways and with varying degrees of success, physicians have influenced the social and cultural life of Britain and its history, as well as contributing to population health both in the UK and globally. The College is marking the occasion of the establishment of the College on 23 September 1518, by a charter granted by King Henry VIII, with a series of celebratory events throughout 2018, and this book contributes to these commemorations.

This book provides a series of illustrated historical impressions, painting a picture of the changing environment of the College and role of physicians over the centuries, within the context of the changes in medicine and medical practice, to complement the other previously published historical narratives. Since its foundation, the primary intentions of the College have been to improve health and healthcare and to assist in the maintenance of the highest standards of medical care. However, in addition, through its library, archives and collections, the College has encouraged learning and the acquisition of knowledge on a much broader front, and these facilities have been used extensively in the writing and illustration of this book.

The editors have compiled the book with contributions from a number of distinguished colleagues: Professor Simon Bowman, Professor Humphrey Hodgson, Dr Henry Oakeley and Sir Richard Thompson. Dr Henry Oakeley also kindly provided additional material for each chapter and assisted in manuscript corrections. Their knowledge and expertise have been invaluable.

The editors would also like to thank many colleagues who have contributed to the production of this book, but especially: the President, senior officers and staff of the Royal College of Physicians, notably the staff of the strategy, communications and policy department and the heritage team; the image researchers, Elinor Pritchard and Giselle Weiss for their search for relevant images; and Third Millennium Publishing, particularly Peter Jones, Susan Millership and Patrick Taylor, and the designer John Dowling, for their attention to detail, content and design. Without the patience, advice and expertise of all these colleagues, the production of this book would not have been possible.

Julie Beckwith, Linda Luxon and Simon Shorvon
London, October 2017

1 Antecedents

...tia 7 vocabulo2 obſcuritate. Quantaue infamia domi/
nis medicis: 7 viris egregis doctis inde eueniat excogi
tari: vir pōt ... rite cōpſita eē egro
ſalutem ꝑmittat. Sperates huius artis artifices diſpē
ſas ſuas ꝑm mentes Meſue diſpenſare. Et ipſi auſu te
merario qd ꝓ quo addunt. 7 tunc medicine virtus di
uerſificat. vt ꝑnceps medico2 ſcribit. Auic. quinto ca
nonis.cap.de tyriaca. Et ꝓr vulgi infamiam apothe/
cario2 ignauia medici incurrūt. Tu.n.ß meo opuſcu
lo nō indiges. Lu3 huius artis tādiu 7 doctrina 7 ex̄pe
rictia cōꝓbatus fueris. Sed volui tibi tāꝗ cariori di/
gniori2 ad corrigendum deſtinare. Quare illū excu/
ties:abijciaſꝗ:ſi qd in eo ſupfluū cōpies:demum illu3
in lucem adire ꝑmittas:vt tuo ingenio libelliꝗ doctri
na rudes te imitari coneuf. Qui ſoles tua ꝓdētia nō
ſolum apothecarios:ſed 7 nouos medicos in ordinā/
do dirigere.Uale diu felix.

℧ Opus qd aggredior in quinꝗ 7 decem diſtinctiōes
erit diuiſum.

℧ Prima erit de confectionibus aromaticis. Et conti
net deſcriptiones.22. Quarum prima eſt.

Lectuariū ð gēmis Meſue cu
ius iuuamentu3 eſt
magnu3 ad egritudines cerebri cordis ſto
maci epatis 7 matricis fridas: 7 nos ſumus
ex̄pti inquit Meſue bonitate3 eius ad tre
more3 cordis:. 7 ſincopim :7 debilitate ſtomachi: 7
qn aliꝗ triſtat 7 neſcit radice3: 7 ei qui diligit ſolitudi/
ne3.7 ſūt eo vſi reges 7 magnates.trahit.n.eos in ꝓñas
bono2 mo2 7 nobilium 7 dilatat aiam 7 facit corporis
odore3 7 colore3 bonu3. ℞.alba2 margaritaru3.3.ij.
fragmēto2 3aphiri iacitbi ſardinis granato2 ſeru3egi.
i.ſmeraldi.añ.3.i.ſ.3edoario do2onigi corticu3 citri ma
cis:ſe.alphelen.ſemiſc.i.o3imi gariofilati.añ.3.ij.corallo
rum rubeo2um karabe limature ebo2is.añ.Э.ij.bebē al
bi 7 rubei:ſunt ꝗdam radices que de armenia defern̄/
tur gariofilo2 3in3iberis pi ... is longi croci ſpice ſolū.be

pidē molare ducere libet vt magis ſubtilis ſit.igit̄ nūꝗ
in triturādo eos ſeſſus ſis.q̄ ꝗto ſbtilio2es tāto pfecio
res exiſtūt. ℧ 3urūbet ñ ē 3edoaria: vt Mattheus ſil
exponit cū Aui.2°.cañ.diuerſa de eis faciat capᵅ. ſ3 3u/
rūbet ē ꝗdā radix ſilis cipo groſſior 3edoariaitus ſub c
trini odore aromatica 7 ſapore acuto.minus tñ 3edoa/
ſ3 ſi caremus ea loco ipſius 3edoaria3 ponimus. ℧ D
aureo pondere ðria eſt inter docto2es de eo 7 magna.
dam dñt vt gentilis ꝗ eſt pondus.3.i.ſ.7 ß affirmat ſi
mó Januen. Alij dñt ꝗ eſt 7ª ꝑs vncie. S3 cōis 7 va
ciſio eſt ꝗ ſi inueniat aureū.i.vt in ß loco 7 iomnibu
alijs medicinis nō ſolutiuis idem eſt qd.3.i.ſ.in medici
nis vo ſolutiuis ſi repit idem eſt qd 7ª partes vncie
plus. ℧ Inſuꝑ q̄ cōfectio ß 7 ſequentes pp laſciuiā
hoium fieri ſolēt in mo2ſellis quantitas ſpēru ad 3uch
ru declāda eſt Jo ad oēm libram.i.3ucha.appói d3.3.
ſpē2 cribellata2.cribellata2 dico pp ſimplicia que cri
bellari nō pñt vt amigdale dactili ſcia oia 7ē.Ad oē3 v
li.i.mellis ſpē2 cribellata2.vt.ß.ℨ.iij.Et ß mó ſaciēd
bñt dñi medici 7 egri virtūte medicina2. a docto2ibᵒ l
mitatā.Secus āt faciunt apothecarij ñri tpis auariti
ducti:ꝗ ignoſcat illis deus 7ē.℧ Nō inſuꝑ ꝗ Meſu
dic ꝓfice cū melle ēblico2: 7 colatura geleniabin. Jo
forte illa facere vis:ſcias ꝗ mel emblico2 ß mó ſit.℞
mirabolano2 emblico2.ℨ.ij.aꝗ cōis lib.ij.Terant ſu
tilr dicti mirabolani 7 infundant ꝑ dies.vij.in dcā aꝗ
poſtea buliāt vſꝗ ad cōſumptione3 medietatis. deinde
colent cū pāno lineo bñ māibus ex̄ꝑmendo:7 in dcā
latura addat mellis boni.lib.i.7 buliant ſil vſꝗ ad con
ſumptōe3 aꝗ 7 coctidem mellis: 7 reſeruet.ß.n.df me
emblico2.Accipe ergo mel. ēblico2:geleniabin.i.me
roſa2.añ.li.ſ.ſupraſcripta2 ſpē2.ℨ.iij.7 ſil miſce: 7 h
bis eiu3 de gēmis in forma liꝗda vt ſcribit meſue.7 h
ſis eſt ab aureo medio vſꝗ ad aureum vnū.℧ De gel
niabin iter docto2es eſt ðria.nam Aui.ſ°cañ.ca°.de cō
ditis dicit.ꝗ geneliabin idem eſt qd roſa cōdita ſiue 7
melle ſiue cum 3ucharo. Et ſic tā 3ucharij roſa. ...

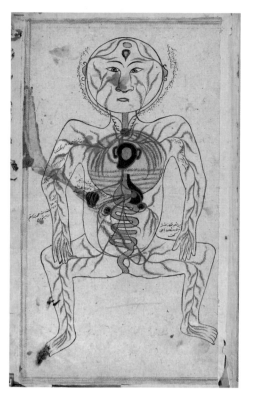

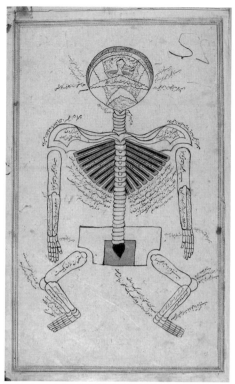

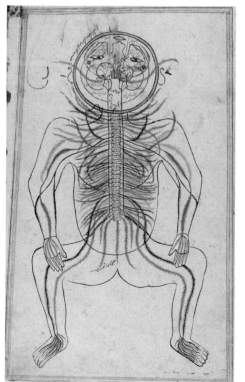

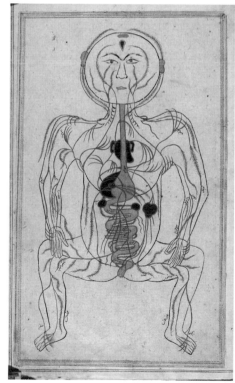

Opposite: The opening page of the *Lumen Apothecariorum* by Quirico de Augustis de Terthona of Milan (fl.1486–1497), published in 1512. It described hundreds of medicines from the Greek and Arabic traditions, and would have been one of the textbooks available to the founders of the College.

Left: Mansūr ibn Muhammad ibn Ahmad ibn Yūsuf ibn Ilyās (Mansūr) was a Persian physician who wrote his anatomy in 1386. It is remarkable for its illustrations, of which these are examples. These were the first coloured anatomical illustrations in the world. This copy is in the RCP's manuscript collection.

Above right: *Punica granatum*, the pomegranate, was called *Malum punicum* in 1543, when this woodcut appeared in Jean Ruel's *Commentaries on Dioscorides*. It is the model for the one on the College coat of arms.

Two thousand years and more of medicine preceded the foundation of the College of Physicians in 1518. During this time, other colleges had come and gone, beliefs and practices had changed (often with imperceptible slowness) and only the importance of diet, exercise and lifestyle had remained a cornerstone of healthcare. The Hippocratic Corpus, named for Hippocrates (*c.*460–370BC), the 'Father of Medicine' (although it is certain that he wrote relatively little of the content), was written between the 5th and 3rd century BC. This text – and in particular the Hippocratic Oath – testifies to the bond that exists between doctors, the loyalty and support they give each other, their duty to educate others in the discipline of medicine, and the ethics of duty of care to patients: to help and not to harm. It was this bond, this unity of belief and purpose, which (at least in part) led to the creation of the College in 1518. This bond has continued to this day through civil war and world wars; through the years when the study of botany, anatomy, physiology, pathology, epidemiology and a host of other '-ologies' overturned the shibboleths of the Doctrine of Signatures and of the four humours, along with the role of evil spirits, magic, divine will, Aristotelian logic and philosophy. All the sciences, from mathematics and chemistry to physics and in particular the pharmaceutical revolution, have contributed to changes unimaginable to our predecessors, but the great names of Aesculapius, Theophrastus, Hippocrates, Dioscorides and Galen – and those less well-remembered, such as Asclepiades, Andromachus, Celsus, Apuleius Platonicus, Nicolaus Salernitanus, Oribasius, Aëtius, Alexander of Tralles, Paulus Aeginetus, Abū Yūsuf Ya'qūb ibn Ishāq

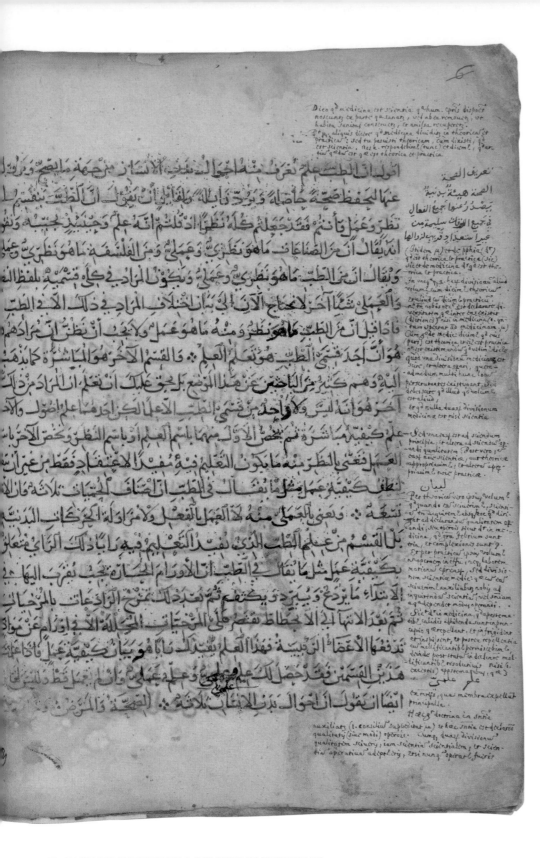

al-Kindī, Rhazes, Avicenna and Mesue – would all recognise the College as their home. Its fellows are the linear descendants of the physicians of Epidaurus, Cos, Salerno, Venice and Padua. Even Imhotep of Egypt, *c.*2980BC, the earliest physician whose name is known, would feel a kinship with Linacre, the first College President, although Imhotep's Step Pyramid at Giza rather dwarfs Linacre's house in Knightrider Street.

This book is an outline of the history of the College, known as the Royal College of Physicians since 1674. It is about the medical milestones, the personages and our contributions to each of five centuries of the College's existence, and what it means for the future. Its fellows are the College, not a hospital, clinic, surgery, health centre or office, but a college of physicians, a guild, a club, a medical freemasonry, a collegium or association, with roots going back to the beginning of time, and now looking forward. As Winston Churchill said when addressing the College in March 1944: 'The longer you can look back, the further you can look forward'. With this benediction the College should feel confident for its future for the next two or three thousand years, because it can look back a very, very long way.

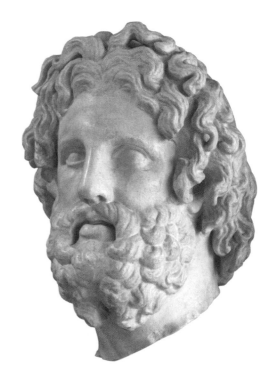

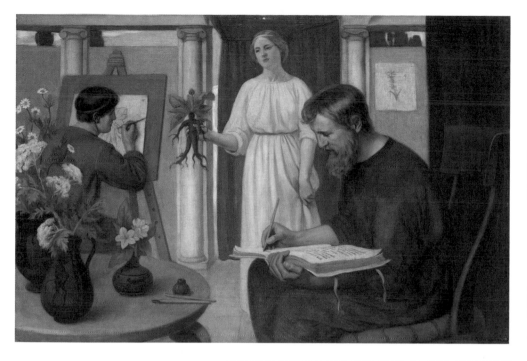

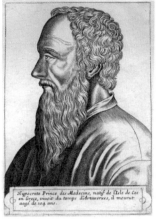

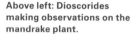

Above left: Dioscorides making observations on the mandrake plant.

Above right: Hippocrates (c.460–370BC) is regarded as the Father of Medicine. His humoural system of medicine persisted from the 4th century BC up to the beginning of the 20th century. Illnesses were distempers, an imbalance between hot, cold, yellow and black humours.

Left: *Platanus orientalis* var. *insularis*, a scion of an ancient tree on the Island of Cos under which Hippocrates taught his medical students, graces the lawn at the College.

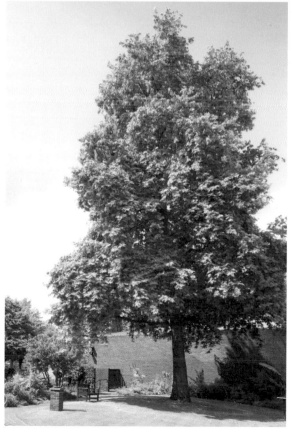

5th century BC to 1st century AD

In the marble atrium of the College, the Lasdun Hall, stands a sculpture – part Roman, part modern recreation, – of Aesculapius and Telesphorus. The former was the Greek god of healing, and although one of his daughters, Iaso, was the goddess of recuperation from illness, the Romans adopted Telesphorus, always a diminutive figure with a woolly hat or hooded cape, from Celtic mythology, to be a son of Aesculapius and the god of convalescence.

The temples of Aesculapius and Telesphorus at Pergamon and Epidaurus in the 4th century BC coexisted, and patients came to both to be healed. In the 2nd century BC the College of Aesculapius and Hygeia was founded in Rome. While it was not a medical college, it had a statute to Aesculapius – as there is in the Lasdun Hall – with an annual dinner to celebrate the emperor's birthday (the RCP celebrates William Harvey instead). It acted as a dining club and had its own statutes.

So while medically orientated social clubs did not practise medicine and have not needed to change much, schools of medicine were struggling to find a way to understand the world and their discipline. If they were to reject the concept that the gods made and ordained everything from mankind to disease, the physicians needed a structure to give them understanding. The four elements of Empedocles (c.490–c.430BC), earth, air, fire and water, united by one force (love) and separated by another (strife), were a workable philosophical hypothesis. Hippocrates (c.460–370BC) extended this to the four humours of which the human body was believed to be composed. Any illness was an imbalance of the humours. The nature of these humours was contested, but certainly it was accepted that the parts of the body could be made up of a mixture of different proportions of the humours. A cold winter's day would cause an increase in the cold, wet, phlegmatic humour represented by the runny nose and phlegm, and was to be treated by hot, red drinks with spices (e.g. mulled wine, or brandy and lemon) to restore the balance. Fevers were treated by removing the excess of the hot humour by bloodletting, or drinking cooling drinks – and pomegranate juice was esteemed for this, which may be the reason for its inclusion on the College coat of arms.

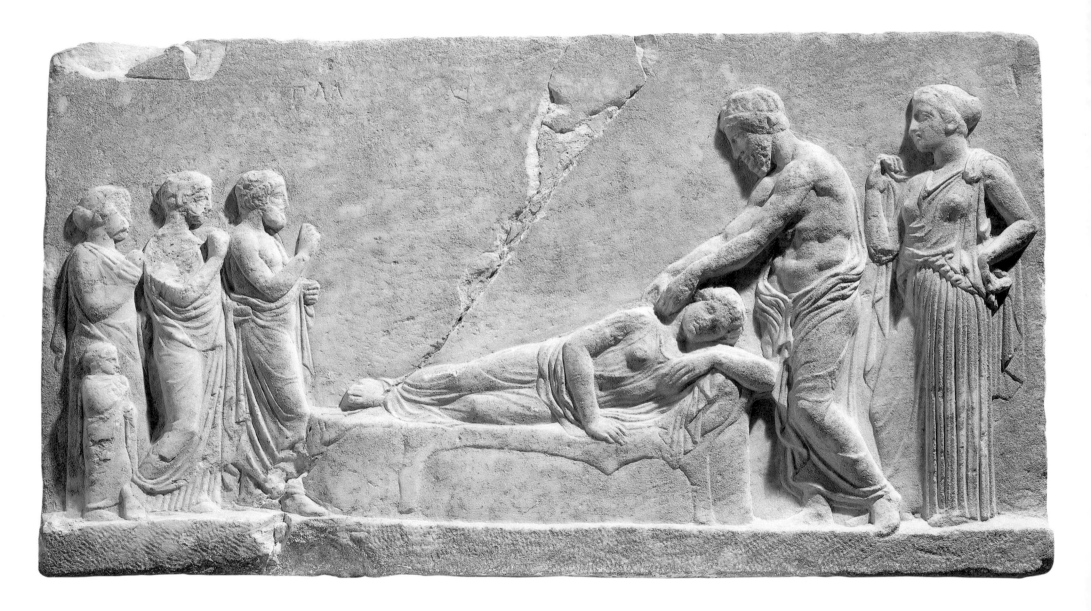

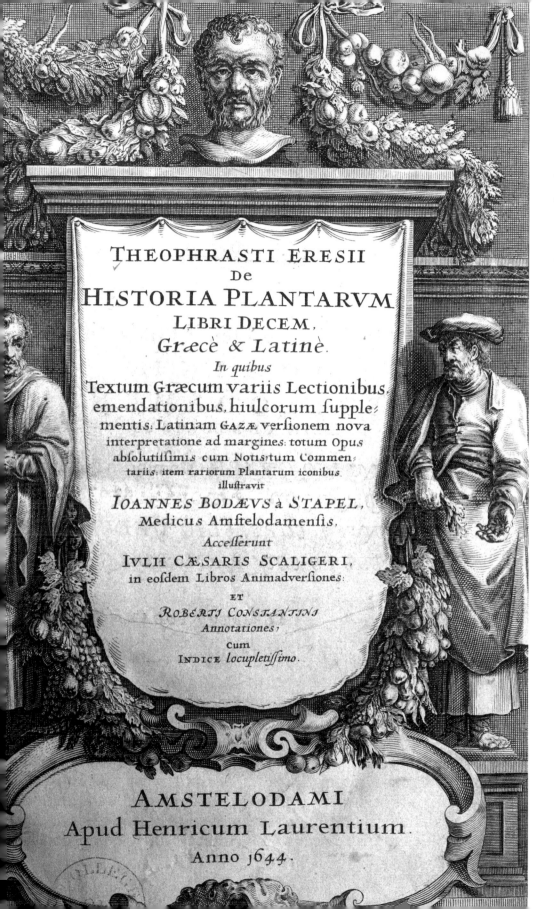

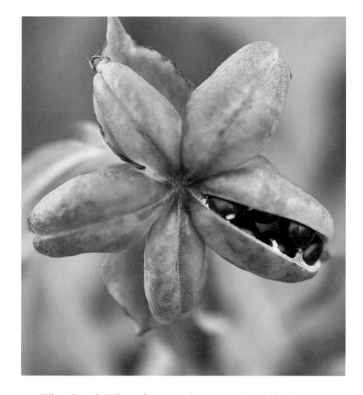

The Greek Theophrastus (*c.*371–*c.*287BC), is known as the Father of Botany because of his monumental *De Historia Plantarum* (The Enquiry into Plants) and *De Causis Plantarum* (The Causes of Plants) in which he described 500 plants, their anatomy and their classification. He was an empiricist, believing in observation, collection and classification – still the basis of clinical medicine.

He is the first to describe how the shape of plants determine their use, a belief system which has since permeated plant-based medicine as the Doctrine of Signatures. He refers to the Doctrine of the Humours, describing plants as 'binding' or 'heating', etc. He describes wrapping up a 'Cnidian berry' in bread, to take as a medicine to avoid it burning the throat – an early enteric coated tablet. He notes the plants that are sedative, poisonous, diuretic, styptic and, among others, those which cause vomiting or purging and those which are good for asthma. These were still being quoted by Pliny three centuries later. Theophrastus should also be called the Father of Pharmacy.

The six books of *De Medicina* of Aulus Cornelius Celsus (25BC–50AD), the only surviving parts of his immense encyclopaedia, are our best source of knowledge of Roman medicine. In book five, his chapter on pharmacy covers stopping bleeding, opening wounds, emollients, etc., with a list of the 'simples' and chemicals used for each condition and symptom. He proceeds to types of medicine: malagmas, plasters, antidotes, etc., which are compound medicines of plants and chemicals, and then to treatments for specific symptoms – and poppy (i.e. opium) is prominent in the ingredients for managing pain. Hippocratic humoural practices are there, but his use of medicines is extensive. His writings in this chapter, in particular his discussion on the treatment of cancer, are wonderfully clear, but his ramblings on bleeding are incomprehensible. Medical students could still learn his four signs of inflammation – *calor*, *dolor*, *tumor* and *rubor* – but it is unlikely that they would do this. His was the first medical book ever printed (in Florence in 1478). It was translated into English by a fellow of the College, Dr James Greive (1729–1773), physician to St Thomas' Hospital and the Charterhouse in 1756. Greive followed Linacre in making classical medicine available to a wider audience.

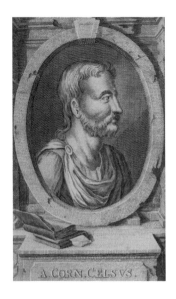

A. CORN. CELSVS

Left: Engraving of Aulus Cornelius Celsus (25BC–50AD), Roman encyclopaedist, who wrote on the history of medicine, pathology, diseases, anatomy, pharmacology, surgery and orthopaedics.

Right: The world's oldest botanical garden was created in Padua in 1545. It is laid out as four squares within a circle, of beds containing medicinal 'simples', surrounded by a high wall to prevent theft. It was founded by the university as a medicinal plant repository. It is now a UNESCO World Heritage Site. This illustration by Filippo Tomasini (1654) shows that the garden – a forerunner of the RCP's own medicinal garden – has not changed much in form to this day.

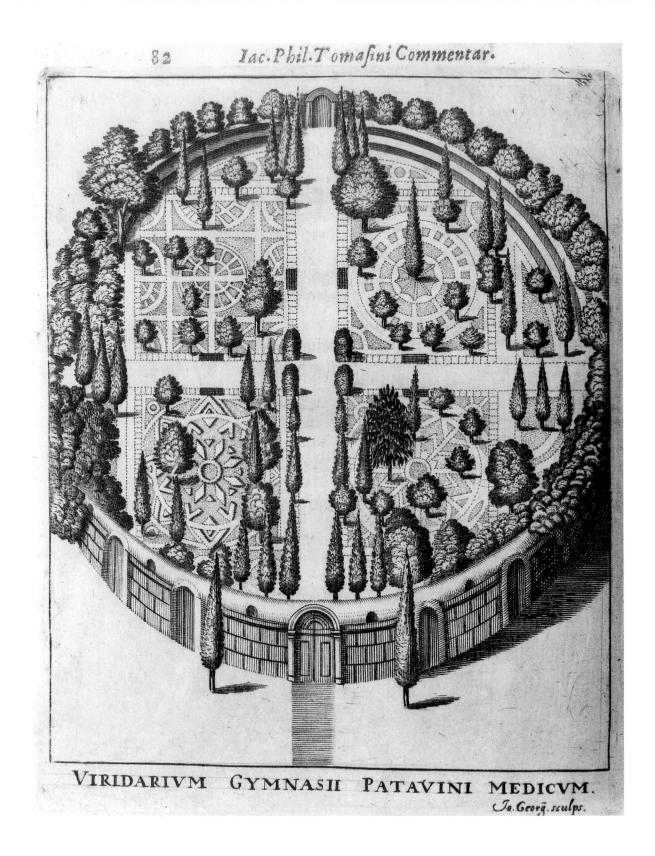

82   *Iac. Phil. Tomasini Commentar.*

VIRIDARIVM GYMNASII PATAVINI MEDICVM.

Jo. Georg. sculps.

'If strength will permit, it is best to let blood, especially if the fever be attended with a burning heat.'

Celsus, *De Medicina*, 50AD

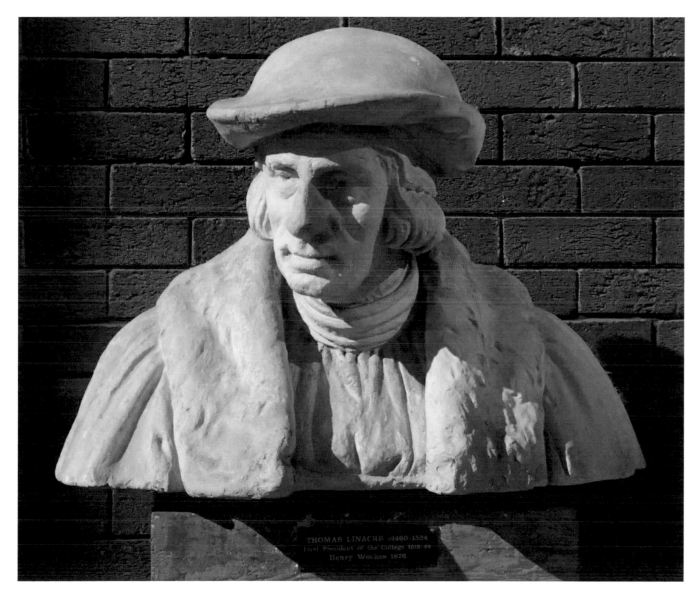

Pedanius Dioscorides (*c.*40–90AD) of Anazarbus (now Anavarza in southern Turkey) and Galen (129–*c.*200/216AD) of Pergamon (now Bergama in western Turkey) are the two dominant forces in medicine from the first centuries of the Christian era. The Dogmatics, Pneumatics, Empirics, Methodists, Stoics, Epicureans, Platonists, Erasistrateans and other medical sects fought over their patients and therapeutic practices, finally merging into the Eclectics under the dominance of Galen.

It is to Dioscorides, however, that medicine – or more precisely, medicines – owes the greater debt. Travelling around the known world in the footsteps of the Roman armies at the time of Nero and Caligula, he collected accounts of 600 plants and their medicinal uses, publishing them in a series of five books, the *Materia Medica* (*c.*70AD) – the Materials of Medicines. Copies were made, translated into Arabic and Latin, and used throughout Europe and Arabia. An illustrated version was made in 515 – the *Juliana Anicia Codex*, with 400 images. It came into print in Italy in 1478 in Latin, and in 1479 in Greek. The heavily illustrated *Commentaries on Dioscorides* by Ruel and Mattioli made them available to the world, and were the basis of herbals for the next 200 years, supplanting Galen in importance.

Galeni

De Optima corporis nostri constitutione,

De Bona habitudine,

De Cibis boni, & mali succi,

Ferdinando Balamio Siculo Interprete.

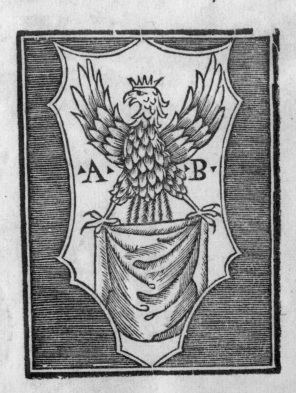

Claudius Galenus, Galen (129–*c.*200/216AD) of Pergamon in Turkey, came from a wealthy family and had a well-rounded education, studying medicine in the sanctuary of Aesculapius, and travelling. He spent four years caring for the gladiators in Pergamon. Aged 33, he moved to Rome to practise medicine. He spent time with the Roman army in Germany, coming back to Rome when it was hit by plagues which killed half the population of the Empire. And he wrote extensively.

With Galen, Hippocratic medicine comes of age, and with bloodletting and other practices he did immeasurable harm. He is a lesson to all authors, for so prolific was he that half of all the writings that have come down to us from the Graeco-Roman era were written by him, and while many are lost it is estimated that he wrote 500 treatises amounting to ten million words, of which three million survive. It is no surprise that the study of his works became the mainstay of the education of a physician for 1,400 years, that his writings became the gospel and that to challenge them amounted to heresy. Medical thought was overwhelmed and suppressed by the tsunami, the sheer volume, of his works and his all-pervading authority.

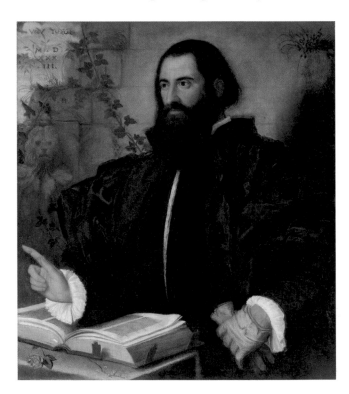

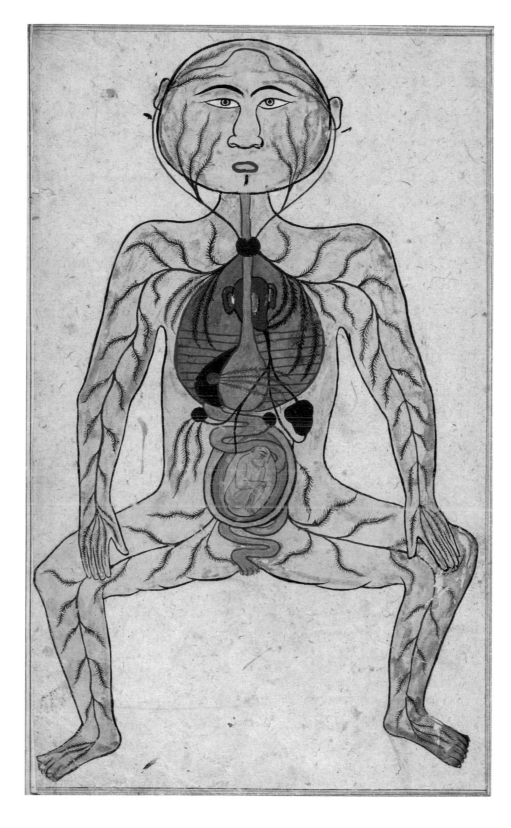

Far left: A classic Galenic treatise on the *Best constitution for our bodies; of Good living; of Good food and the Evils of damp*, translated from Greek into Latin, the common language of educated men, by the Sicilian physician Ferdinand Balamio in 1513. The healthy lifestyles that the College promotes today have not altered in 500 years.

Left: Painting of Pietro Andrea Mattioli by Alessandro Bonvicino (1533). Mattioli was the foremost publisher of commentaries on the works of Dioscorides, with over 50 editions in various languages. His woodcuts were the most important source of illustration and education as to the identity of the plants mentioned in the *Materia Medica of Dioscorides* (70AD) – the main source of knowledge of plant-based medicine for 1,700 years.

Right: An image of a pregnant woman from Mansūr's anatomy of 1386. Unlike all of the other images in the book, this image has no corresponding image in the Latin edition.

There is on the author's bookshelves such a book, a little Galenic work translated from Greek to Latin by Ferdinand Balamio the Sicilian. The book is a typical Galenic treatise on constitution, good living, good food and the evils of damp: nothing earth-shattering; a silent marker of the knowledge of our predecessors. It sits on the shelves, almost smug, as it knows that Balamio was physician to Pope Leo X (a lifelong friend of our founder Linacre), who excommunicated Martin Luther; and it is dedicated to Pope Clement VII, who excommunicated Henry VIII, and published by Antonio Blado in Rome in 1531 using the italic fonts from Ludovici degli Arrighi. While these were not the first italic fonts (the honour belongs to Francesco Griffo), Arrighi's fonts are the basis for modern italics. Blado used them later to publish the seminal works of Niccolò Machiavelli and Ignatius Loyola, the founder of the Jesuits. The greatest names in late medieval politics and theology are here linked to a book, from the greatest name in the practice of medicine, retrieved from a second-hand bookshop below the Croydon overpass next to unfashionable, fading copies of Henty's books for boys – a metaphor for the travels of Galenic medicine around the world and the fate of his philosophy.

Plants as the source of medicines were still important in the post-Galenic era, and the most influential was the 4th-century *Herbarius* of Apuleius Platonicus, sometimes called Pseudo-Apuleius, until the rise of the school of Salerno in the 10th–12th century. The earliest surviving copy is from the 6th century in Leiden, and has illustrations in the style of the *Juliana Anicia Codex*. The text is based on Pliny and Dioscorides. Seventeen manuscript herbals up to the 15th century derived their content from it, but in each of them more and more information accumulated, making it a valuable repository of a millennium of medicines. It came into print in 1481, and, as *L. Apulei De medicaminibus herbarum*, with a commentary by Humelberger, in 1537. It has 128 medicinal plants ('simples'), listed with their names in different countries. It describes the illnesses they treated, as one would expect, but the Renaissance can be detected in Humelberger's commentaries, for there are observations added. Humelberger describes the shape of the flower of Heliotrope (*Heliotropium europaeum*) and its behaviour, calling it a divine flower because it moved during the day to follow the sun, and at sunset the flowers closed.

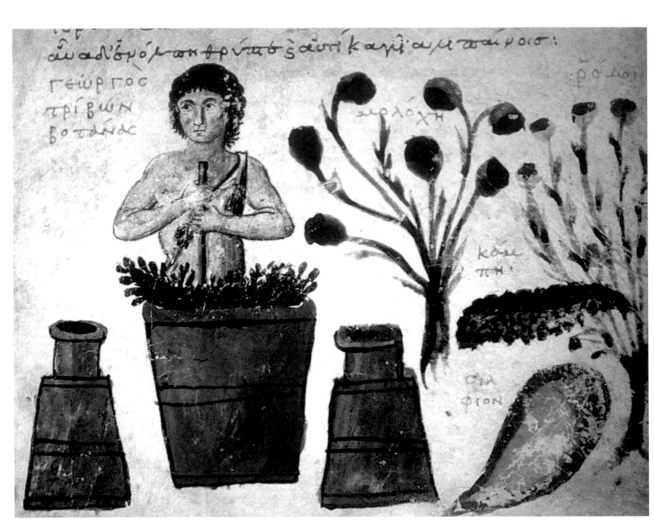

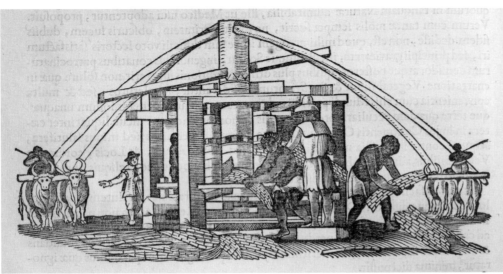

Above: An image from the 10th-century Byzantine manuscript *Theriaka y Alexipharmaka de Nicandro*, a treatise on the treatment of snake bites, showing plants being crushed in a mortar. Nicander of Colophon lived in the 2nd century BC and his *Theriaka* provides remedies for the bites of insects, snakes and wild animals.

Left: Sugar, so necessary for the preparation of Sloane's chocolate drinks and for making medicines palatable, came from the slave plantations in the Caribbean. These images show sugar cane being crushed to extract the juice which was then heated to make crystalline sugar. From Gulielmi Pisoni's *Historiae Naturalis & Medicae* (1658).

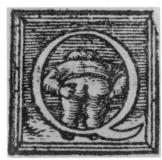

Above: The woodcut letter Q from the *Apuleius Platonicus Herbarium* of Hummelberger (1537). While this edition has no illustrations, it has tiny woodcut letters, 15mm square, for the beginning of each chapter, some wonderfully rude.

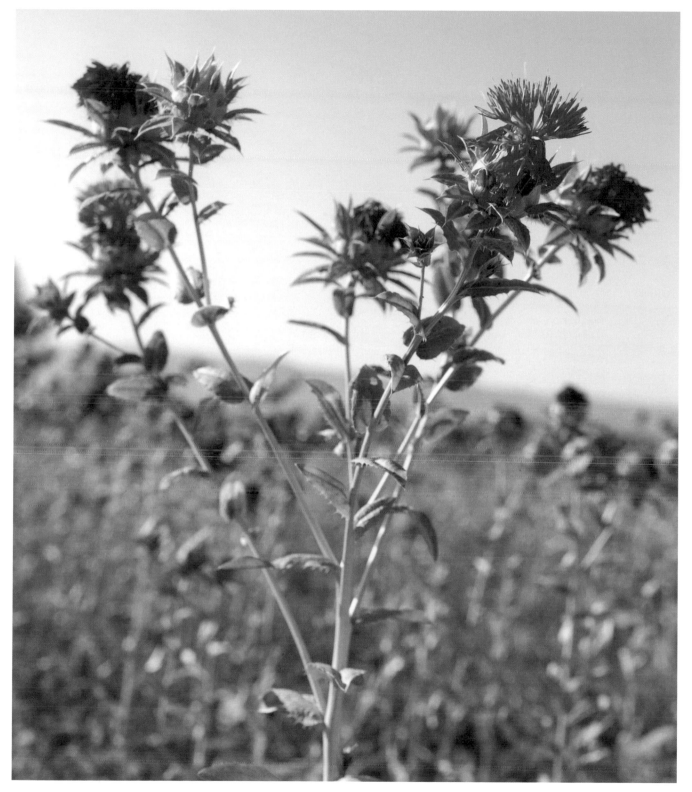

'The science of physic doth not make a man immortal.'

Avicenna, *Canon of Medicine*, 1025

With the Muslim conquests, beginning in the 7th century, Arabic medicine flourished, and with it their pharmacopoeias. One of the great physicians in the Golden Age of science and art in medieval Islam was Al-Kindī (*c.*800–870), in full: Abū Yūsuf Ya'qūb ibn Ishāq al-Kindī. He studied in Basra and Baghdad, became tutor to the son of the caliph, and studied the writings of Hippocrates, Plato, Aristotle, Euclid and other classical authors. In Baghdad, a world centre for science and medicine, he wrote his medical formulary, the *Agrābādhīn of Al-Kindī*. The word means a list of drugs or prescriptions, and this *Agrābādhīn* contains 226 compound medicines with their uses, followed by a list of 319 'simples', from which the medicines were made, exactly like Culpeper's *Physical Directory* (1649) in his translation of the College's *Pharmacopoeia Londinensis* (1618). Dioscorides had no compound medicines, and collected his 'simples' from the Eastern Mediterranean; Al-Kindī's plants included some from a wider area, and he gives different uses.

The *Agrābādhīn* formed the beginnings of European pharmacopoeias and dispensaries and scientifically proven medicines, while Dioscorides's *Materia Medica* was the formative text for the herbals and traditional herbal remedies that continue to be used to this day.

Left: Safflower, *Carthamus tinctorius*, was used by Dioscorides as a purgative and by Al-Kindī in a salve for the skin after a beating with a lash. Genetically engineered versions of this plant have been used to make human insulin.

'Medicine is the science through which one knows the states of the human body, insofar as they are healthy or unhealthy, in order to preserve health when it is present, and to restore it when it is absent.'

Avicenna, *Canon of Medicine*, 1025

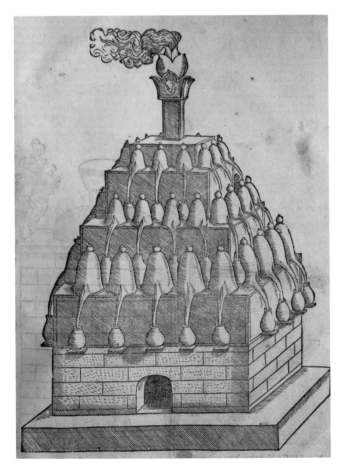

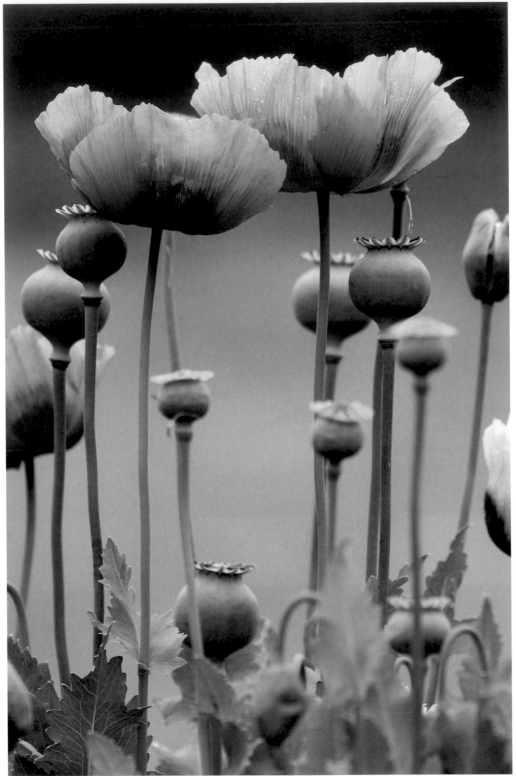

Far left: The distillation of plant material to make medicines was sometimes on an industrial scale, as shown by these furnaces with alembics from Mattioli's *De ratione distillandi aquas ex omnibus plantis* (1569), printed in Venice. Pietro Andrea Mattioli (1501–1577), physician and botanist, was one of the greatest authors and publishers of medical works of the 16th century.

Left: Opium poppy, *Papaver somniferum*. The sap from the seed head contains 13 per cent morphine, which can be absorbed through the skin, and is still used in this fashion in morphine patches. An ingredient of the 'soporific sponge', only a few drops of raw sap are necessary to cause sedation.

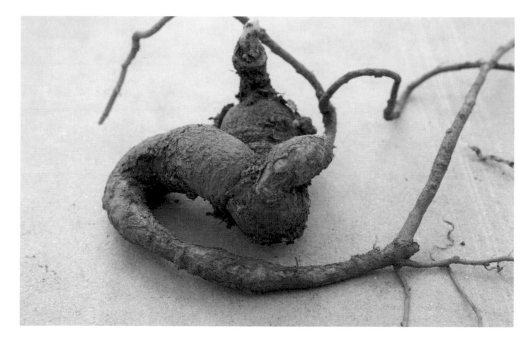

Right: Mandrake, *Mandragora officinarum*, contains tropane alkaloids such as hyoscine (scololamine) and atropine, which are absorbed through the skin and can cause delirium and coma in sufficient dosage.

Below: Henbane, *Hyoscyamus niger*, previously known as *Jusquiamus,* also contains hyoscine and atropine which are used medicinally for sea sickness and as a premed.

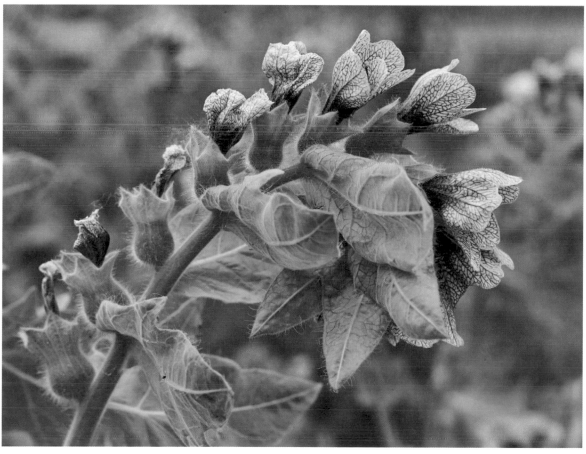

11th century to 16th century

One of the earliest of the pharmacopoeias to be printed in the West was the *Incipit Antidotarium Nicolai* (1471), written by the Italian physician Nicolaus Salernitanus (fl.1140), Dean of the School of Salerno, and printed in Venice.

He tells us for example of the famous *Spongia somniferum*, the anaesthetic sponge: a sponge, fresh from the sea, was soaked in a mixture which contained morphine from *Opii thebaici* (opium of Thebes, *Papaver somniferum*); hyoscine from *jusquami succi* (juice of henbane, *Hyoscyamus niger*) and mandrake (*Mandragora officinarum*), which was used to induce coma in sufficient dosage; along with coniine from the sap of *cicuta* (hemlock, *Conium maculatum*), which has curare-like actions. All of these chemicals were absorbed through the skin, and more readily through mucous membranes. Unripe blackberries with lettuce juice and tree ivy were added. For use, the sponge was moistened with a little warm water and applied to the patient's nostrils, causing immediate sleep. Applying the juice of fennel root to the nostrils would awaken the patient. There seems no reason to deny its effectiveness, as many do today. Its great advantage was that when sufficient of the dose was absorbed, the sponge was removed, and unlike an oral dose, overdose and death was unlikely.

Constantinus Africanus (1020–1087) was the North African who went to the School of Salerno and then to Monte Casino, where he translated the medical books of the great Arabic physicians into Latin, so introducing the advances of medieval Islam to Europe. The prominence of the School of Salerno as the first Christian University is due to Constantinus. He is mentioned in Chaucer's 'The Merchant's Tale' as being the author of a book *Liber de coitu*, which became the earliest printed book on male sexuality.

In the medical school of Salerno in the 13th century, Matthaeus Platearius (d.1261) wrote the (unillustrated) herbal entitled *Circa Instans* (*The Book of Simple Medicines*) from which the *Tractatus de Herbis et Plantis*, *Livre des simples médicines* and the *Grete Herbal* of 1526 derive. The *Tractatus* and the *Livre des simples médicines* were produced with colourful paintings of 200 or so plants, and the *Grete Herbal* had small woodcuts, so becoming the first printed herbal in English. They were grand books, but no more than compilations of earlier works, and were soon to be superseded by the great herbals of the 16th and 17th century and the revolution caused by the invention of printing.

From the School of Salerno, medical teaching moved in the 12th century to the new universities of Bologna, Naples, Paris and Padua (with Oxford and Cambridge trailing far behind) so English students, like Linacre, travelled to continental Europe for their training. The Church, especially the monasteries, dominated the practice of medicine, with regulations on every aspect of its practice – mostly prohibitions. The Holy Roman Emperor Frederick II (1194–1250) introduced legislation regarding the medical training in 1231, with three years studying logic, followed by five of medicine – all very familiar still, including: 'No doctor shall practise after the completion of the five-year period who has not practised for an entire year under the direction of an experienced doctor'. House officer posts are nothing new, but new ideas in medicine were discouraged by the Church. Books were manuscripts, immensely costly to produce, and learning was by listening to lectures and memorising the writings of Galen and Hippocrates. Astrology was regarded as essential for the practice of medicine, urine was examined by all possible senses; physical examination was negligible and prayers essential. However the pulse was felt, and then the wrist was grasped to feel the heat/cold, moist/dry character of the skin – as shown on the College coat of arms – thus assessing the balance of the humours in the patient. Unlicensed medical practitioners with charms, superstitions and toxic nostrums abounded.

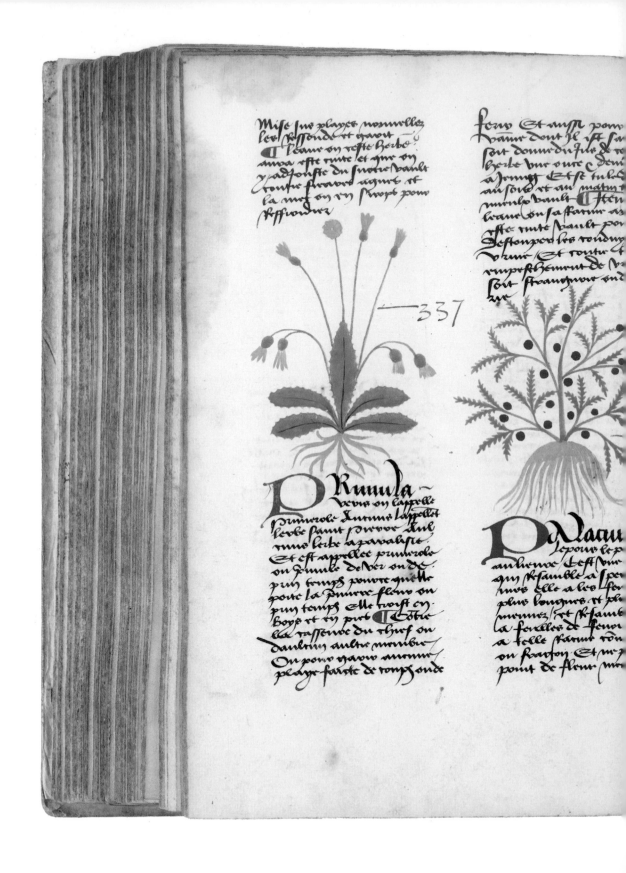

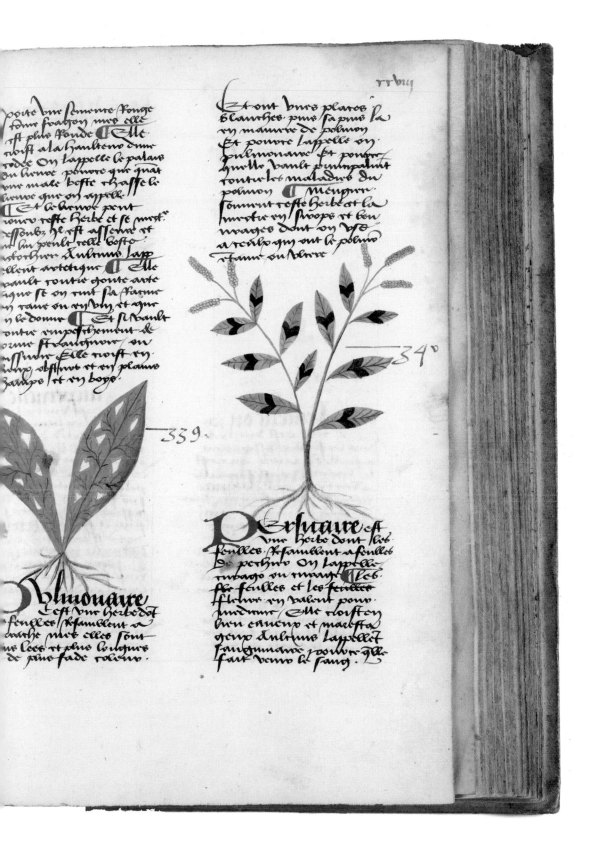

340

359.

'hemp sede if it be taken out of mesure, taketh mens wittes from them … the pouder of the dryed leves of hemp maketh men drounken.'

William Turner (*Herbal* 1568) quoting the 11th-century Byzantine physician Simeon Seth

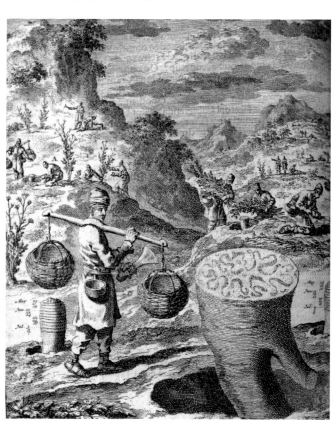

Left: Watercolours and French text from the *Circa instans, seu de medicamentis simplicibus,* an illustrated *Livre des simples médicines*. It was probably produced for the Abbey of Cluny, France in 1480–1500.

Above: The rhizotomists (the root cutters) and plant collectors were the source of the *materia medica* of apothecaries. Their expertise in selecting the correct plant made them an important if much neglected part of the supply chain of the apothecaries and physicians in the 17th and early 18th century. From Engelbert Kaempfer's *Amoenitatum Exoticarum Politico-physico-medicarum* (1712).

> *'Ill diet (as me thinketh) is chief cause of all dangerous and intolerable diseases and of the shortness of man's life.'*

Thomas Paynell, in *Regimen Sanitatis Salerni* (1597), his English translation of the *Regimen Sanitatis* (1480), which was Arnoldus de Villanova's annotated edition of Bernard de Gordon's *Lilium Medicinae* (c.1300)

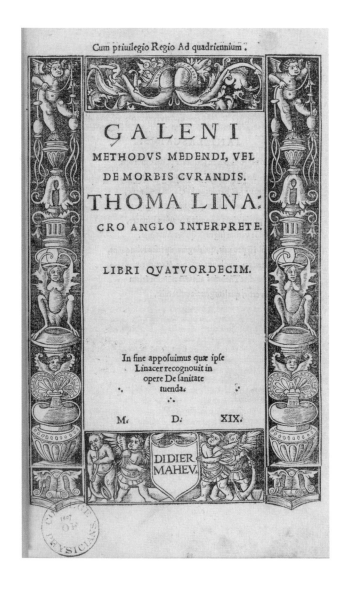

A few notable works emerged from this, our own medical dark ages, prior to the printing revolution. In the Dorchester Library, the College has the Frenchman Bernard de Gordon's (fl.1270–1330, professor of medicine at the University of Montpellier) *Lilium medicinae*, written around 1300, printed in Naples in 1480 (the copy in the College is the edition of 1550). It is a great advance in that it describes plague, tuberculosis, scabies, epilepsy, anthrax and leprosy.

The College also has John of Gaddesden's (1280–1361) *Rosa Anglica* written in 1314, printed in 1492, which belonged to John Chambre, one of the founders of the College (d.1549). It has been reviewed rather unfairly as 'Arabist quackeries and countryside superstitions'. Nevertheless it was the first printed book on medicine by an Englishman and it discusses diabetes and cardiac complaints and shows clinical observational skills.

Gilbertus Anglicus (1180–1250) studied in the school of Salerno and wrote a *Compendium Medicinae* (c.1230), and the College has the first printed edition of 1510. His patronym is given because as an Englishman he lived and worked for much of his life in France. He travelled in Syria, meeting Arabic physicians, and this is reflected in his *Compendium*, which includes a considerable amount of surgery as well as medicine. He attempts the differential diagnosis of fevers, culminating with 21 different types. While we may understand tertian and quartan fevers, epilala, lipparia and synochus causonides are lost to us, but it reflects an intellectual progression to explore the nature of disease, beyond learning the Greeks by heart. Chaucer's *Prologue to the Canterbury Tales* (written c.1387) mentions them all, and others, with descriptions of the practice of medicine at that time.

These, along with the newly discovered Celsus's *De Medicina* appearing as a printed work in 1478, were the basis of the beginning of an advance from the rule of Galen and Hippocrates. The wide distribution of books meant that all literate men could have access to a core of knowledge, which was no longer confined to monastic libraries or scriptoria. Diseases and treatments could be discussed, medical practice standardised and advanced, and unlicensed medical practitioners and apothecaries suppressed.

Over these 300 years the European universities took over medical training; the printed word caused a leap in the dissemination of knowledge unparalleled until the advent of the internet; academic standards could be set and taught; and, in 1518, the College was founded.

Left: Title page of *Methodus medendi: vel, de morbis curandis* by Galen, from the College library, translated by Linacre in 1519. An accomplished Greek scholar, in translating Galen from Greek to Latin he made medical knowledge available to a wider audience who could not read Greek.

Right: Erudition, and the knowledge of books, marked our predecessors in the 16th and 17th centuries. Great authors, including Theophrastus (Latin and Greek), Parkinson's *Herbal* (English, 1640), Ruel (Latin, 1537), Lobel (Latin, 1576), Pliny (English translation, 1634) and Mattioli (Latin, 1569), graced their consulting rooms; pocket editions of Dioscorides (Latin, 1550) went with them on their home visits.

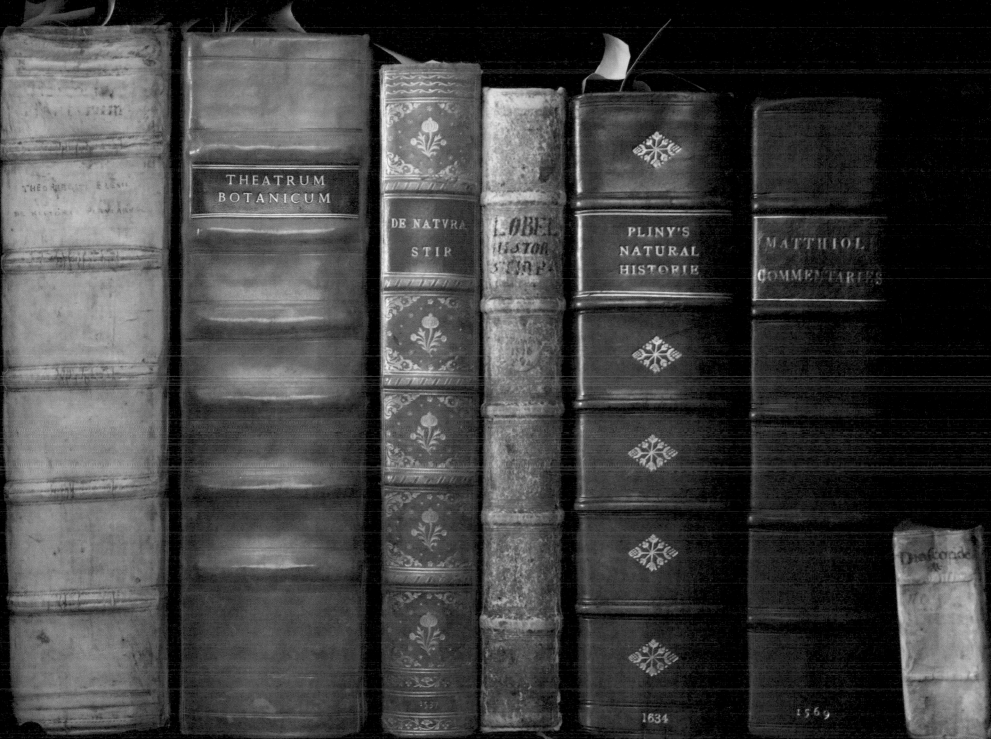

2 Foundation and rise of the College

1518–

1660

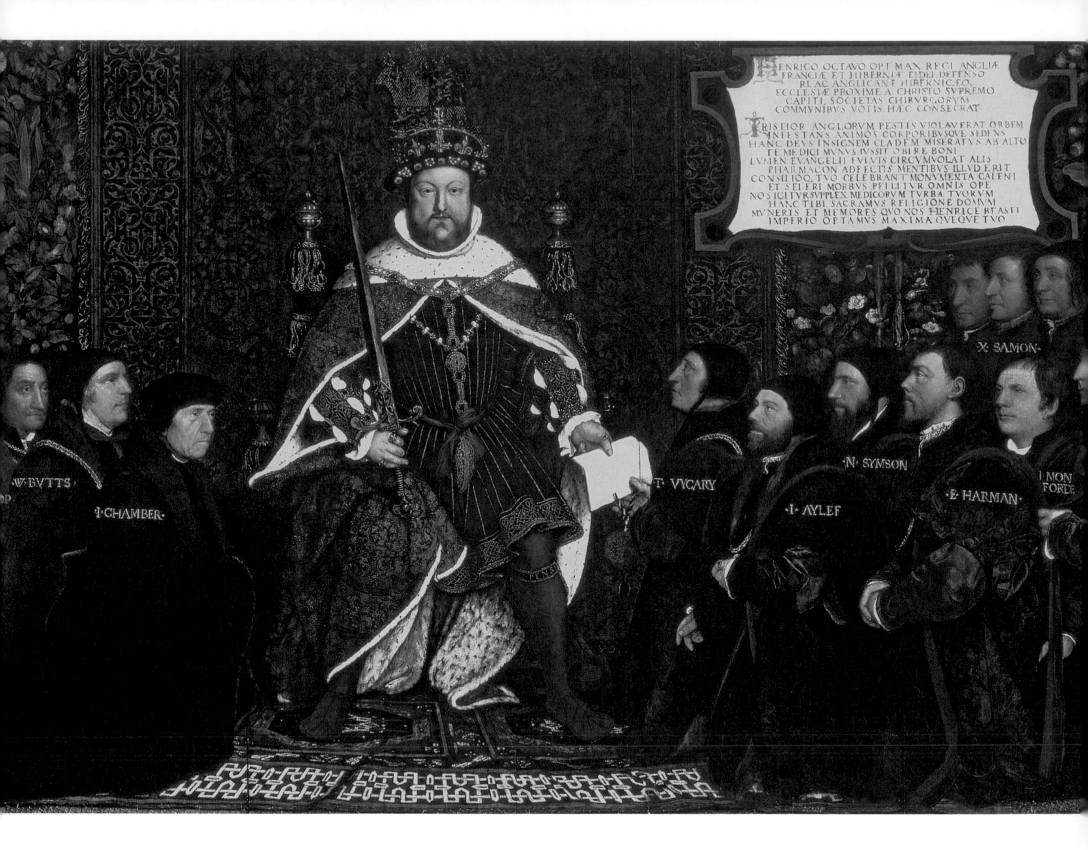

'We have chiefly and before all things necessary to withstand in good time the audacity of those wicked men who shall profess medicine more for the sake of their own avarice than from the assurance of any good conscience, whereby very many inconveniences may ensure to the rude and credulous populace...'

The Royal College of Physicians (then known as the Faculty or Commonalty or College of Physicians) was established, primarily, to protect the public from ruthless practitioners and to regulate the practice of 'physick' – to be differentiated from the barbers, surgeons and apothecaries who were regulated by a guild.

Prior to 1518, the English medical profession was underdeveloped in comparison with those in Italy and France, and had been ineffectively controlled by ecclesiastical authorities. In 1509, Thomas Linacre had been appointed the Royal Physician by Henry VIII and, in 1511, Parliament passed legislation that no one was to practice as a physician or surgeon within seven miles of the City of London, unless examined, appointed and admitted by the Bishop of London or Dean of St Paul's and four doctors of physick or surgeons. The need to reinforce and advance ethical standards in medicine and prevent imposters and charlatans from practice was urgent and, perhaps, fortuitously hastened by the most severe of five outbreaks of the sweating sickness (*sudor anglicus*), which affected both the King and Cardinal Wolsey in 1517–18. Of note, there was an outbreak in Oxford, only seven miles from the Royal Court at Woodstock. In 1523, an Act of Parliament extended the College's authority and licensing powers to the whole of England.

The Royal College of Physicians was founded by the classical and humanist scholar, Royal Physician and cleric Thomas Linacre. Linacre mastered Latin and Greek in the monastery school at Canterbury and continued his education under the greatest scholars of the day: Cornelio Vitelli, at Oxford, where he was elected a fellow of All Souls College in 1484, and then in Italy, with Angelo Ambrogini (Poliziano), who introduced Linacre to the Medici family, and arranged his instruction with the sons of Lorenzo the Great, and Aldus Manutius, the learned Venetian printer.

In 1496, Linacre took the degree of Doctor of Medicine in Padua, 'with the highest applause'. Returning to Oxford, Linacre did not practise medicine, but joined a brilliant group of humanist scholars, teaching such eminent pupils as Erasmus and Sir Thomas More, and counting John Colet, William Grocyn and William Latimer among his intimate friends. In 1501, Linacre was appointed preceptor and physician to Arthur Tudor, Prince of Wales, and in 1509 he became the Royal Physician to Henry VIII, paid £50 per annum from 1516 to 1520. His greatest contribution, however, was the founding of the College of Physicians, before taking priest's orders and becoming Rector of Wigan in 1520. 'In private life he had an utter detestation of everything that was dishonourable; he was … valued and beloved by all ranks … he was reckoned by the best judges a man of a bright genius … one, who by his writings and benefactions, has done great honour not only to his profession but also to his country.'
John Noble Johnson, 1835

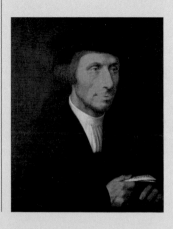

Below: The Stone House, which was Linacre's house in Knightrider Street, south of St Paul's Cathedral. The name distinguished it from the surrounding timber buildings. Two rooms, a meeting room and a library, were the first 'house of the physicians'. Linacre bequeathed the Stone House to the College, enabling two additions: an anatomy theatre and a small rented garden for medicinal plants.

Below right: One of four anatomical tables used for teaching anatomy. They were purchased, or possibly made, by Sir John Finch while studying medicine in Padua. His dissecting skills were renowned and he was appointed Professor of Anatomy in Pisa and then Pro-Rector of the University of Padua. His descendant George Finch donated the tables to the College in 1823.

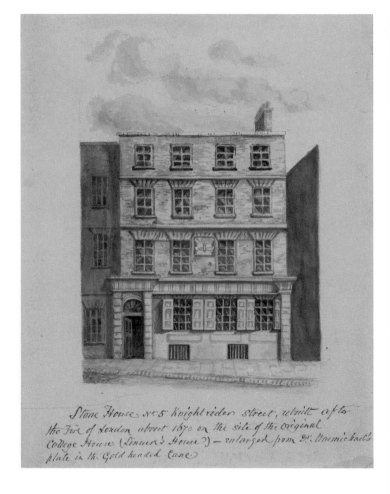

Stone House N°5 Knightrider street, rebuilt after the Fire of London about 1670 on the site of the original College House (Linacre's House?) – enlarged from Dr Macmichael's plate in the Gold headed Cane

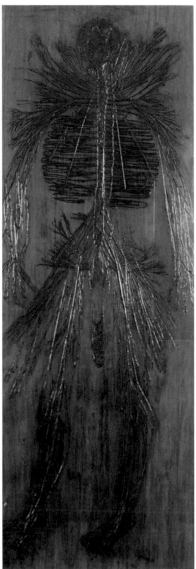

1518

Foundation of the College of Physicians by royal charter of incorporation dated 23 September, enabling the College to license and regulate medical practice within seven miles of the City of London.

1523

On 15 April, an Act of Parliament confirms the charter of incorporation and extends the College's licensing function to the provinces. Eight elects were established and authorised to choose one of their number as President.

1524

First mention of statutes in the *Annals*.

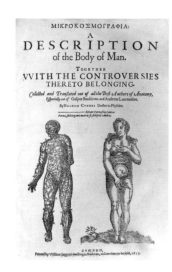

Above: Frontispiece to *Mikrokosmographia, a Description of the Body of Man*, an anatomical textbook by Helkiah Crooke (1576–1648), Court Physician to James I, who became a fellow in 1620 and anatomy reader in 1629. The book was successful but caused controversy, as it was in English, criticised Galen's teachings and contained 'indecent' illustrations of the genitalia.

Right: Queen Mary I performing the 'royal touch' for scrofula. Only the monarch was immune from prosecution for practising medicine without a licence.

The success of the petition made to Henry VIII established the power of medical licensing for a 'corporate Society of Physicians', whose members had the right to 'make such Statutes and Ordinances as they, from time to time, shou'd think most expedient for the publick Service'. Thus, the establishment of the College of Physicians helped to protect the public from unscrupulous practitioners, by examining and licensing physicians, punishing malpractice and pretenders, overseeing apothecaries' remedies and promoting ethical practice. After 1618, apothecaries' remedies were strictly regulated, as outlined in the *Pharmacopoeia Londinensis*.

While the College resembled the guilds, it was distinguished by the long, scholarly education and award of a university degree required for membership, rather than completion of an apprenticeship. Moreover, the terms 'College' and 'President' reflected the scholarship of the Oxbridge colleges. Perhaps not surprisingly, this new authority brought the College immediately into direct conflict with the establishment: the universities of Oxford and Cambridge, which were the only institutions in the country awarding an MD degree, and therefore allowing the holder to practise throughout the country; the Church, which previously had authority to appoint physicians and surgeons; and the guilds, which regulated apothecaries and barber surgeons.

Nonetheless, physicians continued to compete with other licensed practitioners, including surgeons, midwives, apothecaries and quacks, and even English monarchs who generously dispensed the 'royal touch' to heal scrofula, known as the King's Evil.

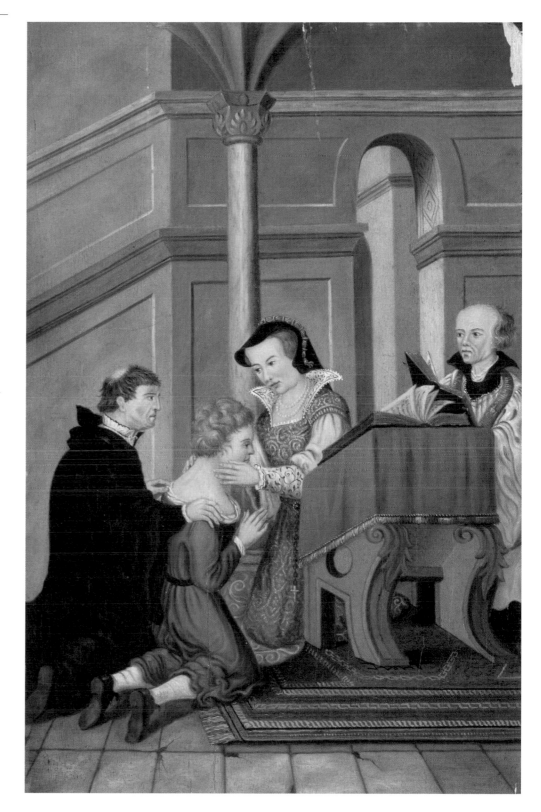

Life in the 16th and 17th centuries was hazardous and, for the majority, staying alive was often an insurmountable hurdle. There was extreme poverty: overcrowded hovels shared with people and animals, open sewers, excrement, decaying refuse, deficient diets eaten with dirty fingers or unwashed implements, no washing facilities and ubiquitous vermin, lice and fleas. In airless, damp rooms, rheumatic and respiratory illnesses and childhood rickets were rampant. There were appalling levels of maternal and infantile morbidity and mortality wrought by the ministrations of the local midwives. Thousands died in epidemics of 'fevers', including smallpox, puerperal fever, measles, 'consumption', scrofula, the sweating sickness, flea- and lice-borne typhus, waterborne typhoid and widespread syphilis, leprosy and endemic malaria. Thomas Sydenham (1624–1689) noted that, in marshlands, dwellers became 'impressed with a certain miasma which produces a quartan ague' and Shakespeare (1564–1616) made frequent reference to the 'ague'. Quarantine was the only remedy for plague, which occurred mainly in cities, was deadliest in summer and was dreaded as a death sentence. Life expectancy was around 35 years, at least one in four died before the age of five, and as many as 40 per cent before they reached adulthood.

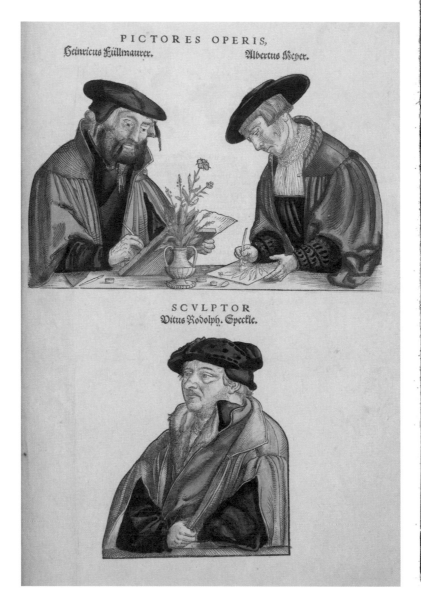

PICTORES OPERIS,
Heinricus Füllmaurer.   Albertus Meyer.

SCVLPTOR
Vitus Rodolph. Speckle.

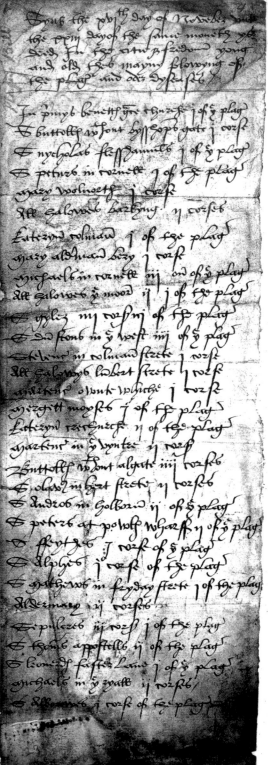

1540

Physicians' Act: physicians are excused civic duties and parish payments in London and the suburbs. Four wise physicians were elected to inspect apothecaries' drugs and College fellows could practise surgery.

1540

The Barber Surgeons of London charter granted by Henry VIII allows the dissection of four executed criminals a year. The physicians taught anatomy and dissection in their Hall.

1541

Proceedings against the unlicensed John Lytster and John Wisdom at Guildhall. Lytster and Wisdom were fined, half each to the King and College. They paid half (£15 and £5), on condition that the suit was dropped.

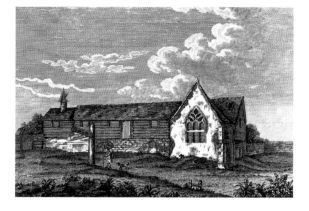

Left: St Petronilla's Hospital in Bury. Various religious orders in England had set up more than 1,000 hospitals, alms houses, hospices for lepers, and hostels for travellers. These were vital to the social structure of the 16th century, and the poor particularly suffered when they were closed in the Dissolution of the Monasteries.

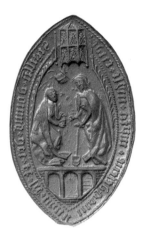

Above: Plaque at Lazar House commemorating the remains of the Leper Hospital of Saint Mary Magdalen. It was founded for male lepers, and later for poor, aged and sick men, by Bishop Herbert de Losigna before 1119. It was closed at the Dissolution in 1547.

Right: Personifications of medicine, pharmacy and surgery. The physician stands centrally on a dais, elevated by his classical scholarship, and gives therapeutic instructions to two subordinate figures. He gives clysters, bloodletting and cupping to the surgeon, on his right, whose body is composed of surgical instruments, and laxatives, juleps and emetics to the apothecary on his left, who is surrounded by pharmaceutical equipment.

Diagnosis and treatment remained unscientific and ineffective. Anatomical dissection was the sole medical discipline, and illness was ascribed to an imbalance of the four bodily humours, as proposed centuries earlier by Hippocrates and Galen, or sin, as pronounced by the Church. A return to health required a 'rebalancing' of humours, with removal of the offending element by the unpleasant and often life-threatening techniques of purging, bloodletting and the use of emetics such as antimony, or by cleansing of the soul. In addition, astrology-based treatments, using specific medicinal plants in specific seasons, were in vogue. Treatment was based on folklore and mistaken hypotheses and the majority relied on the concoctions ('simples' and 'receipts') of apothecaries, barber surgeons, charlatans or the local 'wise woman', but the wealthy who consulted 'licensed' practitioners rarely fared better.

Influenced by his observations of the organisation and self-regulation of medical institutions in Italy, and benefitting from his considerable influence as Royal Physician, Thomas Linacre and a small group of distinguished physicians petitioned Henry VIII, in 1517. These physicians were: John Chambre, a cleric and Censor, and Ferdinand de Victoria, physician to Henry VIII, Doctor of physic beyond the seas, and Censor (both Royal Physicians), together with Nicholas Halswell, a priest, and John Francis and Robert Yaxley, both of whom held office as Consiliarius.

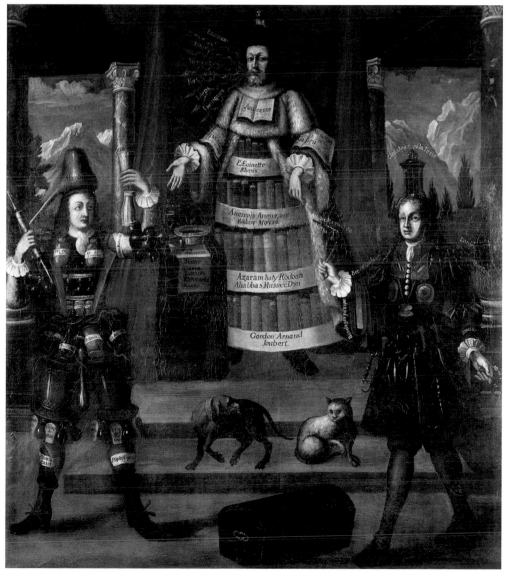

1546

Grant of Arms – received by the College on 20 September.

1554

Simon Ludford is denounced in a letter to his Cambridge college, which refused to interfere. He was re-examined with an Oxford degree and admitted in 1563 – but fined £10 for his earlier misdemeanour!

1555

John Caius elected President for the first time. As a firm believer in ceremony, he insisted on being referred to as '*His Excellency*' and, indeed, the Bedel was required to address each fellow similarly.

1555

The College takes action against a Flemish foreigner, Charles Cornet, who was not 'wholly qualified', resulting in his imprisonment, despite judicial and clerical support.

1556

John Caius presents the President's staff of office, the caduceus, to the College. It was made of silver to show that the President should rule 'with moderation and courtesy, unlike those … who ruled with a rod of iron'.

1559–60

John Geynes is accused of 'asserting to the vulgar that Galen had erred'. Eventually, he acknowledged his error, was examined by and admitted to the College, becoming a Censor and an elect.

The College of Physicians' Grant of Arms was made in 1546 and the elements were stipulated by royal charter. The design shows a golden pomegranate, surmounted by a hand with an ermine cuff emerging from a silver-and-gold cloud to take the pulse on another arm: these elements reflecting the identity and interests of the College. A hand feeling the pulse is a medical examination, but also reflects professional reassurance, while the hand descending from the sky indicates divine authority for both the medical profession and the institution of the College. The pomegranate is a symbol of fertility, wealth and regeneration dating back to classical mythology, and is found in the imagery of several religions. Tradition holds that it 'cures burning agues', but Dioscorides dismisses its use for fevers, while Parkinson (1628) recommends it.

It has been suggested that the pomegranate was selected because of its association with Henry VIII's first wife, Catherine of Aragon, but, by 1546, Henry was married to his sixth wife, Catherine Parr, and it seems more likely to have been chosen for its classical, religious and therapeutic associations. A 1963 redesign showing the correct manner of taking a pulse has never been adopted.

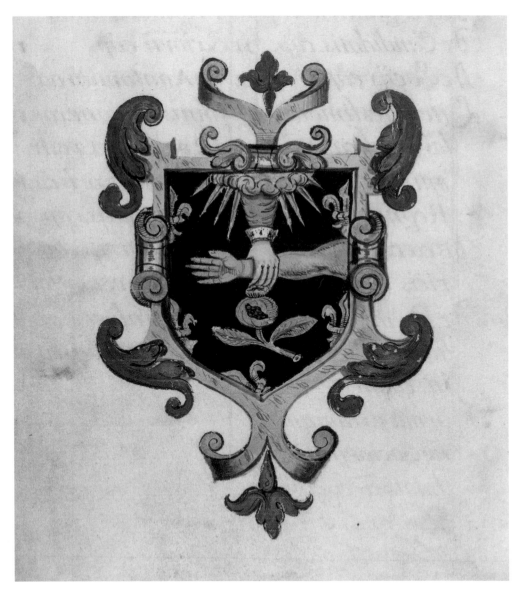

Left: This emblem decorated the College of Physicians' Grant of Arms from 1546. When the College was abandoned in the plague of 1665, the emblem disappeared, presumed stolen. In 1695, it was purchased in a shop by Dr Oliver Horsman and returned to the College.

Below right: The College seal. In 1556 the seal disappeared, and this new seal was commissioned in 1737. The original design, deduced from imprints on documents, shows St Luke with a halo, and wearing an academic skull cap, seated and reading, with a pomegranate at his feet and an image of a hand taking a pulse. The seal is inscribed *Sigillum Collegii Medicorum Londini*.

Far right: The title page from Caius' book of statutes (*Statuta Vetera*), which included the consolidated College statutes, incorporating both Caius' own additions and earlier revisions, with emphasis on the roles of officers, electoral procedures and the principles of the examination for Fellowship. The crimson-velvet-bound book, with ornate silver clasps, was carried before the President at Comitia.

1561–62

Caius' presidency is interrupted for a year by Dr Richard Master. Returning in 1562, Caius reported the 'invasion of empirics' in his absence. An outbreak of smallpox had affected Queen Elizabeth.

1563

John Caius' *Statuta Vetera* dated 1555, but including revisions to 1563, specifies quarterly ordinary Comitia on the day after St Michael's Day (30 September); the day after St Thomas' Day (22 December); the day after Palm Sunday (moveable); and the day after the birthday of St John the Baptist (25 June).

'The caduceus or silver rod indicates that the President should rule with moderation and courtesy, unlike those of earlier days who ruled with a rod of iron. But the serpents, the symbols of prudence, teach the necessity of ruling at the same time with prudence and the arms of the College placed at its summit indicate that these are the means by which the College is sustained.'

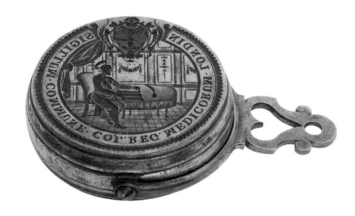

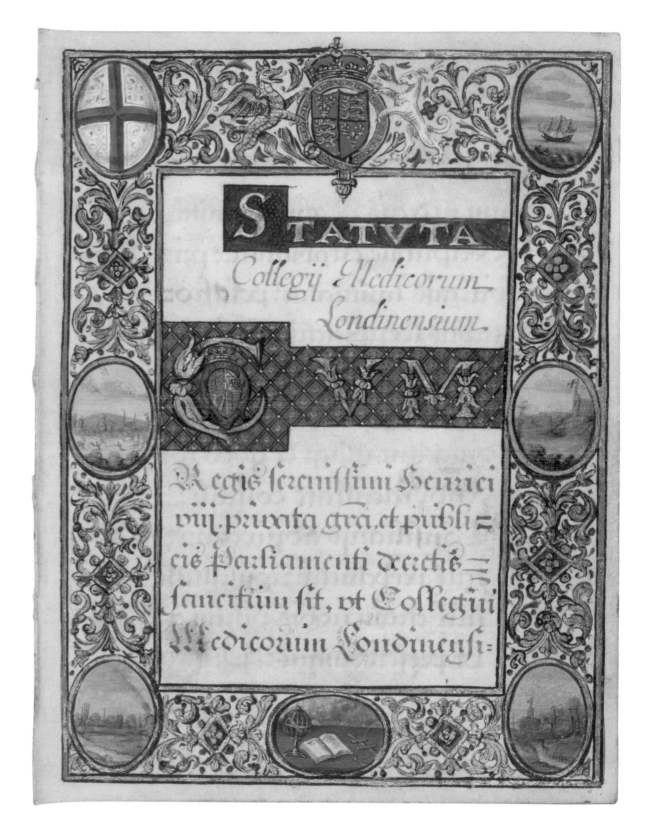

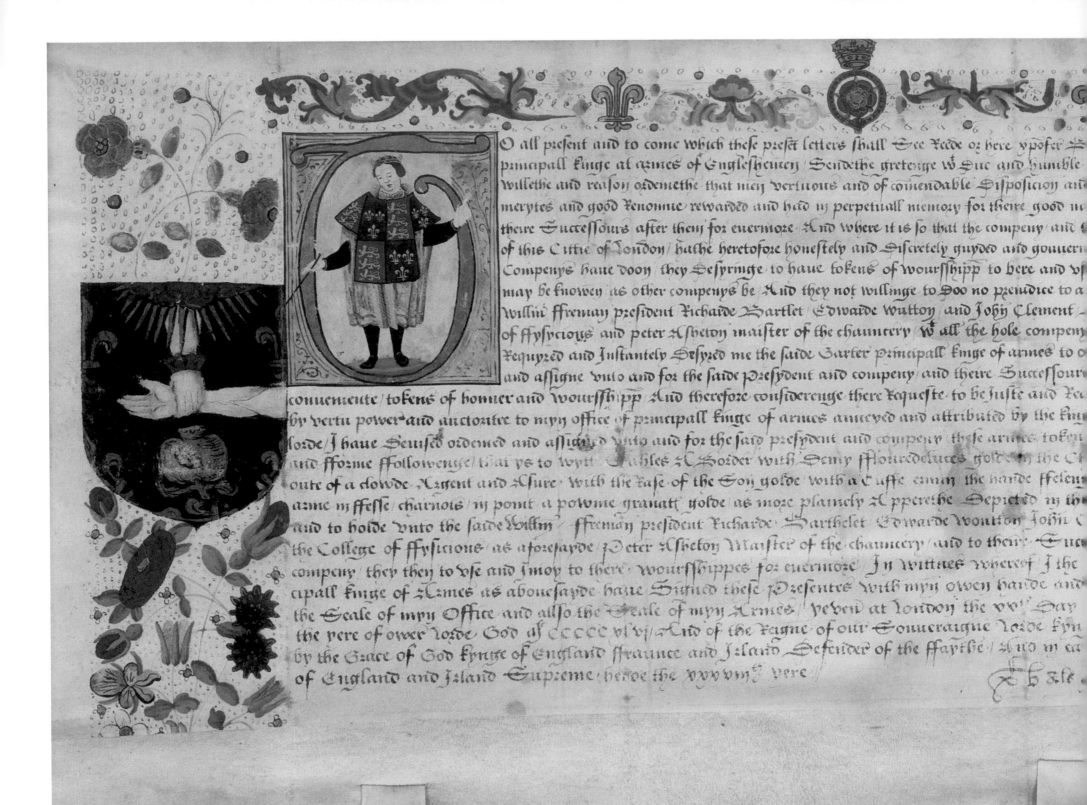

Left: A page from Caius' book of statutes (*Statuta Vetera*).

Below left: Front and back of an English oval gold medal, minted in 1572, commemorating the recovery of Queen Elizabeth I from smallpox, ten years earlier, with only mild scarring. Her servant and nurse, Lady Mary Sidney, was not so fortunate, and was severely disfigured.

Below right: The College's caduceus. Caius was greatly influenced by his time in Padua and adapted the ceremonies of the Italian medical guilds to the English environment. In 1556, he presented to the College the *insignia virtutis*: a silver caduceus with the coat of arms on the head, surrounded by four serpents; a seal; a red cushion of reverence; and the mounted book of statutes.

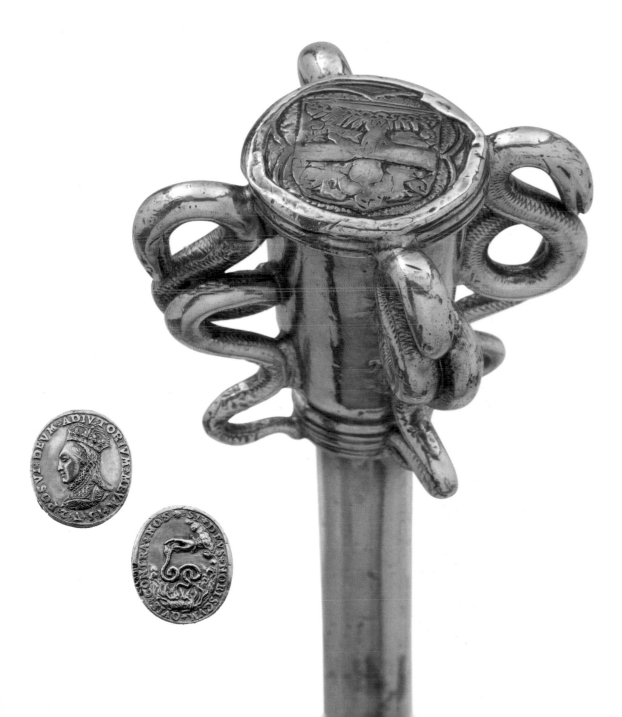

John Caius
1510–1573

John Keys studied divinity at Gonville College, Cambridge and, under the instruction of Montanus and Vesalius, graduated in medicine from the University of Padua in 1541. Returning to England, with some self-aggrandisement he Latinised his name to Iohannes Caius. Like his predecessors, Caius was a man of scholarship: he studied natural history; became the authority on the 'sweating sickness'; wrote a history of the University of Cambridge; was elected President of the College nine times and became Royal Physician to Edward VI, Queen Mary and Queen Elizabeth and Master of Gonville and Caius College, which he had generously endowed, expanded and renamed.

As President, Caius formalised College proceedings and kept detailed records of meetings, prosecutions against unlicensed practitioners and inspections of apothecaries' drugs. He documented College business in the Annals from 1518 and throughout his three presidencies, filling in early gaps from notes and memory. In 1563, he consolidated revisions, including his own, of the statutes and, as President, would read out the *statuta moralia* to new fellows to emphasise the appropriate conduct of their medical practice. Caius was a benevolent philanthropist, erecting a monument to Linacre in St Paul's Cathedral and giving grants to promote the study of anatomy and the development of his Cambridge college.

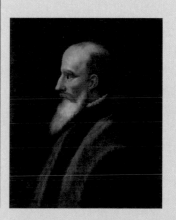

1565

Charter for Anatomies. Under letters patent, Elizabeth I grants the College four bodies of hanged criminals each year to dissect. The dissections were undertaken publicly by the fellows, in order of seniority.

1569–70

Dr Roderigo Lopus (Lopez) refuses to read the anatomy lecture and is fined. This may have been the same Dr Roderigo Lopez who was physician to the Queen's household, and was hanged in 1594 for conspiring to poison her.

1579

Dr Roger Marbeck appointed as the first Registrar. In 1581, he was appointed for life. He was paid 40s a year and 3s 4d for every admission and miscreant fined.

Right: Frontispiece of 1636 edition of Gerard's *Herball*. Gerard was a botanist, herbalist and Master of the Barber Surgeons. He was not a scholar, and his *Herball* (1597) was a translation of Dodoens' *Stirpium Historiae Pemptades sex*, made, with many errors, by a Dr Priest.

Opposite left: This woodcut shows a man smoking a 'tabac', as these giant roll-ups were called. The word 'tabac' gave rise to the word 'tobacco'. It is the first ever illustration of *Nicotiana tabacum*, the source of tobacco, the world's most poisonous plant (from Lobel's *Stirpium Historia*, 1576).

Opposite right: *Nicotiana tabacum* growing wild in its native Peru. From here it was transported to Mexico and around the world.

In 1518, gardens were commonly laid out in royal, religious and lay residences for enjoyment (such as bowling), with fruit trees, herbs, flowers and lawns. The Stone House (see page 30) had insufficient land for a 'physick' garden and, following unsuccessful land negotiations, with a Dr Sackford, the College rented land from Lord Sackville and approached John Gerard for help. He was a surgeon and expert horticulturist, who, in October 1587, 'promised that he would look after the College garden, and agreed to keep it stocked with all the rarer plants for a reasonable charge', although no record of such a garden exists.

When the College moved to Amen Corner, in 1614, the lease from St Paul's Cathedral included a garden of 66 by 100 feet, but lack of funds precluded development. In, 1631, Dr Atkins PRCP unsuccessfully petitioned the King for help, hoping for support in return for advice on the plague.

Finally, in 1651, with Francis Prujean's proposal, which included 'a Repository for simples' – remedies made from only one species of plant – and, with Harvey's subsequent, generous bequest, the tradition of a College 'physick' garden was established. The current home in Regent's Park was transformed in 2004 by the creation of a modern physic garden, bursting with medicinal plants from around the world.

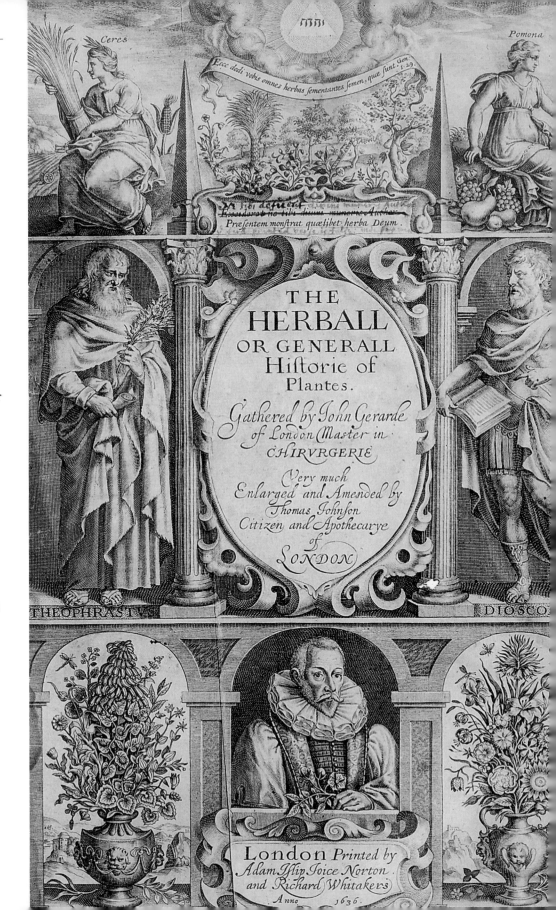

THE HERBALL OR GENERALL Historie of Plantes.

Gathered by John Gerarde of London (Master in CHIRVRGERIE

Very much Enlarged and Amended by Thomas Johnson Citizen and Apothecarye of LONDON

London Printed by Adam Islip Ioice Norton and Richard Whitakers Anno 1636

1582

Founding of the Lumleian Trust and Lumleian lecture on surgery. Named after John, Lord Lumley, who with Richard Caldwell endowed the lectures. Today, the lectures have expanded to cover general medicine.

1583

Dr William Baronsdale appointed as the first Treasurer. The President delegated the duties of receiving revenue, overseeing College property, repairs, paying salaries, dealing with prosecutions and lawsuits and preparing statements of accounts.

1604

Publication of King James I's virulently anti-smoking treatise *A Counterblaste to Tobacco*.

1607

William Harvey becomes a candidate in May 1607 and is elected a fellow on 5 June 1607.

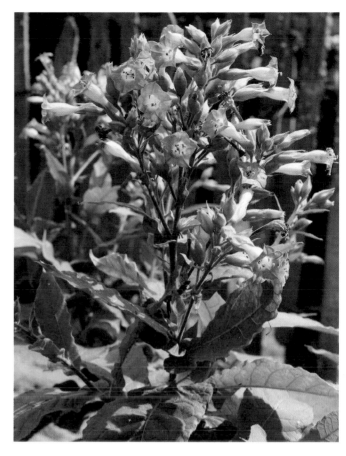

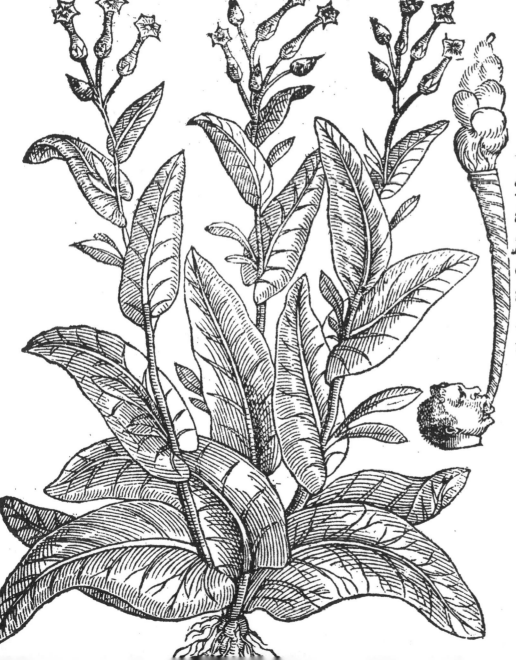

Nicotiana inserta in-fundibulo ex quo hauriunt fumũ Indi & nau cleri.

From its origin in Peru, tobacco was transported to Mexico. In 1518, seeds of tobacco were brought from Mexico to Spain by Friar Ramón Pané, and so the College celebrates its 500-year anniversary in parallel to that of the greatest killer the world has ever known. Francis Drake is said to have brought it to England in 1575 and smoking was then popularised by Sir Walter Raleigh. Many physicians attributed panacea-like properties to the plant, and it was smoked for 350 years before anyone showed that it caused lung and other cancers and predisposed users to vascular disease. Many doctors gave up smoking after the report from Doll and Hill (1954) and, while their deaths from lung cancer went down, their death rate from alcoholism went up. It now causes the premature death of 6 million people annually, ten times more than malaria.

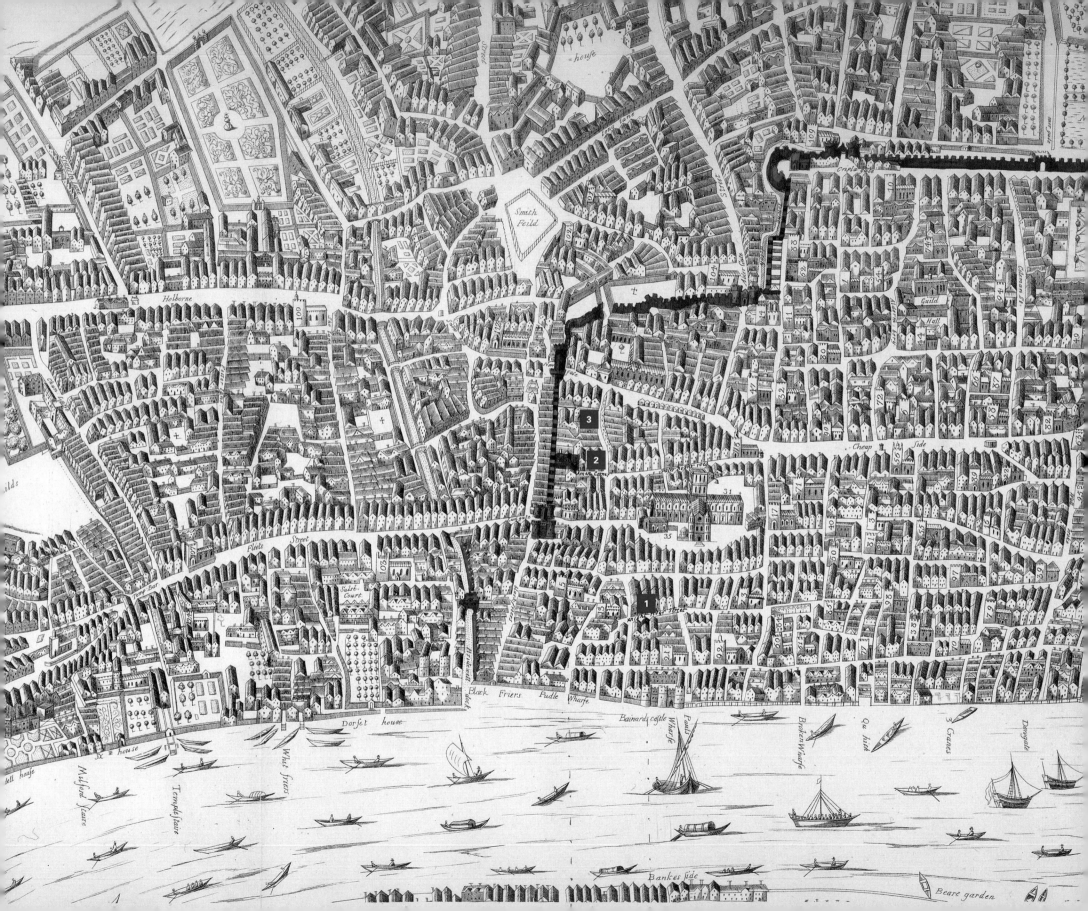

1614

College moves from Knightrider Street to its second home at Amen Corner, just west of St Paul's Cathedral. The building at Amen Corner was destroyed by the Great Fire of London in 1666.

1615–16

William Harvey, appointed Lumleian lecturer in 1615, gave the first lecture in 1616 and retired in 1665. In his detailed lecture notes, he proposed his theory on the circulation of the blood.

1616

Sir Theodore de Mayerne, a Swiss-born physician who treated the kings of France and England, came to England in 1611, following the assassination of Henri IV, and was admitted a Fellow at a specially convened extraordinary Comitia.

1617

James I's charter. This was intended to reinforce the College's powers to prosecute unlicensed practitioners – but was not ratified by Parliament and probably had little effect.

1618

Pharmacopoeia Londinensis first published. Apothecaries were instructed by royal decree to make medicines according to the prescribed formulae.

1624–25

Dr John Bastwick admitted as an extra-licentiate. As he wrote against popery, his licence was revoked, he was fined, imprisoned and 'censured as scandalous, seditious, and infamous'. The charges were eventually rescinded and the College reinstated him, in 1640.

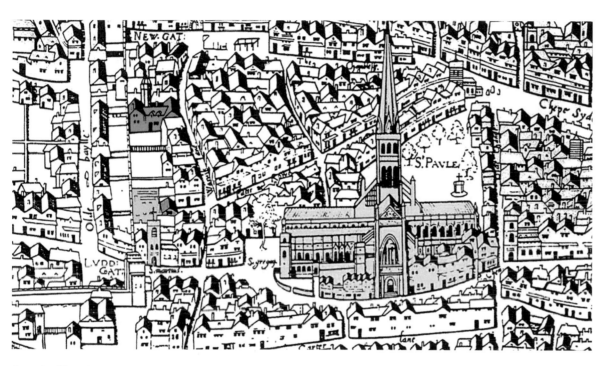

Opposite: Map of London showing the city wall and College sites in (1) Knightrider Street, (2) Amen Corner and (3) Warwick Lane. The red line shows the city wall.

Above and right: An image of Amen Corner and street plan on the Copperplate Map of 1558 showing the position of the College building (pink) at Amen Corner, the garden of the College (green) and the church, St Martin-within-Ludgate (red). In 1614, with an increasing number of fellows, the College leased its second larger home, at Amen Corner, from the Dean and Chapter of St Paul's

Cathedral. During the English interregnum, the building came under threat of confiscation, but, in 1651, was purchased and donated to the College by Baldwin Hamey (see page 43).

Far right: The official advice given in March 1630 by the College to the Privy Council on precautions to be taken against plague. Faced with the risk of a plague epidemic in London, the College organised a commission to investigate preventative procedures and possible cures – sadly all ineffective.

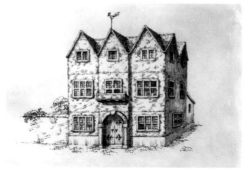

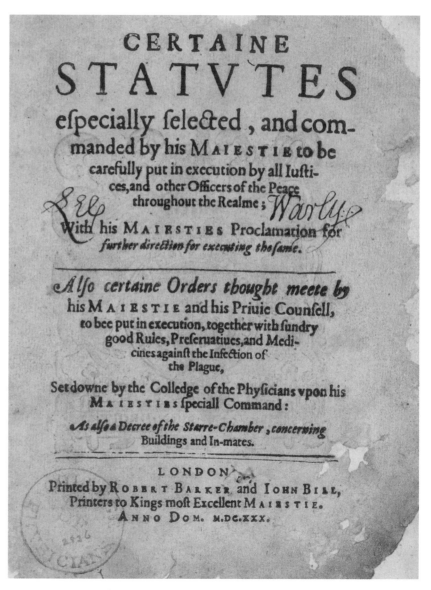

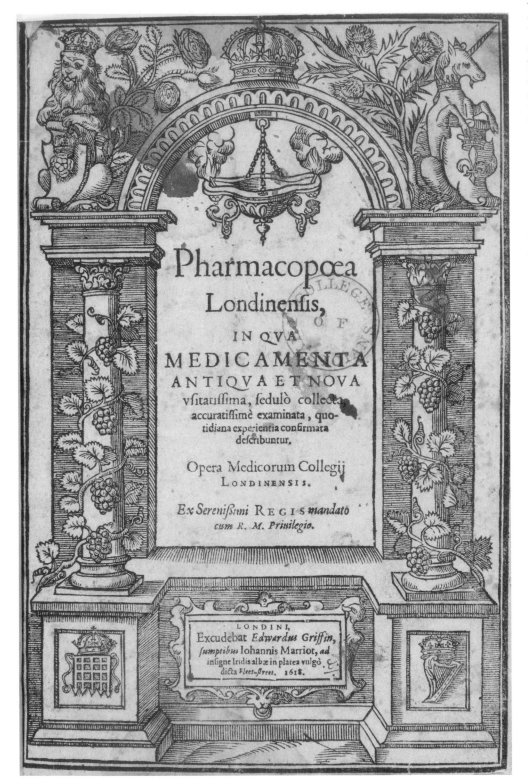

Left: Title page of the first edition of the *Pharmacopoeia Londinensis* (May 1618). This was the most important publication for improving medicine that came from the College of Physicians at the time. The first edition had 712 medicines; the revised edition had 963, but only a few, like senna and opium, had any useful effect.

Right: Nicholas Culpeper (1615–1654), English physician, herbalist and astrologer, took advantage of the abolition of censorship with the disbanding of the Company of Stationers and the Star Chamber, during the interregnum of the Civil War, and published his *Physicall Directory* (1649) in English so everyone could treat themselves, without recourse to a physician.

1626

Sir Francis Prujean becomes a Fellow, then Registrar and President. 'He was a man of elegant tastes, of varied and extensive acquirements, and was respected and trusted equally by the public, as by his own profession.'

1628

Publication of William Harvey's *De Motu Cordis*, in which he describes his theory of the circulation of the blood. Harvey was appointed Treasurer in the same year.

1630

College provides official advice to the Privy Council on precautions to be taken against the plague. Later editions were issued in 1636 and 1665.

The 400th anniversary of the May 1618 publication of the College's *Pharmacopoeia Londinensis* – which ensured that the newly formed apothecaries made their medicines in a standard way – is also celebrated. It was mainly a cut-down version of an existing continental pharmacopoeia, the *Augustana* (1613), with 712 compound medicines and their 680 ingredients – roots, flowers, fruits, etc. Rapidly withdrawn, as the College disliked it, it was enlarged and reprinted in December. Originally written in Latin, Nicholas Culpeper won universal approval from the public and the apothecaries (and the opprobrium of the physicians) by translating it into English in his *Physicall Directory* (1649), giving the use of each medicine.

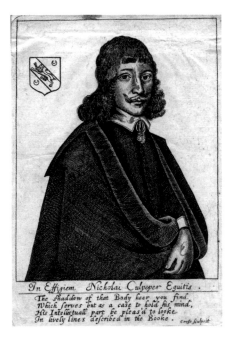

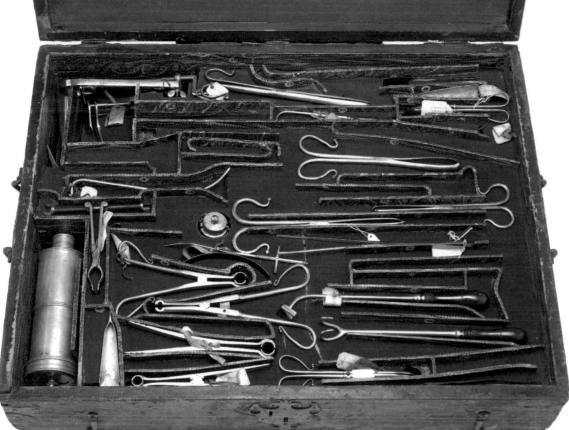

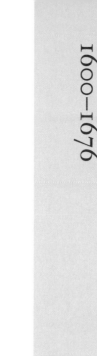

Baldwin Hamey 1600–1676

Baldwin Hamey was a man of many talents: a well-travelled scholar of the classics, philosophy and medicine, an outstanding lecturer, a distinguished physician, a generous benefactor of the monarchy, a faithful member of Church and College, and the most prodigious holder of College office, being repeatedly appointed Censor, Registrar and Treasurer between 1640 and 1666. The son of the eminent Dutch physician Hamey the Elder, who had settled in London, Hamey returned to Leiden to study medicine, graduating in 1626. The mayor of Hastings, intrigued by Hamey's knowledge and conversation, unwittingly saved him from drowning in a shipwreck by delaying his initial voyage.

During the political and religious unrest of the 1640s, Hamey feigned interest in Puritan lectures and sermons by reading Virgil and Aristophanes, disguised as the Bible and Greek Testament, and, despite being a royalist and sending secret donations to the exiled King, he amassed a fortune, as the physician to leading Parliamentarians. Hamey's philanthropy to, and support of, the College were unprecedented: donations included land, the famous bell and the Spanish oak panelling, which now graces the Censors' Room, but his support brooked no competition, and included covertly distributing pamphlets denigrating Charles II's establishment of the Royal Society.

Above: The Prujean chest holds one of the most important collections of 17th-century surgical instruments in the world, including instruments used for obstetrics, gynaecology, lithotomy, trepanation, bullet extraction and amputation.

Right: Controversy surrounded the medicinal use of antimony, which was potentially lethal. Acid in wine, placed in small antimonial cups, leached out the metal and controlled the dose administered; this produced vomiting, diarrhoea or sweating in many disorders. Baldwin Hamey purchased this antimonial cup and leather case, from a 'quack', Reverend John Evans, in the 1630s, to confiscate them and/or initiate a College discussion.

Below right: Hamey's bell. As President, Hamey used the bell to call Comitia to order and donated it to the College when he demitted office. After his death, the interior of the bell was inscribed *'Mortuus est, tamen hic Auditor Hamaeus'* (Though he be dead, yet in this place Hamey is still heard).

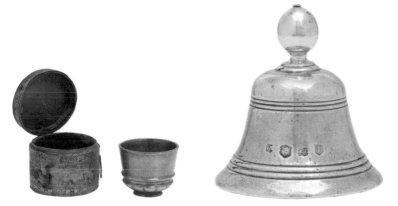

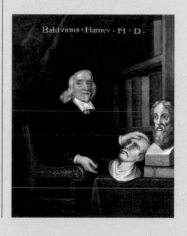

In the College tradition, Harvey was educated in Canterbury, Gonville and Caius College Cambridge and the University of Padua, graduating with distinction in medicine, in 1602. On returning to London, Harvey became a Fellow and Treasurer of the College, physician to St Bartholomew's Hospital and Lumleian lecturer at the College, giving lectures for 40 years from 1616. He was appointed physician to Charles I, who encouraged Harvey's circulation research by providing deer for experimentation. Harvey was a royalist, accompanying the King during the Civil War and returning to London only after the fall of Oxford in 1646.

Harvey's interest in circulation developed in Padua, under Colombo and Fabricius ab Aquapendente, who had, respectively, described the movement of the blood from the heart to the lungs and the valves of the veins. In 1628, after 26 years of additional experimentation, Harvey published *De Motu Cordis*. His theory of circulation brought acclaim, but was challenged and only fully acknowledged when Marcello Malpighi, with the benefit of the microscope, described capillaries in 1661. Harvey's legacy to the College is unsurpassed, but, importantly, he exhorted the Fellowship to 'search and study out the secrets of nature by way of experiment'.

The esteem in which Harvey was held is evidenced by this portrait being the only major artwork from the College that was preserved during the Great Fire of London in 1666. This splendid image still hangs in the College's Dorchester Library.

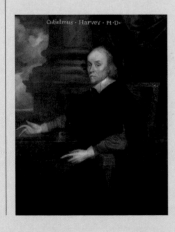

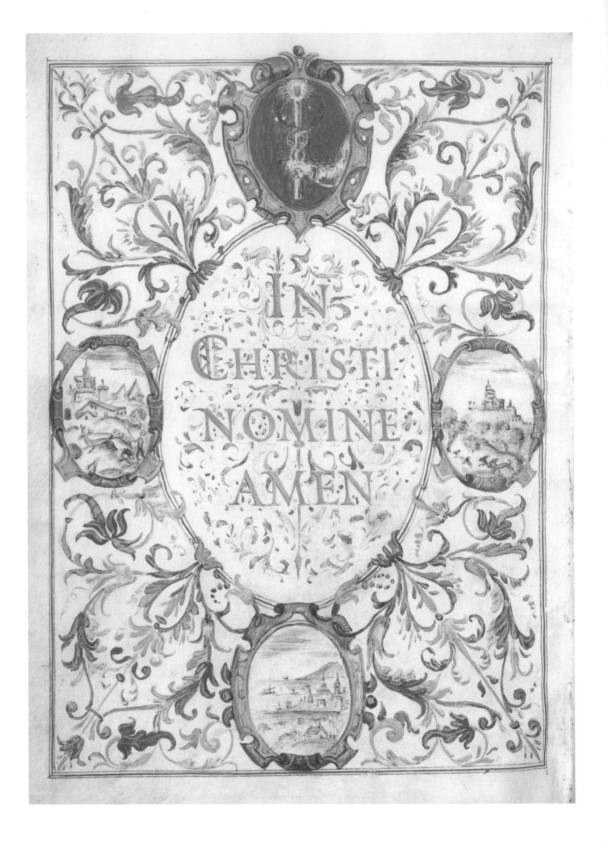

Opposite: Diploma of Doctor of Medicine presented to William Harvey by the University of Padua on 25 April 1602. Padua was the most celebrated school of medicine in the world. He was taught by Fabricius ab Aquapendente, professor of anatomy, John Thomas Minadous, professor of medicine, and Julius Casserius, professor of surgery, who observed his outstanding scholarship. He graduated with the highest honours and returned to Cambridge, where his degree was incorporated.

Below left: Harvey's interest in circulation began in Padua, and was facilitated by Charles II's provision of royal deer for experiments on circulation. He refined his ideas in his annual Lumleian lectures, and these resulted in the publication of *De Motu Cordis* 1628.

Below right: An illustration of Harvey's circulation experiments (1628), demonstrating the function of valves in the veins in taking blood from the peripheries towards the heart.

1632

Foundation of annual Goulstonian Lectures. Dr Theodore Goulston (1574–1632) leaves a bequest of £200 for a lecture by one of the youngest doctors, if possible on a corpse, between Michaelmas and Easter.

1633–34

Dr Baldwin Hamey the Younger elected FRCP. He went on to hold several offices including Censor, Registrar and Treasurer, and was one of the College's most generous benefactors.

1643

During the Civil War, the College, struggling to pay a £5 weekly levy on the 40-year Amen Corner lease to the Dean and Chapter of St Paul's, tries to free itself from this commitment. The College 'volunteered' three fellows to serve in a medical capacity in the parliamentary army.

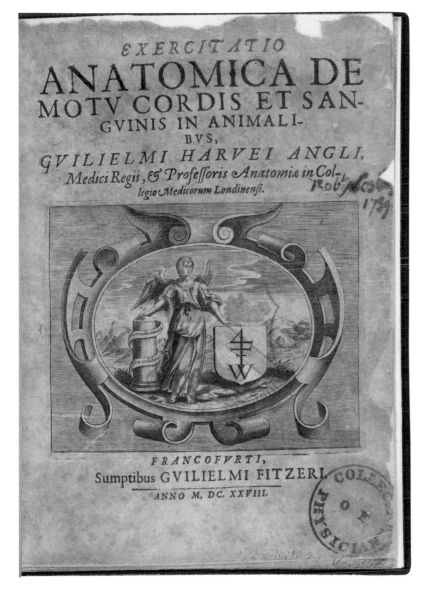

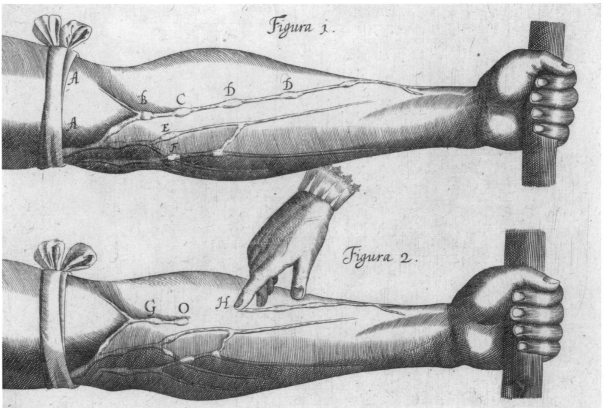

'*If I can procure one, that will build us a Library, and repository for Simples and Rarities, such a one as shall be suitable and honourable to the Colledge, will ye assent to have it done, or no?*'

Prujean, 4 July 1651

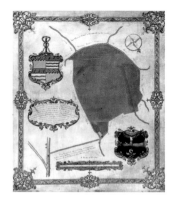

Above: Map illustrating Harvey's patrimonial Burmarsh estate, in Romney Marsh, Kent. Harvey was a great benefactor of the College. In 1654, he donated the estate to endow the new College library, the *Musaeum Harveianum*, an oration and 'once every year a general feast' to encourage 'friendship between the members of the said College'.

Right: Design for the proposed *Musaeum Harveianum* by John Webb. On 4 July 1651, Prujean, as President, asked the Fellowship for their views on the acquisition of a new library building to support the increasing collection of books, manuscripts and papers, ranging across many medical and non-medical topics, as befitted the scholarship of physicians. The response was a resounding agreement.

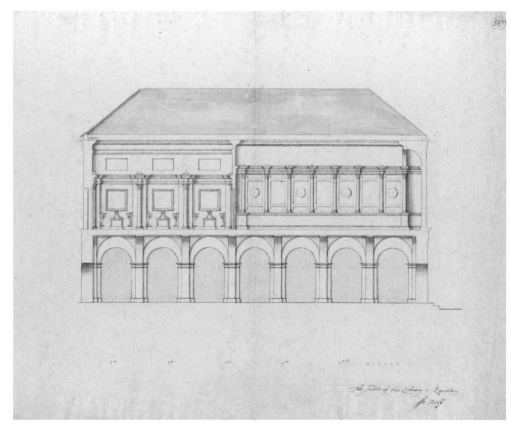

The founding physicians of the College were polymaths and humanists, distinguished by their classical and scholarly education, and a library to continue their scientific pursuits, both within and beyond medicine, was considered essential. Linacre donated his own library in the Stone House to the newly founded College and numerous major donations followed, including 680 volumes from a German physician and surgeon, Matthew Holbosch, in 1629. By 1632, the books were housed in a dedicated library in Amen Corner, and could be borrowed, provided the fellow pledged twice the value.

In 1651, Francis Prujean, as President, highlighted the importance of a new library, and, in 1652, announced funding by an anonymous donor. As a supporter of Charles I, branded 'a malignant' by Parliament and exiled from the College, Harvey had been discreet about his donation, but, in 1654, the library was named after him in recognition of his endowment of the family estate of Burmarsh in Kent to fund the library, as well as an annual oration and dinner.

In 1660, Merret (sometimes spelt Merrett), the first Harveian Librarian, catalogued 1,278 titles in the library, including texts on geometry, physics, cosmology, astronomy, geography, music, optics, natural history, 'voyages to the more remote regions of the Earth' and medicine, to befit physicians of great scholarship and learning, as required by Harvey in his instructions for the *Musaeum Harveianum*.

Over five centuries, the College library has amassed many treasures, including Plutarch's *Lives* (1476 edition); a copy of the first book printed by William Caxton (Bruges, *c*.1474); the only recorded copy of *L'art et l'instruction de bien danser* (Paris, *c*.1490); 120 books which belonged to John Dee, the Elizabethan mathematician, astrologer and alchemist; and a manuscript of Chaucer's *Canterbury Tales* (*c*.1440–50).

1649

Nicholas Culpeper publishes *A Physicall Directory*, an unauthorised translation of the College's *Pharmacopoeia*. His second book, no longer a translation, *The English Physician*, was published in 1652. Later editions of this became known as *Culpeper's Herbal*.

1650

Sir Francis Prujean elected President. Dr Francis Glisson publishes *De rachitide, an account of infantile rickets* and Dr Thomas Willis described the fourth cranial nerve.

1651

Dr Baldwin Hamey buys the house and garden at Amen Corner and gives it 'in perpetuity' to the College. It had been confiscated during the Commonwealth as part of the property of the Church, to be sold at auction.

1655

Hamey presents his silver bell to the College. It is a rare piece of pre-1665 College silver, as much of the silver was stolen from the Amen Corner College safe during the plague.

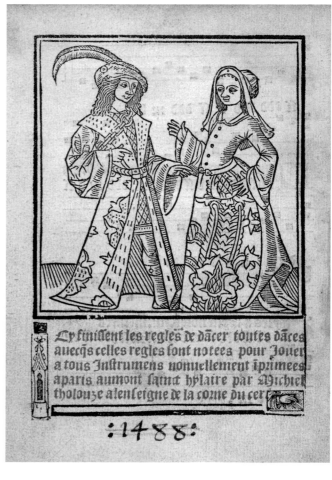

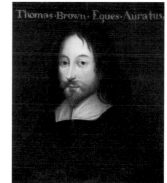

Above: Illustration from *L'art et l'instruction de bien danser*.

Left: Sir Thomas Browne (1605–1682), physician, philosopher, collector and polymath, saw the extraordinary in the ordinary, and introduced over 700 new words to the English language, while inspiring literary greats such as Virginia Woolf and Edgar Allan Poe. His collection of artefacts, books, plants and natural objects reveals a fascinating perspective on 17th-century scientific and medical research.

Far left: Extract from the book belonging to John Dee with his annotations in Latin and drawings.

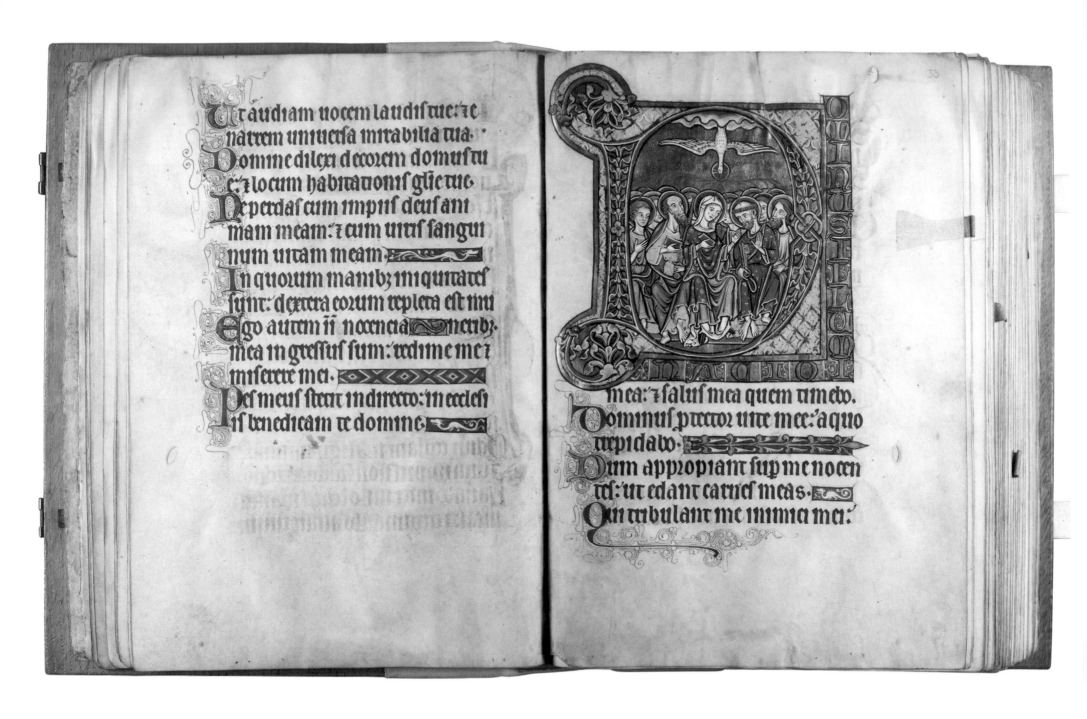

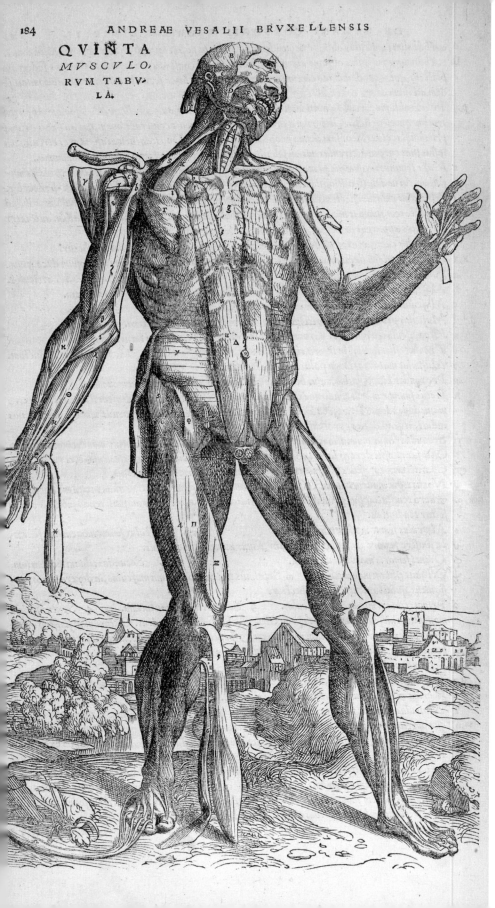

QVINTA
MVSCVLO.
RVM TABV-
LA.

'Nature can do more than physicians.'

Oliver Cromwell

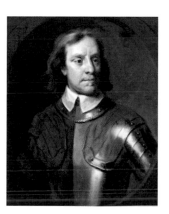

Above: Oliver Cromwell, Lord Protector, who issued letters patent to the College.

Left: Andreas Vesalius, *De humani corporis fabrica* (1543). Following the Black Death, the papacy had relaxed its prohibition on the post-mortem examination of bodies. In 1537, anatomical dissection was approved. The Flemish scholar Andreas Vesalius (1514–1564), having studied in Louvain, Paris and Padua, introduced scientific observation into dissection and wrote one of the most influential books on human anatomy, with unsurpassed anatomical illustrations by Jan Stephan van Calcar.

This period of history was marked by the union of Scotland, England and Ireland under King James I, followed by the Civil War and the execution of Charles I in 1649, Cromwell's Protectorate and the restoration of Charles II in 1660. During this long and turbulent period, the College nominally remained neutral, but affiliations were somewhat unreliable, changing to suit the current political situation.

Charles I was unpopular with the College because of taxes imposed to pay for wars with France and Spain and for approving the Church of England to license physicians. Nonetheless, many of the early fellows were physicians to the royal family and court, and throughout the Civil War remained staunch royalists, including Harvey, who was expelled from the College as a papist, and Baldwin Hamey the Younger, who, while caring for the Parliamentarians, harboured royalist loyalties. Meanwhile, the College sought and obtained letters patent from 'Oliver, Lord Protector' to ensure its position and, in 1643, sent three fellows to provide medical services to the Parliamentary army.

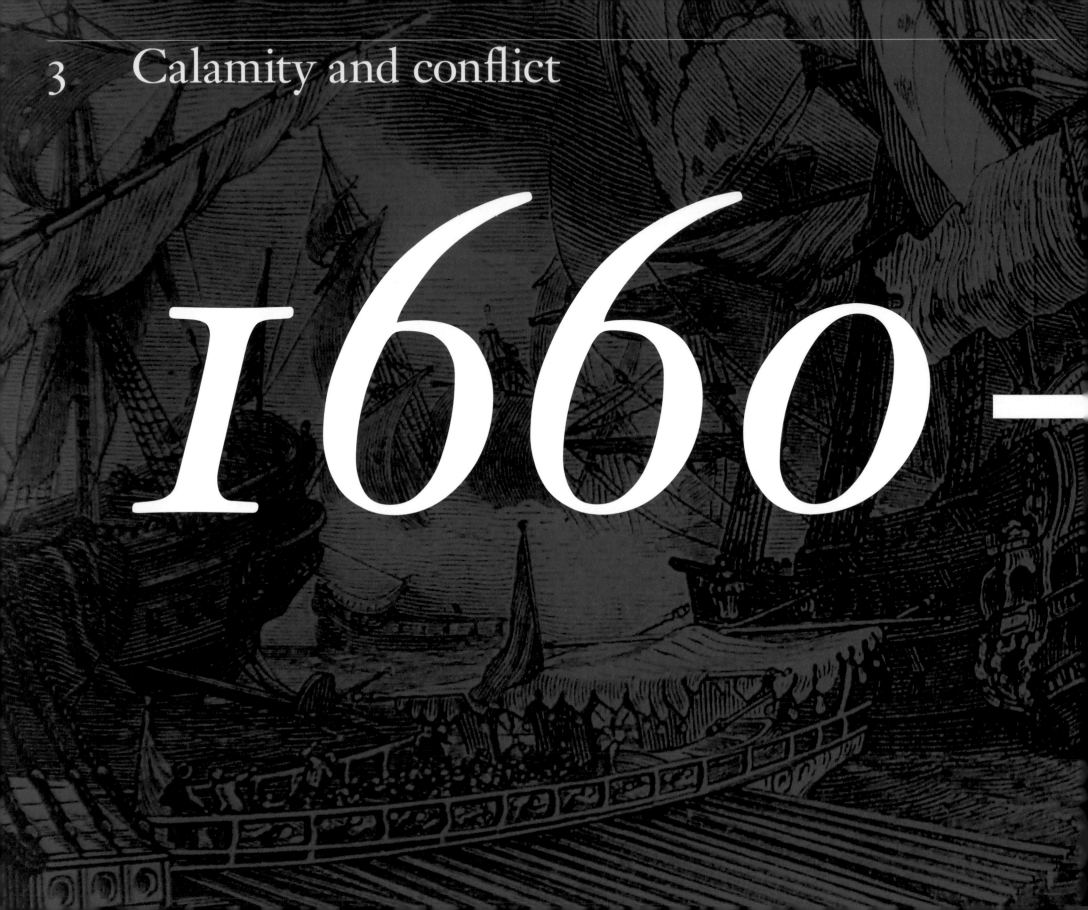

1660–

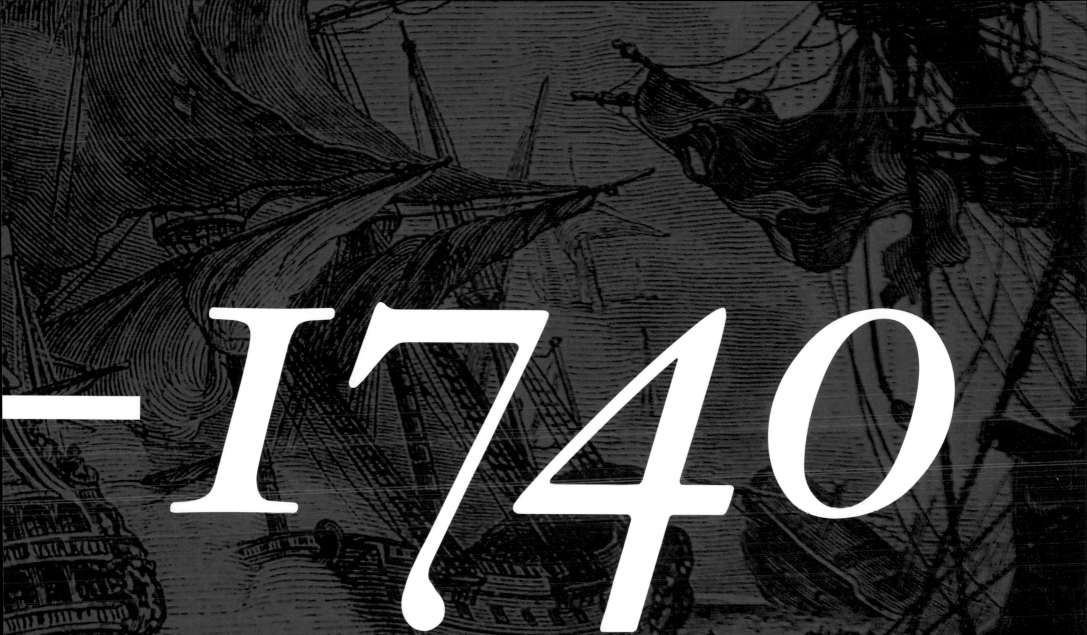

–1740

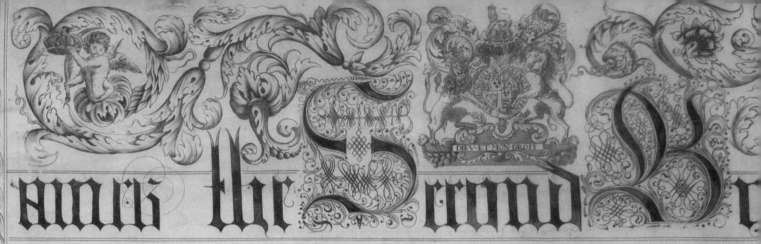

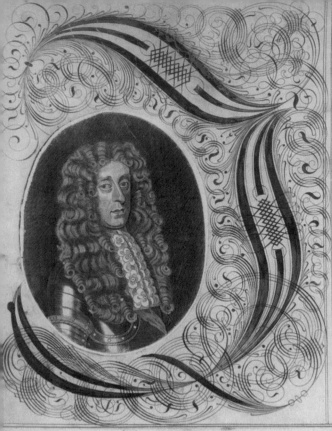

James the Second

by the grace of God of England Scotland France and Ireland King defender of the faith &c To all to whom these presents shall come greeting Whereas our most noble and renowned predecessor henry the Eight late King of England by his letters patents bearing date at Westminster the twenty third of September in the tenth yeare of his Reigne did Erect found and establish a perpetuall Colledge Comonalty and Incorporacon of Phisitians in the Citty and Suburbs of London and for seaven miles every way in distance from the same with power Annually to Elect a President of the same Colledge or Coialty and did thereby give and grant unto the sayd Colledge or Coialty divers Liberties Priviledges Imunities powers and authorities aswell for the advantage of the said President Colledge or Coialty and their Successors as for the suppressing and restrayning of illiterate persons from being Practizers in the said faculty as by the same Letters Patent remayning of record amongst other things therein conteyned more plainly and fully doth and may appeare which said Letters Patent and every Article Grant and thing therein conteyned were by Act of Parliament made in the Parliament begun at London in the fourteenth yeare and prorogued to Westm in the fifteenth yeare of the reigne of our said Noble Predecessor King henry the Eight approved ratified and confirmed And by severall other Acts of Parliament divers other Priviledges powers & authorities are and were afterward given granted and confirmed to the said President Colledge or Corporacon of Phisitians and their Successors as by the same severall Acts of Parliament thereof made more fully and at large also it doth and may appeare And whereas neverthelesse our Royall Grandfather James the first of ever blessed memory late King of England perceiving abuses not then sufficiently provided for did dayly encrease through the unskilfulnesse and fraud of Phisitians Apothecaries Druggists and such like by his Letters Patent under the Great Seale of England bearing date at Westm the Eighth day of October in the fifteenth yeare of his Reigne over England did ratify allow approve and confirme unto the said President Colledge or Coialty of Phisitians and their Successors the said Letters Patents of our said Noble Predecessor King henry the Eight herein before mencioned and every Grant Article and thing therein conteyned and not altered by the said Letters Patents of our said Royall Grandfather And further our said Royall Grandfather did by his said Letters Patents give and grant unto the said Colledge or Coialty and their Successors divers other Liberties Powers Priviledges abilities and authorities not onely for the benefitt of the aforesaid President and Colledge or Coialty and their Successors but also for the more certaine speedy and easy discovery punishment and restraint aswell of illiterate & unskilfull Practizers of the faculty of Phisick as likewise the frauds and deceipts of Apothecaries Druggists & others as by the same Letters Patent remayning of record among other things therein conteyned doth and may appeare And whereas our dearest Brother Charles the second late King of England of ever blessed memory in his great wisdome and prudence finding the many and great Liberties powers & priviledges aforesaid unto the said President Colledge & Coialty given granted and confirmed by the said Letters Patents & Acts of Parliament ineffectuall for the purposes intended was graciously pleased to the end that all frauds abuses and defects might be more easily remedied and supplied by his Letters Patents bearing date at Westm the twenty sixth day of march in the fifteenth yeare of his reigne to give and grant unto the said President & Colledge or Coialty that they from thenceforth forever should be continue and remaine one Perpetuall Body Corporate and Politick in deed fact and name by the name of the President Colledge and Comonalty of the Kings Colledge of Physicians in the Citty of London And by the same Letters Patents did likewise give and grant unto the said President fellowes or Coialty divers Liberties Priviledges and Immunities powers abilities and authorities aswell for the good government of the said Colledge or Coialty as for the surveying restraining and punishing unlicenced and unskilfull Practizers in the faculty of Phisick and all dealers in corrupt medicines and Druggs or other things to be used in Phisick as in and by the said Letters Patent of our said Royall Brother remayning of record amongst many other things therein conteyned more fully and at large it doth and may appeare **Know yee** that wee graciously designeing and zealously affecting nothing so much as the safety and honour of our Kingdome and the publique good and Comon benefitt of all our loving Subiects and seriously intending to remedy and prevent the great abuses frauds and Enormities frequently practized and comitted by divers Apothecaries Druggists and others in the said Citty of London and to punish and suppresse all ignorant unskilfull and unlicenced Empericks who have in open defiance and Contempt of authority dared publickly to professe and practise Phisick and have yett evaded the Just and condign punishment provided & intended by the Charters and Acts of Parliament aforesaid for such presumptuous offenders and to give all due encouragement to the Iudicious learned and experienced Professors of so noble and necessary a faculty of our especiall grace certaine knowledge and meer mocion at the humble Peticon of Sir Thomas Witherley Knt now President of the said Colledge or Coialty one of our Physitians and of divers other learned Doctors of the said Colledge or Coialty **Have** willed ordeyned given granted and confirmed And by these presents do for us our heires and Successors will ordeyne give grant and confirme unto the said President Colledge or Comonalty that they from henceforth forever hereafter shall bee continue and remaine one perpetuall Body Corporate and Politick in deed fact and name by the name of President Colledge or Coialty of the faculty of Phisick in London and that they shall have perpetuall Succession and a Comon Seale to serve and use for all the affaires causes and things whatsoever of them and their Successors And that they shall be capable by the said name of President Colledge or Coialty of the faculty of Phisick in London of purchasing having holding a leuing and disposeing land tenement goods and chattell and of impleading and being impleaded answering and being answered in any Court before any person or persons and in any suits causes or demands whatsoever And Wee have further of our like especiall grace certaine knowledge and meer motion willed ordeyned given granted ratified allowed and confirmed and by these presents do for us our heires and Successors will ordeyne give grant ratify approve allow and confirme unto the aforesaid President Colledge or Comonalty and their Successors forever the said Letters Patents of our said Noble Predecessor King henry the Eighth and of our said Royall Grandfather King James the first and of our said Dearest Brother King Charles the second herein beforemencioned and all and singular the Articles Clauses Gifts Grants franchises Liberties Priviledges Immunities powers and authorities therein mencioned or conteyned and not hereby altered in as full and ample manner as if the same were herein perticularly and at large recited and granted And the said President Colledge or Comonalty and their Successors by the name of President Colledge or Comonalty of the faculty of Phisicke in London shall and may forever hereafter have receive take retayne keepe use exercise enioy all and singular rights titles Liberties Priviledges Immunities Abilities powers authority and other things as by the said Letters Patents or by any Acts of Parliament are or were given granted or confirmed or were thereby mencioned or intended to bee Given Granted or Confirmed Notwithstanding the not useing misuseing abuseing or surrender of the same or any of them And that these presents and the aforesaid Letters Patent and every Article and Clause therein conteyned shall bee adiudged taken and construed most benignly and favourably to and for the best Benefitt and advantage of the aforesaid President Colledge or Comonalty and their Successors Any Ordinance Custome usage or other matter or thing to the contrary in any wise notwithstanding And for the better execucion of our will and pleasure herein declared Wee have named Constituted and appointed and by these presents do for us our heires and Successors name constitute and appoint Our Trusty and welbeloved Subiect Sir Thomas Witherley Knight Our Physician Sir George Ent Knight Sir Charles Scarborgh Knight Our Cheife Phisitian Doctor Walter Charlton Doctor George Rogers Doctor Thomas Burwell Doctor John Betts Doctor Peter Barwick Doctor Samuel Collins Doctor Nathaniel Hodges Sir Thomas Millington Knight Doctor John Lawson Doctor humphrey Brooke Doctor John Bidgood Doctor Nicholas

1660
The restoration of the monarchy, and the College recovers from the Civil War. The College has its first audience with the King.

1663
The College is granted its new royal charter. It had been the only learned society outside the universities to be granted a royal charter until 1662, when the Royal Society was also awarded its charter.

1665
The first royal visit to the College.

1665
George Ent is knighted by the King – the only example of such an honour conferred within the premises of the College.

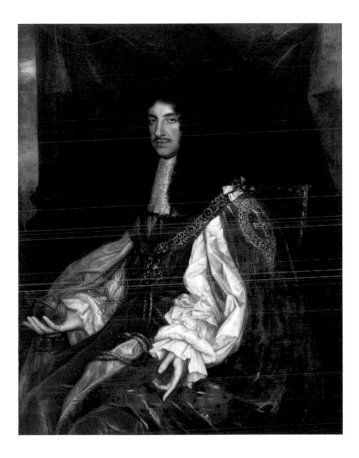

The College, perhaps surprisingly, survived the Civil War, the Commonwealth and the Protectorate in reasonably good health. Despite being immersed in politics, and embattled on various fronts, its fellows negotiated the changing fortunes of the opposing sides, and trod the political tightrope with skill and guile. Several fellows were influential in Cromwell's government and army, and the then President John Clarke was a trenchant Roundhead whose landed estates increased greatly during Parliamentary rule. However, in a supreme volte-face, the College quickly shed itself of Parliamentarian sympathies when Charles II ascended to the throne and robustly enthused about the restoration of the monarchy in 1660, referring to Cromwell's henchmen as 'seditious tribunes of the people and ill-conditioned scoundrels'. Perhaps this adjustment was not too difficult, as the fellows must, as a body, have found the elitist and traditional nature of monarchy more to their taste, and the return to the *status quo* rather a relief. Many fellows left London during the period of turmoil, but others stayed, hiding their royalist credentials, and some such as Hamey indeed made their fortunes in London during Parliamentarian rule. Others adroitly changed allegiance – George Bate for instance, who had been one of Cromwell's personal physicians, assumed the same position after 1660 in the service of Charles II.

Within a few months of the Restoration, the College acted to make clear its royal allegiance. The President, Dr Edward Alston, and a select band of fellows were granted audience with the King, and presented him with a golden unicorn horn, provided to the College by Hamey. A unicorn horn was known for its medicinal powers, as well as aphrodisiac properties, and this perfectly aimed dart seemed to hit its target successfully. The King was addressed by the President, who was knighted there and then for his pleasant sentiments, and as a reward for its political alacrity the College was granted a new royal charter in 1663. This extended the College's (and its President's) power, its jurisdiction spreading to an area of seven miles from the City of Westminster as well as the City of London, but also put it more under the scrutiny of the King's privy seal. Relationships were then further strengthened in April 1665, when the King made the first royal visit to the College, listened to an anatomy lecture by George Ent and knighted him on the spot in the Harveian Museum after the lecture.

Opposite: The royal charter of 1663, signed by Charles II. The College was referred to as the 'Kings College of Physitians in the Cittie of London'. The charter confirmed and extended the powers of the College, including its powers over the apothecaries which it viewed in an increasingly hostile manner. However, it was not confirmed by Parliament so its provisions could not be adopted officially.

Left: Portrait of Charles II, by John Michael Wright. The Restoration was an event of great importance to the College. The hedonistic Charles II proved a good friend of the College. Initially known as the College of Physicians, it was only from 1660 onwards that it started referring to itself consistently as 'Royal' – a sign that its officers demonstrated their debt to the monarchy.

1665

The Great Plague of London. Many fellows of the College are criticised for fleeing the capital and leaving its citizens without physicianly assistance – although it has to be said that available treatments were largely futile.

1665

The College publishes its *Directions for the Cure of the Plague*.

1665

Nathaniel Hodges, a candidate of the College, remains in London during the plague and later publishes a book of his observations.

Below left: Plague book title page. On 13 May 1665, the Privy Council asked the College to provide advice and 'such your directions to be speedily prepared and printed as possible can be', and eight days later the 'Certain necessary directions' (the plague book) was prepared and printed. It gives advice on public health and treatment.

Opposite: The angel of death gloats over the desolate scene in London, holding an hourglass in one hand and a spear in the other. This woodcut by an unknown artist was published in *The Intelligencer* on 26 June 1665.

'This day, much against my will, I did in Drury Lane see two or three houses marked with a red cross upon the doors, and "Lord have mercy upon us" writ there; which was a sad sight to me, being the first of the kind that, to my remembrance, I ever saw. It put me into an ill conception of myself and my smell, so that I was forced to buy some roll-tobacco to smell to and chaw, which took away the apprehension.'

Samuel Pepys

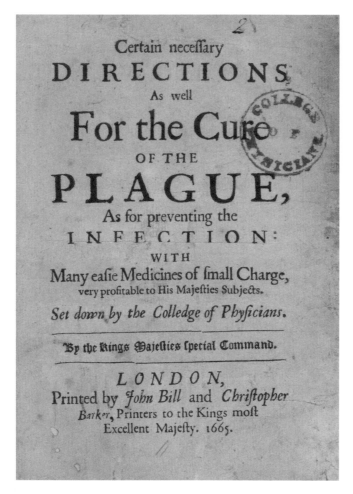

For the College, the pleasure of basking in the light of royal approval after the referendum proved to be only a short-term respite. A few months later, in the winter of 1664, as a bright comet was seen ominously in the skies over London, the first victims succumbed to what became known as the Great Plague. This was the last major epidemic of bubonic plague in Britain, caused as it has now been shown by the bacillus *Yersinia pestis*, which had recurred sporadically over previous centuries. The Black Death of 1347 was the greatest pandemic, affecting much of Britain and Europe, and in 1603 and 1625 smaller epidemics afflicted London and elsewhere, but the 1665 outbreak was termed the 'Great Plague', as it was the most devastating. It is estimated that 100,000 Londoners died, nearly a quarter of its population, its victims being largely the poor, as the richer citizens had rapidly fled the city. The royal court moved to Salisbury and then to Oxford, and most of the physicians also left. This flight of the fellows was a source of much criticism later, especially from the apothecaries, who largely could not afford to leave. However, not all physicians were so timid, and 17 fellows stayed in London, including Baldwin Hamey and Francis Glisson.

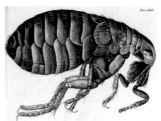

Left: The rat flea – *Xenopsylla cheopis*. The cause of the Great Plague was finally firmly identified only in 2016, with DNA analysis of a skeleton from the plague pits in London, showing this to be the bacillus, carried by the rat flea.

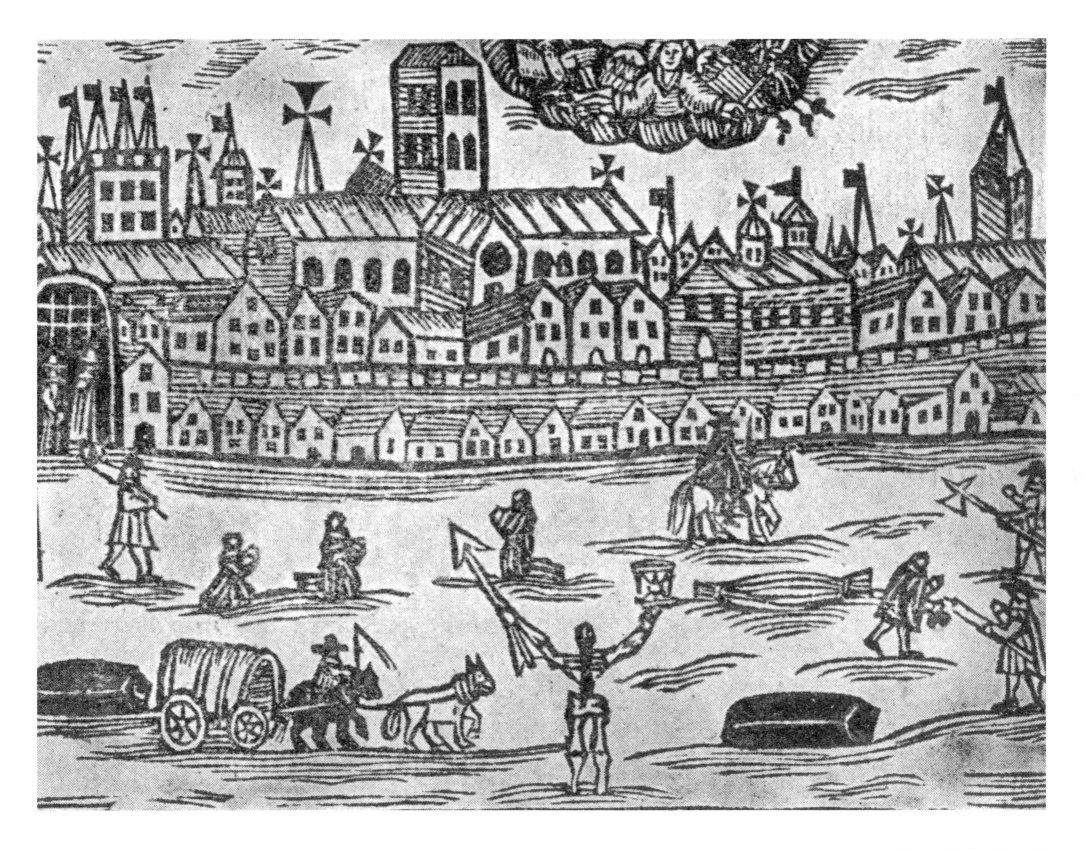

1665

The deserted College buildings are burgled. All its cash and most of its treasures are stolen from a specially secured safe. The thieves are not apprehended and neither the money nor the stolen goods are restored.

1665

The start of the long and acrimonious dispute between the College and Christopher Merret.

Right: Johannes de Ketham's *Fasciculus Medicinae* (1500) is a printing of six late-medieval manuscripts, a beautiful edition of which was acquired in 2015 by the College. This illustration shows a doctor treating a plague victim, holding a cloth to his mouth and burning lamps to try and keep the 'bad air' away.

Far right: Ancient precautions against plague included: closing windows against the infectious south wind, fumigating rooms with herbs like bay or hyssop, keeping a wood fire burning to clarify the air, confessing sins, washing regularly with rose water or vinegar, avoiding bad smells such as dead bodies and stagnant water, and avoiding crowds of people (*Regimen contra pestilentiam*, 1487).

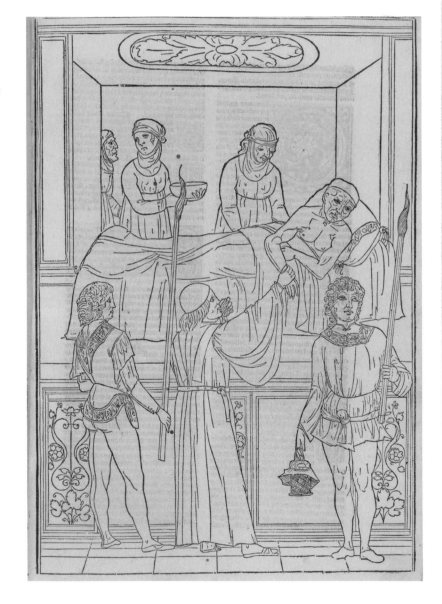

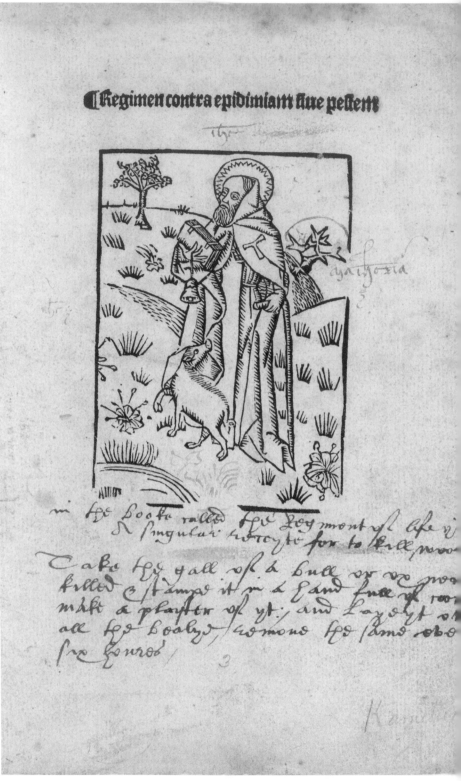

The College Censor Peter Barwick achieved fame and honour for remaining in a heavily infected area and prescribing for the poor without charge. It must be admitted though, that flee or remain, physicians and apothecaries alike had little influence on the disease itself, and no effective treatments. Their ministrations were confined to diagnosis and words of comfort. Isolation was then enforced, with the wretched victims left to their fate.

The middle years of the 17th century were not auspicious ones for the College. During the plague, thieves broke into the College's empty building and relieved it of most of its silver and treasures, and all of its cash. The money was stowed away in what was considered an impregnable deposit room and chest, but this proved not to be the case. Rumours were that this was an inside job, and Merret himself was at one time suspected.

Right: This was probably the iron chest that was broken into during the plague.

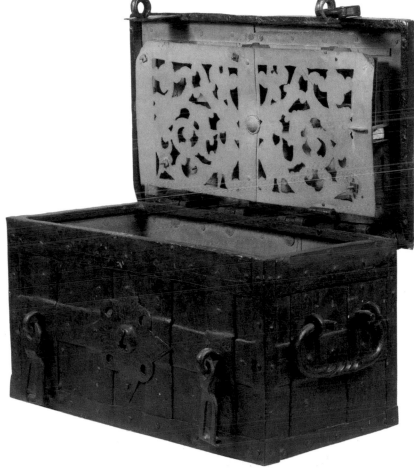

Peter Barwick
1619–1705

Censor at the College in 1674, 1684 and 1687, and elect in 1691, Barwick was admired for staying at his post during the Great Plague, where he administered to the sick and the clergy and daily attended the services at St Paul's, where his brother was Dean. He was a professed royalist, and during the Commonwealth attended the proscribed services of the Church of England, read by his brother, in the presence of friends. On the Restoration, he was appointed physician in ordinary to the King. After his home burned down in the Great Fire he moved to Westminster, taking up charity work and writing. Munk provides an engaging image:

He was a man of a very comely person, equally remarkable for the solidity of his learning and for a wonderful readiness as well as elegance in expressing it. His piety was sincere and sublime, his reputation absolutely unspotted, his loyalty exemplary, and his modesty almost without example. In all stations of life he was admired and beloved, and he was of a cheerful and serene mind in all situations. He was happy in the universal approbation of all parties, as he was himself charitable to all, and never vehement but in the cause of truth.

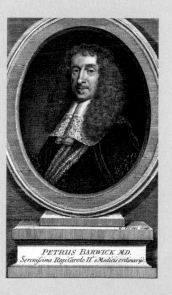

PETRUS BARWICK M.D.
Serenissimo Regi Carolo II.ᵈᵒ Medicis ordinarius

1666

The Great Fire of London destroys the College's building in Amen Corner – the final straw in a series of catastrophes for the College.

1669

The College buys a new site in Warwick Lane for £1,200 and starts rebuilding after the fire.

Then, in the autumn of 1666, further catastrophe struck. The Great Fire of London spread through the city between 2 and 5 September, gutting its medieval centre. The fire consumed and completely destroyed the College and its contents in the mid-afternoon of 4 September. It seems that only two fellows were present to try to prevent the calamity, Dr Christopher Merret and the Bedel. They managed to save about 100 of the books from the library, as well as manuscripts, charters and treasures from the College museum, including the caduceus, which had evaded theft the year before, but all else was reduced to ashes. According to the testimony of his son, Merret acted bravely and without concern for his person, and saved College treasures and books at the expense of his own private library, which was sacrificed in the fire. As his son wrote, 'All the Cheifest of ye books and Things of Value in & abt ye sd Library and College were brought in to ye sd College yard in readiness to p'serve ym, and he bravely attempted his salvage despite fire bursting out all around him'. The fire and the burglary brought the College to the edge of bankruptcy.

Right: A painting by Lieve Verschuier (1627–1686), a renowned Dutch Golden Age artist famous for his maritime subjects. The ferocious nature of the fire and its devastating effects are well caught by the artist.

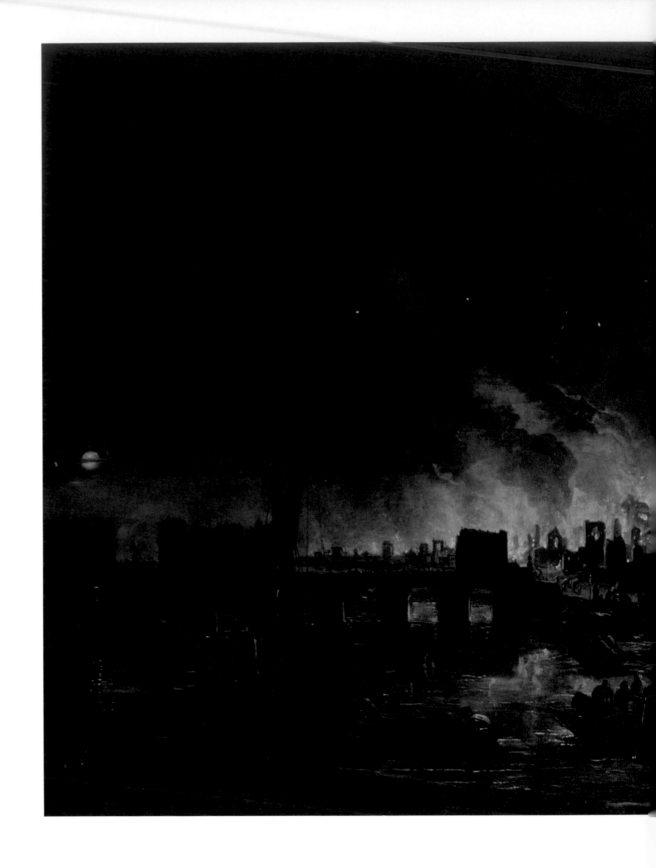

Christopher Merret
1614–1695

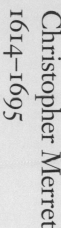

Merret's rise and fall in relation to the College make interesting reading. He was, on Harvey's nomination, keeper of the new library and museum which Harvey had donated and its first Harveian Librarian in 1654. In 1660, he was also a founder member of the Royal Society. A brilliant man, he presented papers to the Royal Society on diverse matters, including a method for making wine sparkle, in effect creating champagne years before this method was rediscovered in France. His reputation was at its height when the Great Plague struck and he fled London to the safety of the countryside. He seems to have been responsible for the security of the College, and during his absence the College was burgled. Merret had placed all its silver plate and cash into a heavy iron chest which he locked in a specially secured room, but the thieves still managed to break in, and all the contents of the safe were stolen. It seemed to be an inside job, and Merret was initially under suspicion. Then further calamity occurred, and the Great Fire totally destroyed the College and its library. In the following years, Merret became entangled in complex litigation with the College and his Fellowship was rescinded and four years later the Royal Society also expelled him for being in arrears. He died an embittered man, a feeling which might have been assuaged had he lived to see a genus of algae named *Merrettia* by S.F. Gray years later in recognition of his greatest work: *Pinax rerum naturalium Britannicarum* (1666), a catalogue of British plant and animal species.

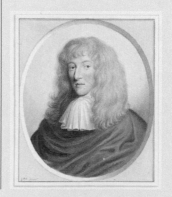

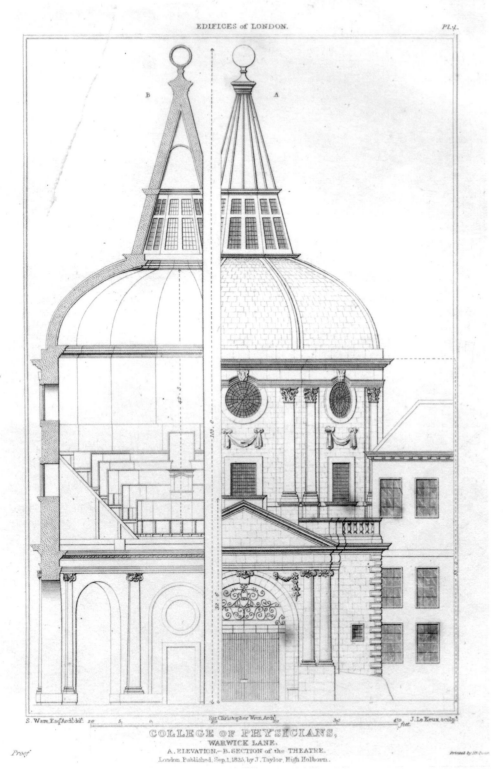

EDIFICES of LONDON.   PL. 4.

B   A

COLLEGE OF PHYSICIANS,
WARWICK LANE.
A. ELEVATION.—B. SECTION of the THEATRE.
London Published Sep.1, 1825, by J. Taylor, High Holborn.

S. Ware Esq. Archt. del.   Sir Christopher Wren Archt.   J. Le Keux sculpt.

Proof   Printed by M. Queen.

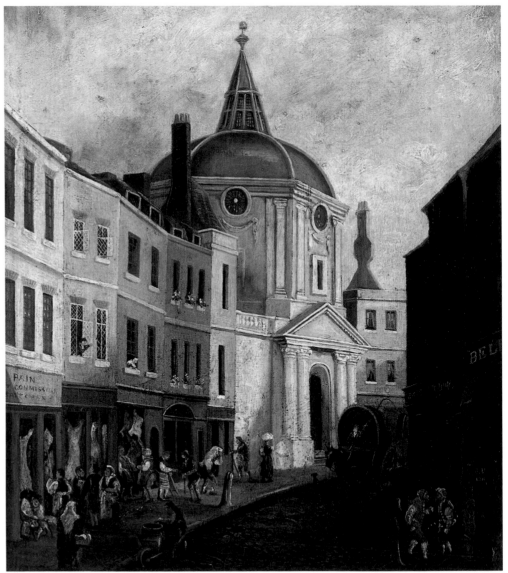

1674

Sir John Cutler decides to
provide funds for the building of
an anatomy theatre. The Warwick
Lane building opens.

1677

Third revision of the *Pharmacopoeia
Londinensis* is published. For
the first time the title of 'Royal'
(*Regalis*) appears, affixed to the
College's name.

1678/79

The College's fortunes begin
to turn. The Cutlerian Anatomy
Theatre is completed.

After the fire, new premises were needed. A series of complex financial arrangements resulted in the purchase of land in Warwick Lane, a much larger site than that previously occupied. New buildings were designed by Robert Hooke, who had had no previous architectural experience, but his buildings for the College were highly praised. Hooke decided upon a design with five-storey buildings on four sides around a large rectangular courtyard, and with an impressive gateway. On the first floor of the range, opposite the gateway, a long gallery was created, which was to be the centre of College ceremonial. This room was decorated with fine Spanish oak panelling, financed by Baldwin Hamey, and this panelling has been preserved and today lines the walls of the current Censors' Room. The large courtyard was decorated on its long side with plasters and pediments, swags and a niche, in which was wisely sited a statue of Charles II.

A striking feature of the new ensemble was the Anatomy Theatre, a last-minute addition to the building, paid for by a large donation from Sir John Cutler. The Anatomy Theatre was built over the gateway, and was a magnificent and striking structure, with a large dome, perfectly lit and arranged to allow the steep banking of seats for the onlookers. On its back wall was a niche for a statue of Cutler, facing King Charles himself, magnificent above the main doorway across the courtyard.

There had been no theatre at Amen Corner, but an anatomy theatre was the only part of the Barber-Surgeons' College building to survive the fire, and perhaps competition between the two colleges was a factor in the physicians' desire to own one. It was one of Hooke's greatest works, and was described at the time as a 'perfect study of acoustical and optical architecture'. On the outside of the theatre was placed the inscription 'Theatrum Cutlerianum', but in 1699 relations soured when Cutler's executors demanded £7,000 from the College, claiming that the donation was a loan rather than a gift. A settlement of £2,000 was made and the College, in revenge, obliterated the inscription 'Omnis Cutleri cedat labor Amphitheatro' on the wall of the theatre. The elegant classical assembly soon became a tourist destination, with visitors paying three pence each to be shown around.

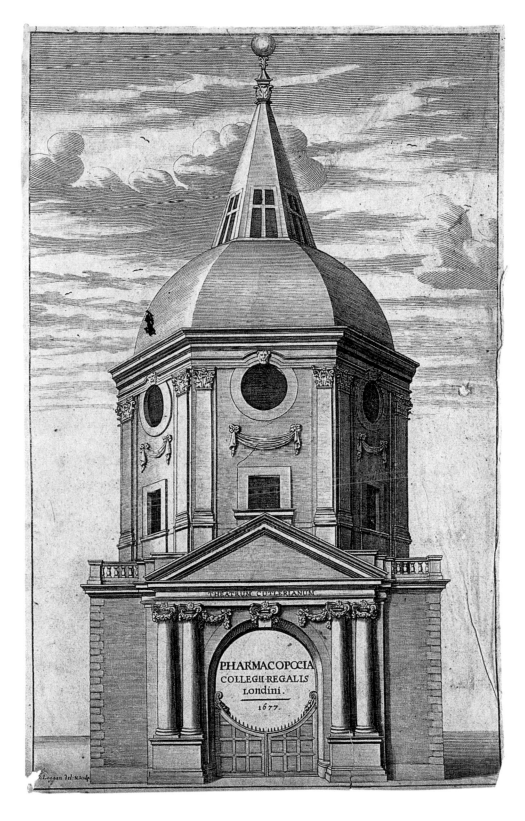

Far left: This splendid engraving by J. Le Keux, after an original by Samuel Ware, of the Warwick Lane Anatomy Theatre, was made in 1825. It shows the entranceway to the College's new buildings and the Anatomy Theatre in elevation.

Middle: Warwick Lane, buildings by Robert Hooke. This painting shows the crowded nature of the site of the new building, which looks wholly out of place in the higgledy-piggledy Warwick Lane. One can detect the confident mood of Hooke and Wren as they endeavoured to move London's architecture away from its medieval past.

Left: The Warwick Lane Anatomy Theatre, engraved by D. Loggan in 1677. This plate is said to be based on an original by Robert Hooke, the architect of the building. It is the frontispiece of the 1677 edition of the College's *Pharmacopoeia Londinensis*.

Sir George Ent was 'an ornament of his age', serving as College Censor for 22 years, Registrar for 15 years and President for eight years at various times between 1670 and 1684. He was a scholar and anatomist, and founder member of the Royal Society. He qualified in medicine in Padua and was incorporated in the University of Oxford. He wrote in a beautiful Latin style, was a powerful orator, and author of many books, including his *Apologia pro circulatione Sanguinis*. This was a defence of Harvey's theories on the circulation of the blood and was an influential document in its time. Ent was, throughout his life, a close friend of William Harvey. In his *Apologia pro Circulatione Sanguinis, contra Æmilium Parisanum* (1641) he 'learnedly defended Harvey against his opponent, and gave a rational account of the operation of purgative medicines' according to Munk. He also edited and published Harvey's *De Generatione Animalium*. All admired his intelligence, and his friends inscribed his coat of arms with the motto *'Genio Surget'* (genius rises), an anagram of his name (with 'George' spelled as *'Georgius'*).

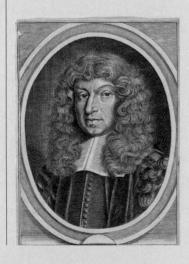

Below: Sir John Evelyn's plans, showing the proposed position of the College of Physicians in a map made by Walter Harrison. Evelyn's ambitious and modernising plan to rebuild London after the Great Fire was never realised. The College of Physicians (#6) was to be rebuilt close to its original position west of St Paul's Cathedral.

Opposite: Warwick Lane, buildings by Robert Hooke. This wood engraving (signed WHP) shows the interior quadrangle of the College's buildings in Warwick Lane, with their elegant and classical façades – imparting a sense of dignity and seriousness which no doubt the College wished to convey to the public and to the court. Interestingly the niche with the statue of the King is missing – perhaps this was an earlier design, or a mistake.

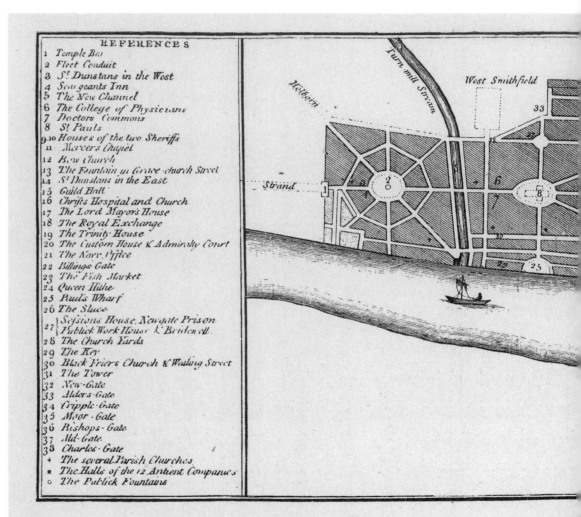

REFERENCES
1 Temple Bar
2 Fleet Conduit
3 St Dunstans in the West
4 Serjeants Inn
5 The New Channel
6 The College of Physicians
7 Doctors Commons
8 St Pauls
9.10 Houses of the two Sheriffs
11 Mercers Chapel
12 Bow Church
13 The Fountain in Grace-church Street
14 St Dunstans in the East
15 Guild Hall
16 Christs Hospital and Church
17 The Lord Mayors House
18 The Royal Exchange
19 The Trinity House
20 The Custom House & Admiralty Court
21 The Navy Office
22 Billings Gate
23 The Fish Market
24 Queen Hithe
25 Pauls Wharf
26 The Sluce
27 { Sessions House, Newgate Prison, Publick Work House & Bridewell
28 The Church Yards
29 The Key
30 Black Friers Church & Watling Street
31 The Tower
32 New-Gate
33 Alders-Gate
34 Cripple-Gate
35 Moor-Gate
36 Bishops-Gate
37 Ald-Gate
38 Charles-Gate
+ The several Parish Churches
* The Halls of the 12 Antient Companies
o The Publick Fountains

Sir John Evelyn's Plan for Rebuilding the Ci

1680

On his death, Lord Dorchester announces the bequest to the College of his enormous library of 3,200 volumes, one of the most renowned in Europe.

1682

The College describes itself as the 'Royal College of Physicians of London' in its *Annals* of 1682.

1682

The first nominal Roll of the College is published, listing licentiates as well as fellows.

1684

The worst frost on record, and the Thames freezes over in the winter of 1683/4. The Thames froze 24 times between 1408 and 1814, but this was the most severe.

1685

King Charles II dies. Nine fellows of the College draw up an address of condolence and congratulation to his brother, James II, whose hand they kiss.

1685

Daniel Whistler, who had been President of the College, and who had died the year before, was found to have embezzled money from the College.

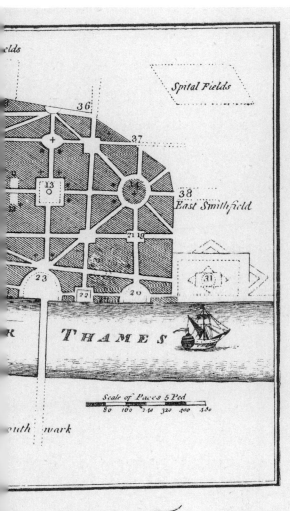

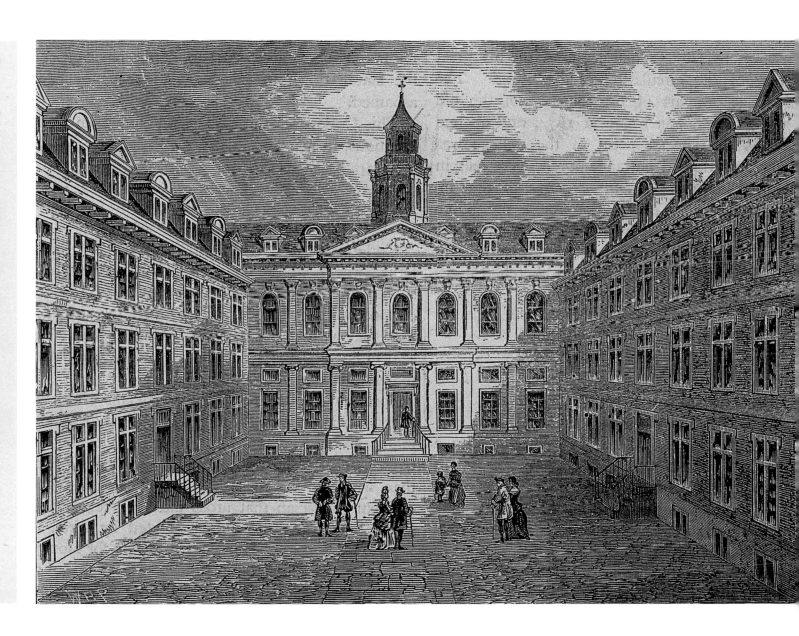

1687

A new royal charter is granted by the new King, extending the College powers especially over licensing. It is written in English. The maximum number of fellows permitted in the College rises to 80. Both Hans Sloane and John Radcliffe are admitted as fellows.

1688

The Glorious Revolution weakens the College's power over the apothecaries and surgeons and causes many legal problems.

1688

A custom-built library built by Sir Christopher Wren is opened to house the Dorchester collection.

1689

After the Glorious Revolution, the College reports the names of seven fellows to the House of Lords who were papists, reputed papists or criminals.

1689

Mary and William succeed to the throne and the College exclude obvious Catholics from the Fellowship.

1694

The College is involved in legal wrangles with the licentiate Johannes Groenvelt, and this, with the William Rose case a few years later, damages its public reputation.

Medical practice in the 17th century was very different to that of today. There were by then three types of recognised practitioner – physicians, surgeons and apothecaries.

The physicians were the 'first class of medical practitioner in rank and legal pre-eminence', often learned, and the most fashionable. Their role was to diagnose and to prescribe drugs. They treated only the wealthiest patients, and in London therefore had the opportunity to become very rich. Many had made great fortunes and the richest lived in the style of the aristocracy.

The surgeons were considered essentially craftsman, and to be of a lower social order. They were joined with the barbers into the Company of Barber Surgeons by Act of Parliament in 1540 and remained so until 1745, when they then formed their own livery company, the Company of Surgeons.

At the bottom of the pile were the apothecaries, who had been formed into the Society of Apothecaries in 1617, when they broke away from the Grocers Company to which they were previously assimilated. Their role was to prepare, make up and dispense drugs on behalf of the physicians. Traditionally, and by act of Parliament, they were not allowed to prescribe or to practise medicine – this was the province of physicians. However, in London, as the urban poor who had no contact with physicians grew in number, the apothecaries increasingly made diagnoses and acted as doctors.

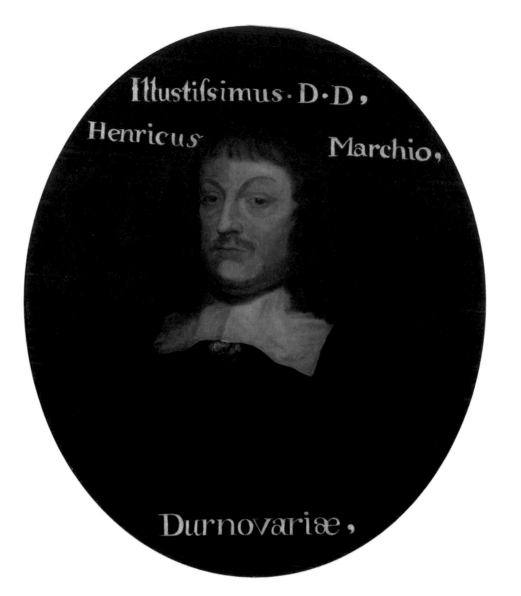

Illustissimus · D·D, Henricus Marchio, Durnovariæ,

Left: Henry Pierrepont (1606–1680), the 1st Marquis of Dorchester, left his library of over 3,200 volumes to the College on his death. He was an honorary fellow of the College and an amateur physician. His library was considered the finest philosophical library in Europe, and contained books on 'Physique, Mathematique, Civile Law, and Philology', as well as works of fiction and the classics. Sir Christopher Wren adapted the College buildings to accommodate the library.

Opposite: This satirical drawing by Hogarth, entitled *The Company of Undertakers, or the Consultation of Physicians*, shows 12 pompous and animal-like physicians sniffing their pomanders and examining a flask of urine. They are presided over by three notorious quacks of the time: Joshua 'Spot' Ward, Mrs Mapp and the Chevalier James Taylor. The inscription translates 'And the many images of death'. The whole is set in a mock coat of arms, the explanation of which starts *Beareth Sable, an Urinal proper*.

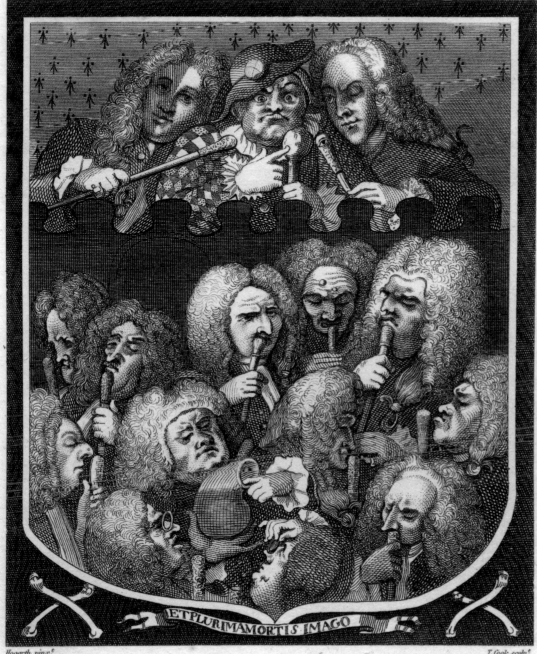

ET PLURIMA MORTIS IMAGO

Hogarth pinx.t   T.Cook sculp.t

CONSULTATION OF PHYSICIANS.

In addition to these three classes of officially recognised practitioners there was also a very large body of quacks and charlatans, who had no affiliation to any guild or college. They operated entirely independently, and their activities were wholly unregulated. In practice, it was the quacks and charlatans who provided the medical care for the poorest in society who had no opportunity to consult a physician or even a surgeon or apothecary.

In the second half of the 17th century there was an increasing clamour for change. Apothecaries were far more numerous than physicians, and they were also becoming more professionalised. Their role had *de facto* expanded beyond the mere formulation of medicines, and they prescribed and treated patients as well. The cowardly behaviour of physicians during the plague enhanced the apothecaries' position, and as the population of London grew, so too did the need for more equitable medicine. The new charters granted to the College by Charles II and James II gave the College new powers of regulation over the apothecaries. Clashes between physicians and apothecaries over rights of practice became frequent and acrimonious with raids on apothecaries' shops by the College Censors, the imposition of punitive fines by the College, the publication of hostile pamphlets and tracts, and the occasional law suit.

The temperature was further raised when the College moved into apothecary territory by opening its own 'Dispensary', providing free medicines for the poor. The feud intensified, much to the amusement of the satirists and playwrights of the period, and it was only in the 18th century that relationships improved, and with the passage of the Apothecaries Act of 1815 and the Medical Act of 1858 that their relative roles were finally accepted.

1696

The College statutes are translated from Latin into English. This seemingly innocuous move results in contention and tumult.

1697

The College reopens its dispensary, inflaming relations with the apothecaries.

1699

Samuel Garth publishes his poem 'The Dispensary', and the College becomes the centre of much public banter.

1701

Settlement is reached with the estate of Sir John Cutler over a dispute about the building of the Anatomy Theatre. £2,000 is paid in damages.

1702

A second dispensary is opened, in Cornhill.

1704

The senior judges of the House of Lords rule in favour of the apothecary William Rose in his legal battles with the College. This landmark case allows apothecaries to practise 'medicine', and the central aspect of the privileges of the physicians is removed.

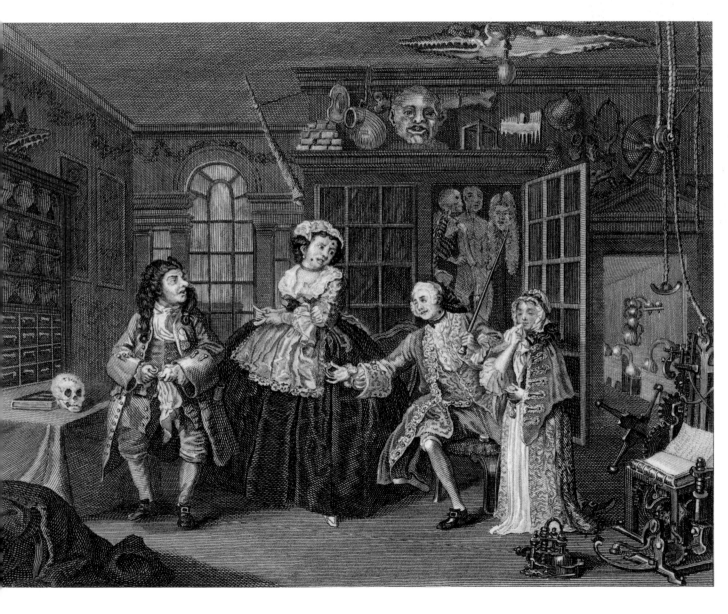

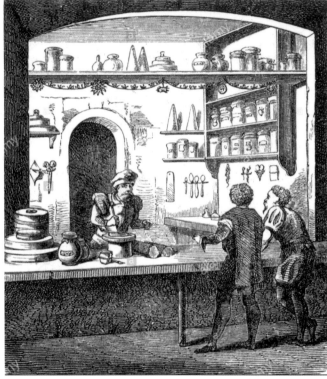

'Medicine itself is sick. This Art, of all others the most useful, knows not how to help itself while rather from mock Physicians, than diseases, this country suffers … Here an operator mounted on his pyed horse, draws teeth in the streets; another is so obliging as to be at home at certain hours to receive fools; another pores in urinals, and if he finds no disease there, he makes it up; another still, draws together a crowd by the help of rope-dancing; he comes, he sees, then rushes forth upon the multitude and murders without mercy. Yet not with weapons do these swarms of mountebanks inflict wounds, but with some nostrums more dangerous than any weapon.'

Samuel Garth, *Oratoria Laudatoria* (1697)

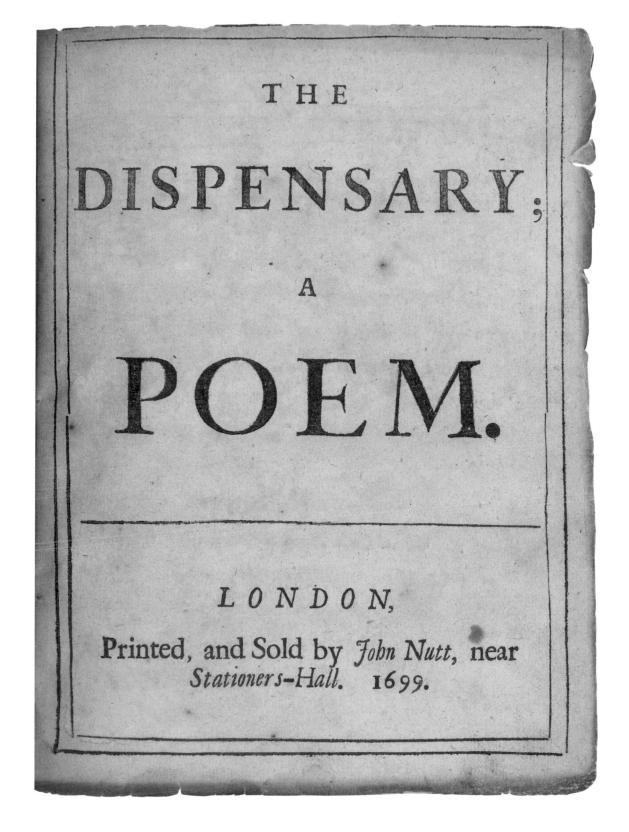

THE

DISPENSARY;

A

POEM.

LONDON,

Printed, and Sold by *John Nutt*, near *Stationers-Hall.* 1699.

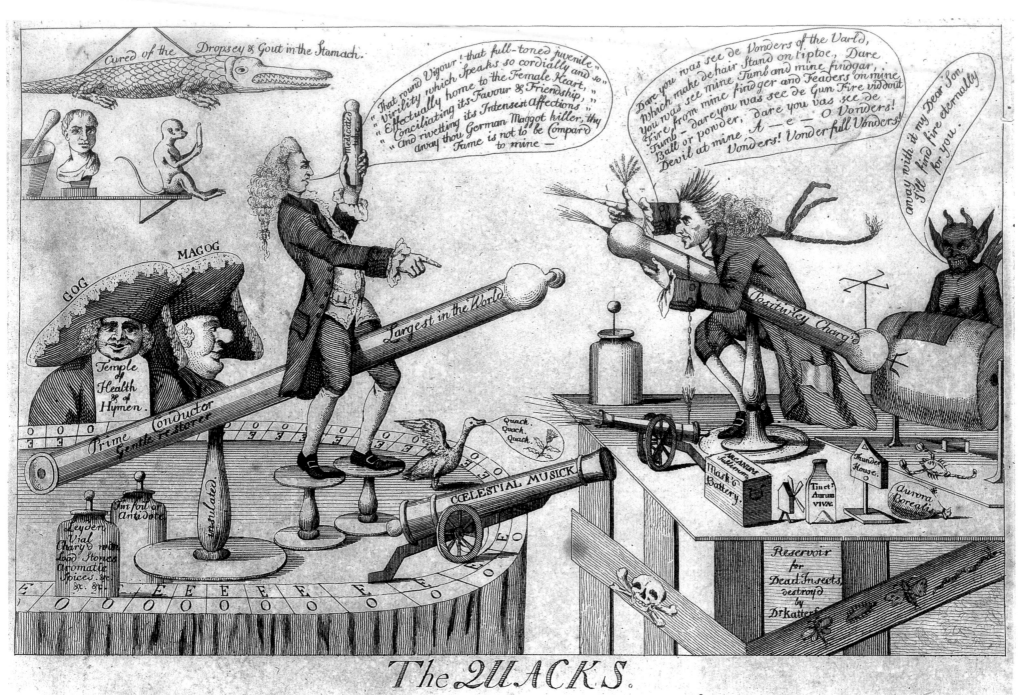

Opposite: James Graham was a notorious quack who specialised in sexual disorders – with cures for venereal disease and methods for improving sexual vigour. His electromagnetic treatment was particularly popular, as was his 'Great State Celestial Bed'. This nine-foot bed could be hired out at £50 a night. There were various accoutrements designed to intensify the ardour of the bed's occupants, including erotic paintings, mirrors, flashing lights and 'celestial sounds' from organ pipes in the bed frame triggered by rhythmical movement. This satirical etching, showing him battling with his competitor Gustavus Katterfelto, another famous London quack, was published in 1783.

Right: Francis Glisson (1599–1677), physician and anatomist, College President 1667–70, and Regius Professor of Physic at Cambridge from 1636 until his death. He is remembered also for remaining in London during the plague. He was one of the first to describe rickets, published detailed work on various other conditions and was elected as a member of the Royal Society. He was active in natural philosophy circles and an important figure in 17th-century medicine, where he represented the modern scientific generation at the College.

Below: Thomas Rowlandson's *Death and the Apothecary or The Quack Doctor* shows Death peering at the living in the apothecary shop.

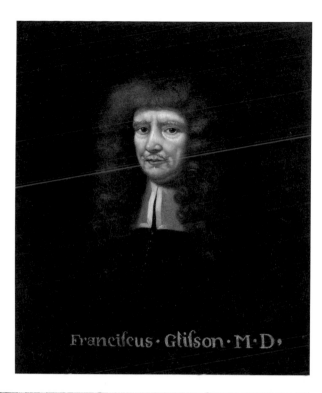

Francifcus · Glifson · M·D·

In the late 17th century, medicine was still embedded in the classical tradition, although leading practitioners like John Radcliffe were renowned for their diagnostic and prognostic skill. The physicians at the top of the pile earned huge fortunes and were not keen to forego their privileges. Medicine, though, was beginning to change, and the hegemony of classical learning was threatened by what became known as the Scientific Enlightenment. The appointment of Sir Hans Sloane as President in 1719 was a turning point for the College. He held the post for 16 years, and during his time the College engaged with the modern scientific awakening. Influenced by his friends and colleagues Robert Boyle, Thomas Sydenham and Isaac Newton, Sloane espoused the revolutionary Natural Philosophy and the new approaches to science and medicine being promulgated by the Royal Society, of which he was later president. He transformed the attitude of the College to science and scientific method, and under his leadership the College's traditional reactionary Galenic conservatism melted away. The new theories and practices of scientific medicine were espoused particularly by Sloane's friend Thomas Sydenham, whose publications were to mark the reawakening of academic interest in the College. Under Sloane's guidance, an agreement was also concluded with the Society of Apothecaries in which the Chelsea Physic Garden was leased to them on the understanding that the garden would supply the Royal Society with 50 good herbarium samples a year, an agreement that effectively ended the longstanding hostility between the College and the apothecaries.

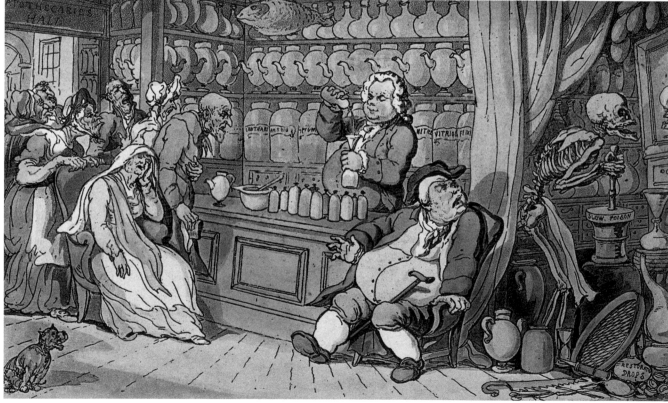

1704–18

ʜe College goes through a period of relative neglect. Five presidents come and go without making much of a mark.

1719

Sir Hans Sloane appointed President of the College, ushering in a period of enlightenment and the promotion of natural philosophy and national science.

1721

Revision of the *Pharmacopoeia Londinensis* is published, showing the influence of Sloane.

1722

Sloane leases the Chelsea Physic Garden to the apothecaries, marking the beginning of the end of conflict between the physicians and apothecaries.

1724

The College dispensary at Warwick Lane closes.

1725

The College petitions the government on the evils of 'distilled spirituous liquors' (gin).

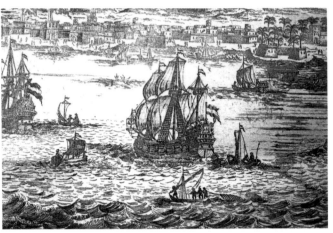

Of all the specimens in the College's herbarium, quinine may be considered the most important. It comes from the bark of the Peruvian *Cinchona* tree. It was introduced to England in 1655 as Jesuit's Powder, and Robert Talbor, an apothecary, popularised its use in 1672. Sloane had cornered the market in Peruvian bark, at a time when malaria killed more people than any other transmissible disease. The appearance of quinine in the *Pharmacopoeia Londinensis* in 1677 was a landmark event, for here for the first time was a cure. Talbor treated a member of Charles II's court, was given a knighthood and appointed King's Physician, to the disgust of the College. Quinine remained the mainstay for anti-malarial treatment thereafter until the advent of artemisinin in the 1990s.

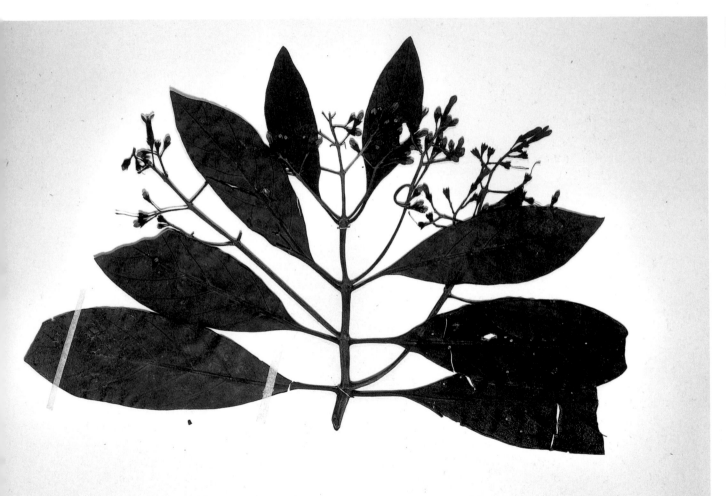

Discovered by Mr R. Thomson in the central cordillera of the Colombian Andes

Cinchona "negra" Cultivated, Bogota Mr R. Thomson

'The knowledge of Natural-History, being Observation of Matters of Fact, is more certain than most others, and in my slender Opinion, less subject to Mistakes than Reasonings, Hypotheses, and Deductions are … These are things we are sure of, so far as our Senses are not fallible; and which, in probability, have been ever since the Creation, and will remain to the End of the World, in the same Condition we now find them.'

Sir Hans Sloane

Opposite left: The search for the species of *Cinchona* with the greatest content of quinine occupied plant hunters for 300 years. Specimens were sent back to the Pharmaceutical Society in London for analysis, and their herbarium, now at the College, contains numerous specimens like that of *Cinchona officinalis*. Quinine is still extracted from the bark.

Opposite right: In the 17th and early 18th century, ships like these great galleons transported plants and resins from every corner of the known world for the flourishing trade in exotic medicines in Europe. From Engelbert Kaempfer's *Amoenitatum Exoticarum Politico-physico-medicarum* (1712).

Right: *Cinchona officinalis*, the source of quinine, grows wild in Peru, and here in the highlands near Huánuco in the Andes, the bark has been harvested for treating fevers by the Quechua from before the Spanish conquest, and was used in England beginning in 1655.

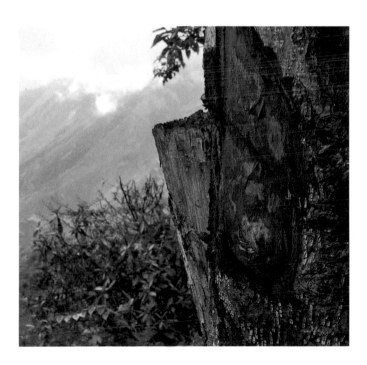

One of the most significant public figures of the period in England, Sir Hans Sloane was a scholar, scientist, physician, philanthropist and public benefactor. He had a very large medical practice amongst the upper classes, including, it is said, 16 dukes and ten earls, but every day also treated the poor without payment. He was appointed physician to Queen Anne and George I and then a physician in ordinary to George II, 'having been before constantly employ'd about the whole Royal Family, & always honour'd with the Esteem & favour of the Queen Consort'. He promoted and popularised the practice of inoculation in England, not least by inoculating the entire royal family in a blaze of publicity. He brought quinine into England, prepared from 'Peruvian bark', and recommended it for 'intermittents, fevers of other denominations, nervous disorders, and gangrene and hæmorrhages'. He acquired fortunes in Jamaica by cornering the market in Peruvian bark and from his recipes for milk chocolate, and he died an enormously rich man. He was elected president of the Royal Society in 1727 and left his huge collections of books, manuscripts, prints, drawings, flora, fauna, medals, coins, seals, cameos and other curiosities to the nation on his death. This collection, with the royal library of George II, was opened to the public as the British Museum in 1759, and much of the collection later became the foundation for London's Natural History Museum.

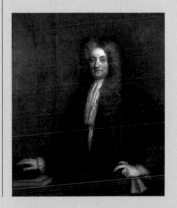

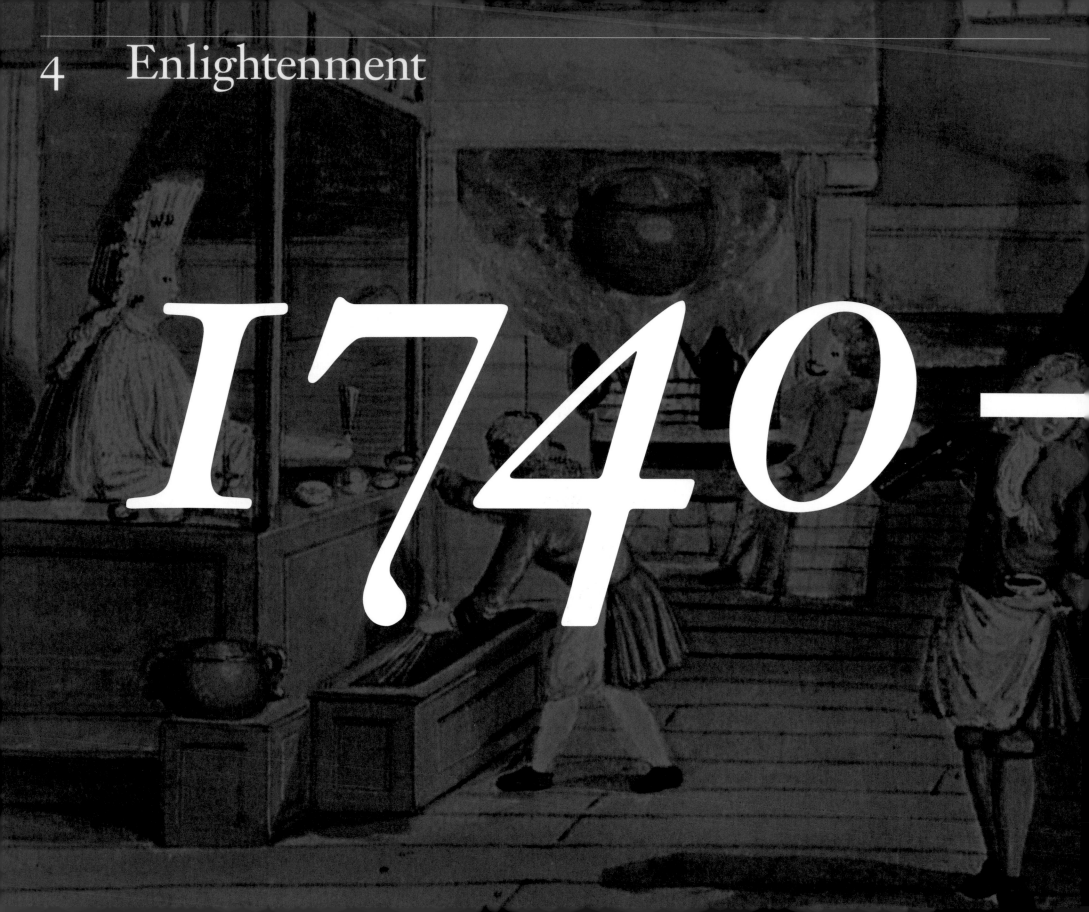

1740–

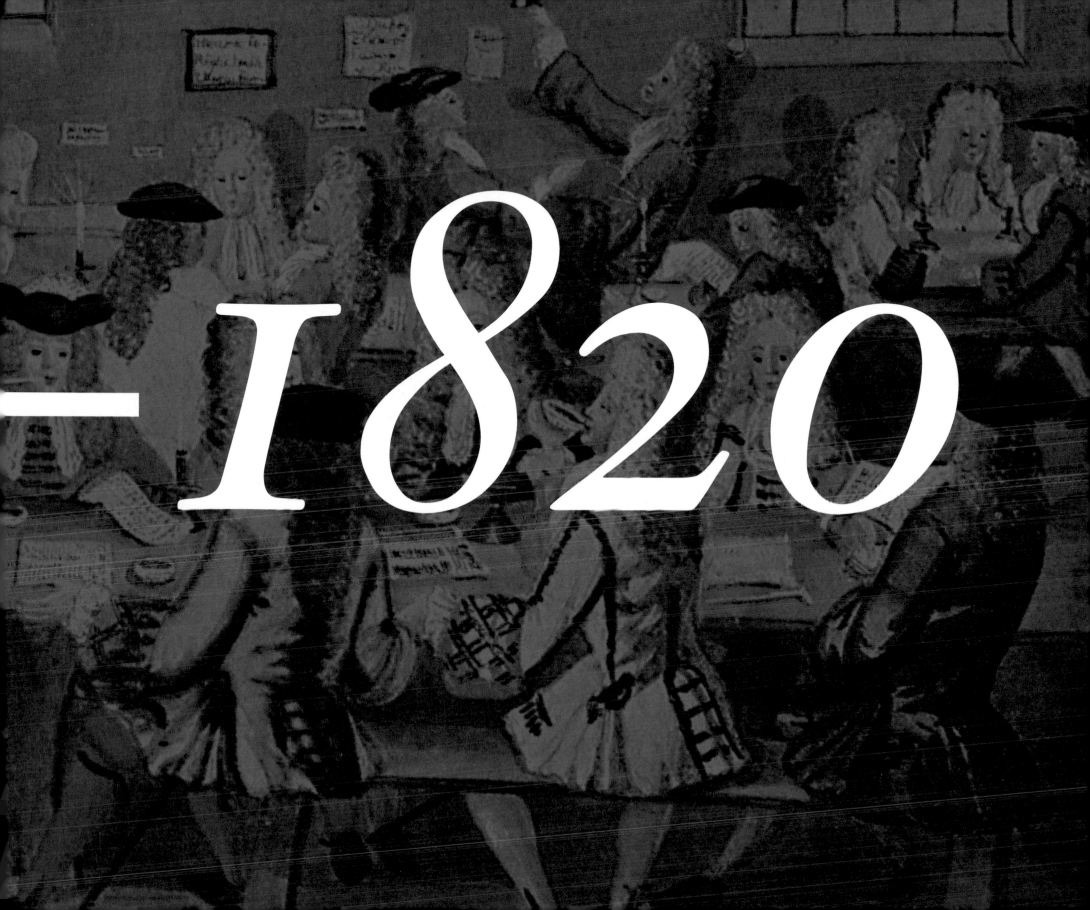

−1820

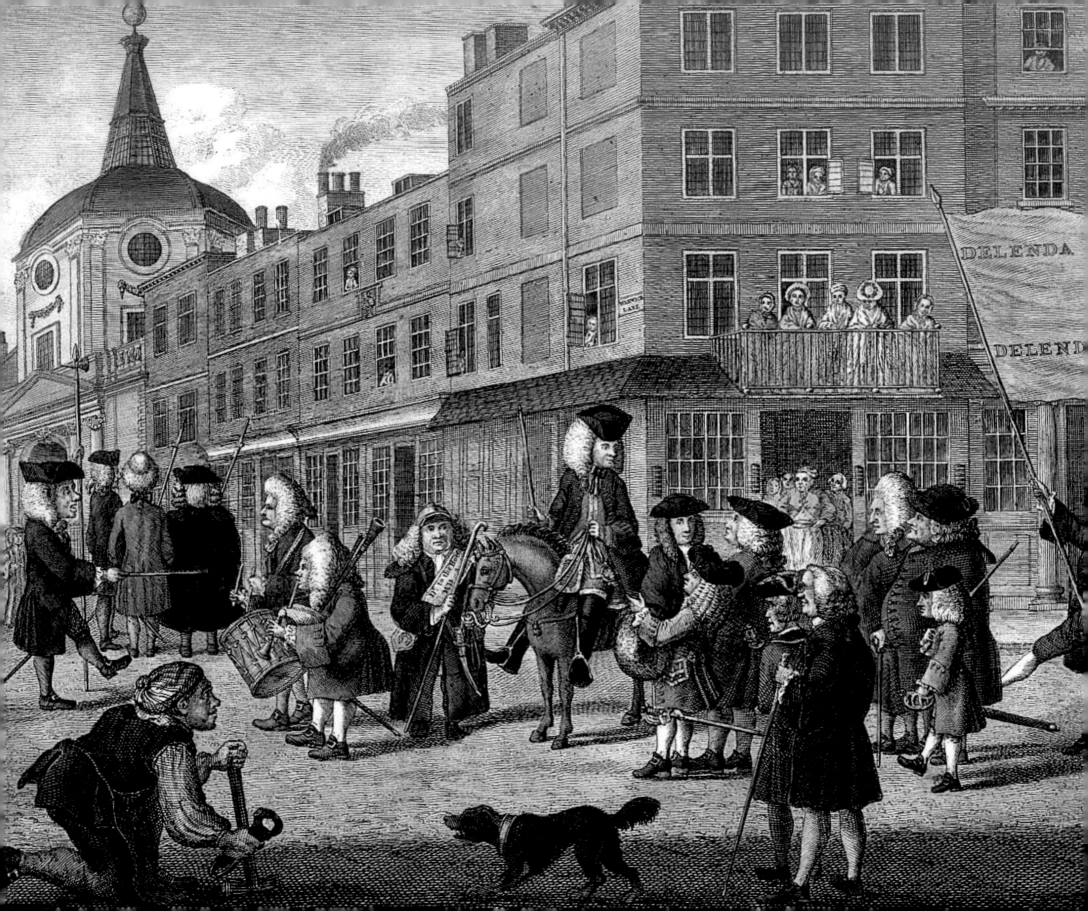

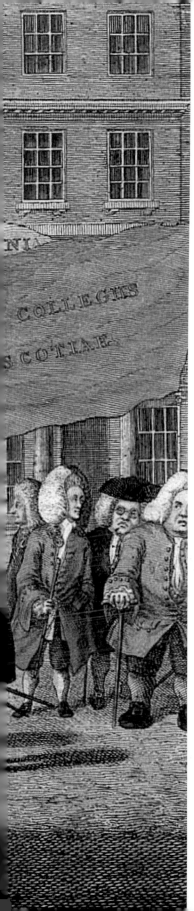

1740

After the War of Jenkins' Ear, the College is asked for advice by the government about what liquor the navy could use as a substitute for French brandy. This marked the beginning of the role of the College as advisor on medical matters.

1741

The beginning of the litigation of Isaac Schomberg against the College (proceedings were resolved only in 1771).

1744

Richard Mead is elected President of the College but declines to take up the office. Mead and Sloane represented the new world of natural philosophy movements and epitomised the advanced thinking of the Scientific Enlightenment. Both accumulated magnificent collections of books and manuscripts.

1744

The first Edinburgh graduate, John Fothergill, is admitted to the College as a licentiate.

Left: *The March of the Medical Militants to the Seizure of Warwick Lane Castle.* **In September 1767, a group of licentiates stormed a meeting of Comitia, having hired a gang of ruffians from a local public house. They used sledgehammers and crowbars to force their way in and the resulting brawl caused great amusement amongst the public and cartoonists alike, and damaged the already poor reputation of the College.**

Right: **Frontispiece of** *The Expert Doctor's Dispensatory* **(1657) allegedly translated and edited by Nicholas Culpepper [sic] from Pierre Morel's** *Methodus praescribendi ...* **(1630), showing a doctor's dispensary and an apothecary's shop in the 17th century.**

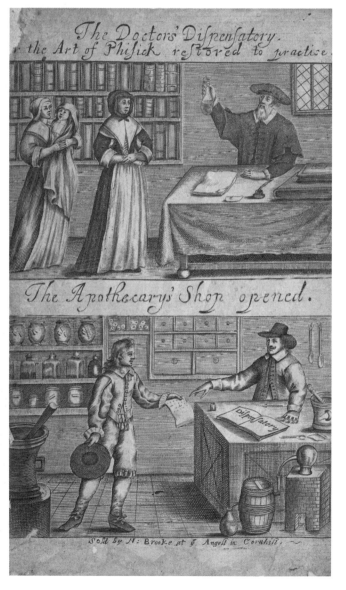

The two main functions of the College traditionally were the encouragement of learned practice and the licensing of physicians in London, as enshrined in its royal charter. The licensing of doctors outside London was in the hands of other authorities, usually the local clergy, but it was in London that medical practice was most lucrative and most desirable, and it was there that the College exerted its powers. Conflicts over rights to practise in London, though, were never far from the surface. In the 17th century, the conflicts were mainly with the apothecaries. Guided by the inducements and emollient hand of Sloane, these faded away but they were replaced in the 18th century by a series of spectacular rows between the fellows of the College and the licentiates of the College over the rights and privileges of the latter. The rise in scientific medicine was the crowning achievement of this period, and it ended in reform, long overdue, and the slow erosion of regulatory powers of the College, which had for too long been exercised with too great a degree of self-interest. The changes in the College reflected changes in English society and in its power structures and institutions.

Richard Mead was one of the leading scientific physicians of the age. He trained partly in Padua and in Leiden and became a close friend of Boerhaave. In 1702, he published his *Mechanical Account of Poisons,* which was rightly acclaimed. He was elected to the Royal Society in 1703 and appointed physician to St Thomas', and then in 1713 was named vice-president of the Royal Society by Isaac Newton. He published *A Short Discourse Concerning Pestilential Contagion, and the Method to Be Used to Prevent It* in 1720. He was elected FRCP in 1707 and rose in the ranks of the College, being offered the presidency in 1744, which he declined. He was the finest physician of his age, with a brilliant mind, and he accrued an enormous fortune – it is said amounting to £5,000–£6,000 per year. He attended Queen Anne on her death bed and was physician to George II. He had a magnificent house in Great Ormond Street, in which he created a gallery for his huge collection of statues, coins, gems, drawings, prints and books. His library is said to have comprised over 100,000 volumes, which took 56 days to auction after his death. He was known to all the literati of Europe and renowned for his scholarly and refined taste. He was also a philanthropist, helping to create the Foundling Hospital, and it was Mead who persuaded the wealthy citizen Thomas Guy to bequeath his fortune towards the foundation of the hospital which bears his name.

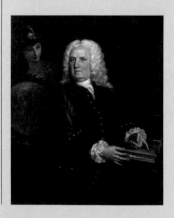

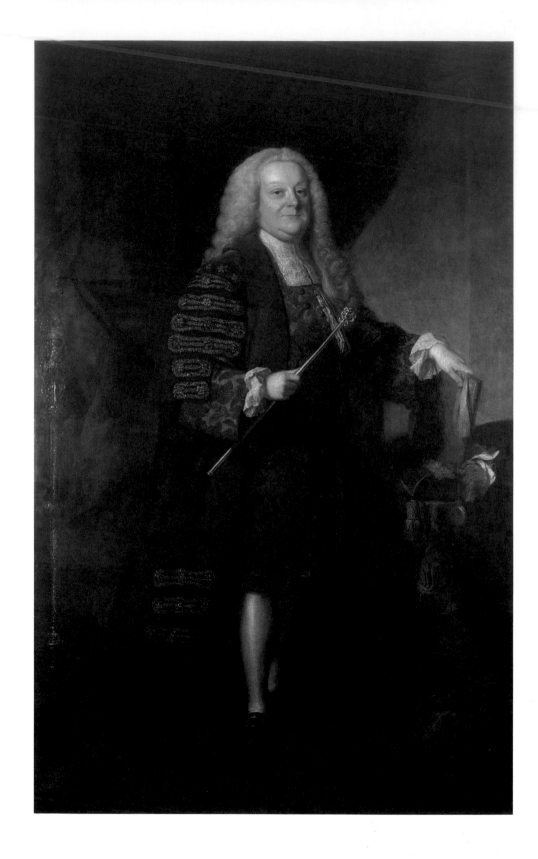

1746

New edition of the *Pharmacopoeia Londinensis* published. This was a major revision, in which much of the pharmacopoeia was modernised.

1747

New battles begin between the College fellows and the licentiates, which continue to erupt periodically over the next three decades.

1752

The licentiates protest against their exclusion from College affairs.

1757

A complete catalogue of the College library is printed for the first time – *Bibliothecae Collegii Regalis Medicorum Londinensis Catalogus.*

1764

The College Club is formed, as a dining club, and part of a general societal movement for the creation of such informal groupings.

1765

Sir William Browne assumes the presidency of the College.

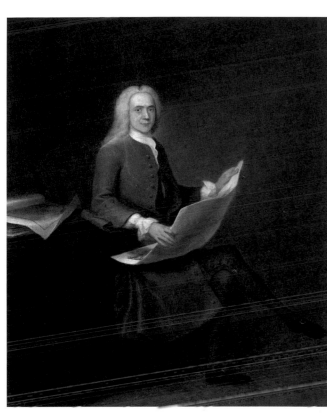

Left: Sir William Browne, President of the College during the Siege of Warwick Lane, was Fothergill's principal opponent, yet after the siege Browne proposed him for the Fellowship. Although the butt of much satire during the period, he was in fact a generous and humourous person. In this portrait, Browne is holding the caduceus, wearing the presidential robes and has his hand gently laid on the College statutes.

Above: Dr John Fothergill was a brilliant physician, a Quaker and a follower of radical causes. Although the portrait has an air of austerity he was in fact amongst the richest doctors in London. A leading licentiate, he was at the centre of the dispute with the College and participated in the Siege of Warwick Lane.

At the top of the College hierarchy was of course the President. He (and it was always a he) was elected by a small group of senior fellows known as the 'elects', and chosen from their number. The elects also nominated the Censors, whose main duties were to conduct the Fellowship Examinations and to police College rules. The President chaired the Comitia, which was the College's governing committee, on which all fellows were entitled to sit. Indeed, attendance was expected, and there were penalties for those absent from meetings. The Comitia decided, for instance, who should be admitted to the College, and oversaw in their generality College policy and affairs. At the bottom of the pile were the licentiates – doctors who were licensed by the College to practise medicine in London, and who paid a substantial annual fee for the privilege, but were not allowed any of the privileges of the fellows, and were not members of Comitia.

The foundation charter limited the number of fellows to 40 at any one time, and although this was increased temporarily to 80 persons in the charter of James II, the numbers of fellows hovered between 40 and 50 for most of the 18th century. There was only a small number of licentiates until the 1760s, when their numbers began to increase, and by 1795 had exceeded 100. There was a further category of honorary fellows, dating from the early 1660s, when 60 were created largely to shore up the failing finances of the College (although the resulting monies were lost in the 1665/6 burglary), but they were then progressively phased out. In 1784, a further category was created, the extra-licentiates, who were doctors licensed by the College to practise outside London.

Fellows were admitted only after passing an examination by the Censors, and Fellowship was restricted only to those who were English citizens and had a doctorate awarded at, or incorporated by, the Universities of Oxford or Cambridge, and who professed the Anglican faith. Fellowship was prohibited to foreigners, dissenters, nonconformists, Roman Catholics, non-Christians and those who practised surgery or midwifery. Once elected, a fellow could expect a lucrative practice and many honours, and Fellowship was a jealously guarded honour. However, by the 1740s these rules, which had been established in the 16th century, were seen as increasingly inappropriate, and began to be the source of bitter argument. A particular grievance was felt by the Scottish physicians, who were excluded on grounds of nationality and also education, despite the fact that excellent schools of medicine had by then arisen in Edinburgh, Glasgow, St Andrews and Aberdeen. Those holding degrees from the renowned medical schools in Europe, including the great schools in Montpellier, Bologna and Leiden were also excluded, and their feeling of insult was greater not least because the only two English schools of medicine, at Oxford and Cambridge, were by then seen as increasingly backward, stuck as they were in the grip of classical learning. The power of election, vested as it was in the hands of a small number of Censors who conducted the examinations, was open to great abuse, and the examination process was in practice extremely arbitrary. It was indeed possible that a medical degree could be, and sometimes was, bestowed on persons with no medical knowledge at all.

1765

The College is taken to court over its failure to admit an obstetrician, Dr Letch, creating a lengthy legal battle with the licentiates. The College wins the case in 1767 but its restrictive practices are heavily criticised by the Judge, Lord Justice Mansfield.

1765

New College Statutes written, and for the first time are not kept secret but are distributed to all fellows and licentiates.

1766

The College publishes the work of William Harvey.

1767

Foundation of the Society of Collegiate Physicians, which agitates for amendments to the Fellowship rules of the College.

1767

Evening meetings for the reading of scientific papers initiated and a committee formed to select papers for publication in the *Medical Transactions* of the College.

1767

The Siege of Warwick Lane, which has been called the single most embarrassing episode in the history of the College.

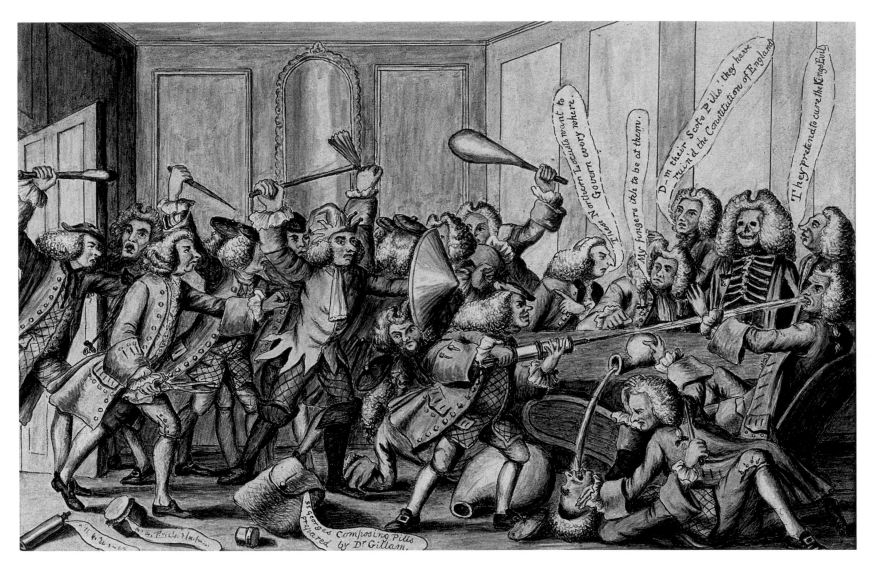

Left: The invasion of the council of the College of Physicians, known as the Siege of Warwick Lane. The siege was enjoyed by the public and the cartoonists and newspapers of the day, who were amused at seeing the physicians, often considered arrogant and self-interested, being brought down to size.

Trouble was bound to arise, and so it did. One of the first skirmishes was with Dr Isaac Schomberg, a licentiate who became embroiled in a long legal wrangle with the College over its protracted refusal to admit him as a fellow, despite his clearly adequate qualifications. The argument started in 1741, and it was only in 1771, after several lawsuits, that he was admitted as a fellow. It was an uncomfortable episode, for it appeared that the College prevented appointment on personal prejudice rather than a professional basis. Other cases followed, and in 1752, the licentiates as a group protested at their exclusion from College affairs and were rudely rebuffed. In 1765, further actions in the law courts were brought by the licentiates against the College. One such action concerned Dr Letch, who was refused Fellowship on the basis that he had practised obstetrics, and although the judge found in the College's favour, he commented that the College's rules were so highly restrictive that they would have 'excluded even the great Herman Boerhaave'. The College hierarchy however refused to make changes.

Tensions increased in 1767, when a group of licentiates established a new organisation, the Society of Collegiate Physicians, the main function of which was to agitate for an amendment of College rules. Amongst their number were celebrated doctors such as William Duncan, John Fothergill and William Hunter, excluded from Fellowship by virtue of Scottish degrees or nonconformist views, and on 25 June 1767, a violent confrontation broke out between the new society and the College. The trouble started when Hunter and eight other licentiates turned up at the College Comitia and tried to take part in the proceedings. They were asked to leave but refused to do so, and Hunter was reported to have declared that 'If any Man or Constable offered to lay hands upon him to turn him out of their House (adding for this is our House) he would run him through the Body'. A small riot followed and the council meeting was dissolved.

There then followed a bizarre event, which became known as the Siege of Warwick Lane, much to the amusement of the public, and the cartoonists, whose field day this turned out to be. On 24 September 1767, when the next meeting of the Comitia was due, the President, Sir William Browne, discovered that a 'great number of Licentiates' had been drinking at the nearby Queens Arms Tavern, and became concerned that the Comitia was to be disrupted. The gates of the College were ordered to be locked and guarded, but soon after Sir William Duncan, William Hunter and about 20 other licentiates arrived with a group of men hired at the tavern. The doors were broken down with sledgehammers and crowbars, windows were broken, and the distinguished doctors entered the council meeting and sat down. A fight broke out and the council meeting was again abandoned. Sir William Browne described the scene in florid prose: 'With inhuman violence they broke into this very senate, like swimming sea monsters in our medical ocean.'

The siege resulted in the resignation of Sir William and, slowly over subsequent years, measures were taken to reform what were seen as injustice and a lack of fairness. Increasingly exceptions were made to the College's Fellowship rules, and as a result the Society of Collegiate Physicians ceased functioning in 1798. Nevertheless, it was not until 1836 that the College formally changed its regulations to open its doors to graduates of universities other than Oxford or Cambridge, and several of the most skilful doctors of the period remained excluded from College Fellowship.

Right: A document in the College archive by Sir William Browne, who presided over the Comitia during the fiasco of the 'Siege of Warwick Lane', venting his fury at Scottish doctors.

'Sir William Browne, *a man of strong feelings, extraordinary garrulity, and utterly void of discretion, was wholly unfit at such a crisis to occupy the presidential chair.'*

Munk's opinion about the President of the College at the time of the Siege of Warwick Lane

The existence of the College depended on its learned nature – and it was this that distinguished its fellows from the surgeons, quacks and apothecaries who purported to offer medicine to the citizenry. The first royal charter mandated the institution of 'a perpetual College of learned and grave men', but it has to be admitted that by the early 18th century, the academic reputation of the College had sunk to a very low level. Its salvation proved to be the revolution that was the scientific enlightenment. This promulgated a new approach to science and natural philosophy, in which reason and experimentation replaced tradition as the basis of learning. The scientific enlightenment in medicine was centred in Oxford and in London at the Royal Society, and amongst the College's learned fellows were many who also were members of the Royal Society, such as Sloane, Latham, Baillie, Saunders, Pegge and Pemberton, and other celebrated physicians such as Richard Mead and William Heberden, who managed to span the divide between physic and natural philosophy. By the end of the 18th century, for the first time, scientific method and scientific discovery were applied to medicine and the College had repudiated its Galenic traditions.

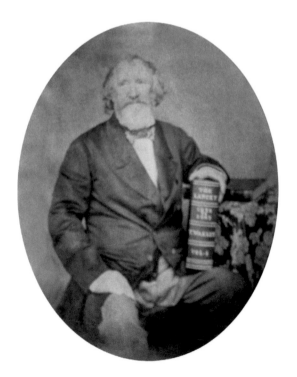

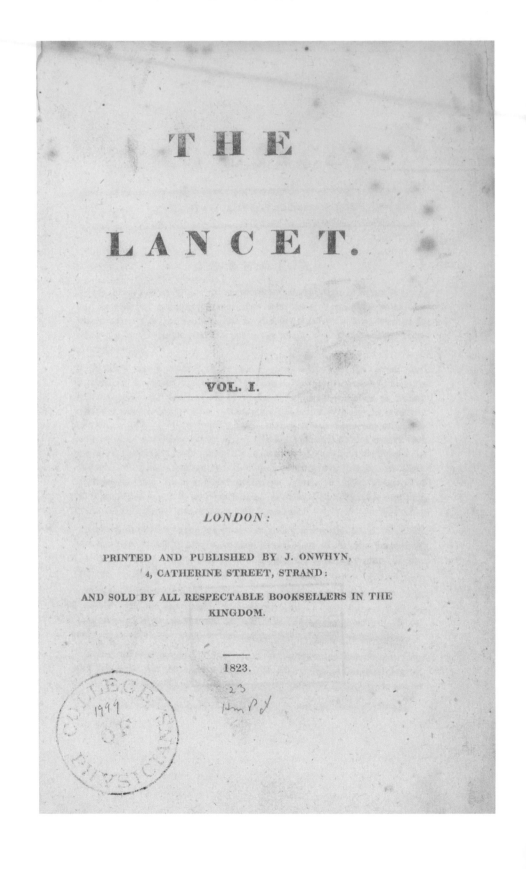

THE LANCET.

VOL. I.

LONDON:

PRINTED AND PUBLISHED BY J. ONWHYN,
4, CATHERINE STREET, STRAND:

AND SOLD BY ALL RESPECTABLE BOOKSELLERS IN THE KINGDOM.

1823.

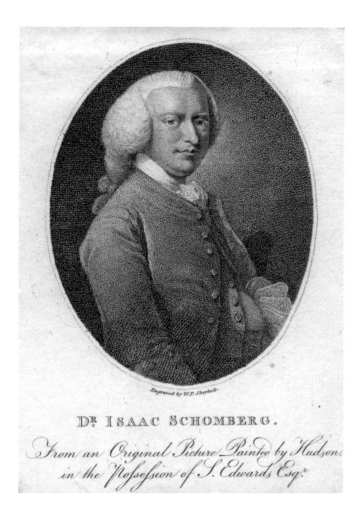

Dᴿ ISAAC SCHOMBERG.

From an Original Picture Painted by Hudson, in the Possession of S. Edwards, Esqᴿ.

Above: Isaac Schomberg (1714–1780) was engaged in a bitter dispute over his eligibility for admission as a fellow of the College from 1749 to 1771. He was the victim of prejudice and arrogance and the public arguments contributed to the College's deteriorating reputation. He was said to have a generosity of character and 'warm benignity of soul', which won him many friends including William Hogarth.

Right: Anthony Askew (1722–1774) was a physician and book collector, a protégé of Mead and a fellow of both the Royal Society and the RCP. On his death, his library included 7,000 books, which took 19 days to sell at auction, according to Munk. Some were sold to George III including the Second Folio of Shakespeare now in the King's Library of the British Museum.

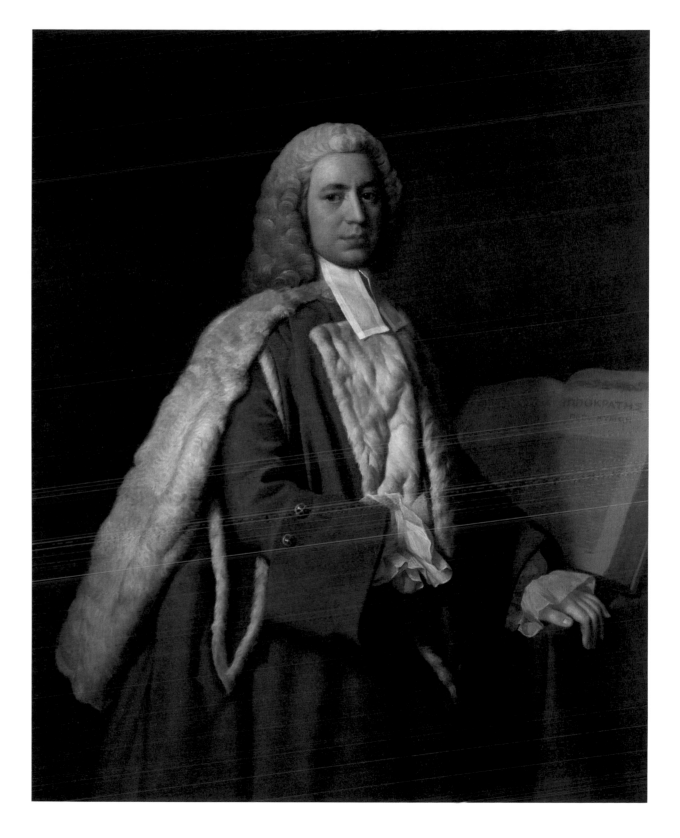

1768–71

Further litigation between the College and the licentiates resulting, in 1771, in advice by Lord Justice Mansfield about revision of the statutes, starting a slow process of reform.

1768

The first volume of the *Medical Transactions* published by the *College of Physicians in London* is produced.

1771

Final resolution of the Schomberg case.

1771–78

Rapprochement with the licentiates and the end of the long professional disputes which had disrupted relationships with the College for three decades.

1774

The College given the responsibility of licensing 'Private Madhouses', marking a new phase in the role of the College in general health policy.

1779

The first *Medical Register* published by Dr Simmons. This was an unofficial work, and had no claims to be comprehensive, but was revised over subsequent years, and became a landmark in professional affairs.

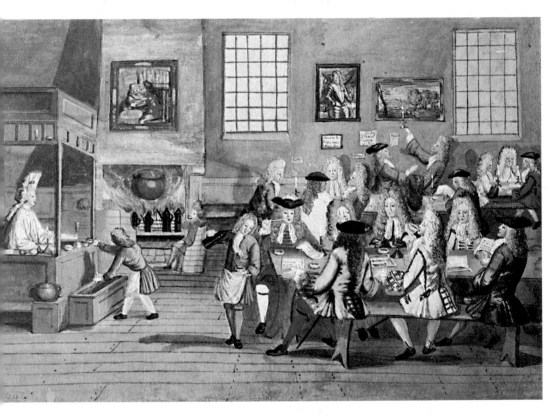

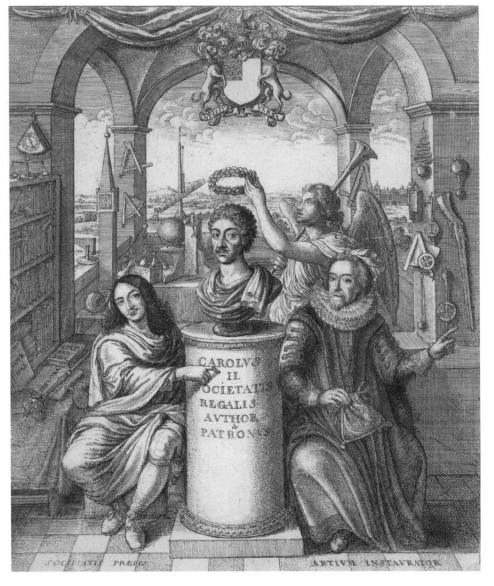

Above: An illustration of the Royal Society, with Boyle, Hooke and Wren at a coffee house. It is probably the new coffee house opened by Arthur Tillyard, an apothecary, which became a meeting point for the Oxford Coffee Club, a precursor of the Royal Society.

Right: Frontispiece of Thomas Spratt's *History of the Royal Society*, showing Charles II and Francis Bacon, 1667.

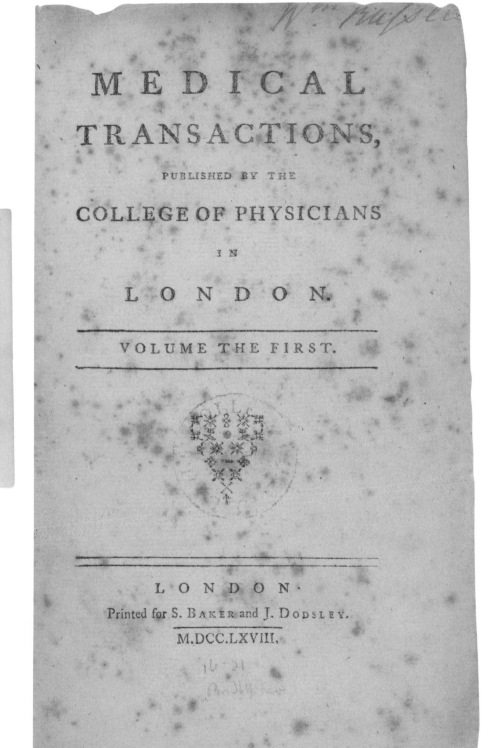

A
Short Account
OF THE
PROCEEDINGS
OF THE
College of Physicians, *London*,
In relation to the
SICK POOR
Of the said
CITY and SUBURBS thereof,

With the Reasons which have induced the College to make Medicines for them at the Intrinsick Value.

LONDON, Printed in the Year 1697.

MEDICAL
TRANSACTIONS,
PUBLISHED BY THE
COLLEGE OF PHYSICIANS
IN
LONDON.

VOLUME THE FIRST.

LONDON·
Printed for S. BAKER and J. DODSLEY.
M.DCC.LXVIII.

Stimulated by the publication of the *Medical Observations and Enquiries* (as it was said, executed in the Hippocratic method and recommended by Lord Bacon) by the Society of Physicians in 1757, the College decided that it should have a publishing arm. In 1764, a committee was formed first to publish the works of Harvey, which it did in 1766, and then in 1768, the first volume of the *Medical Transactions Published by the College of Physicians in London* was produced. Heberden led the production of this, with a style, format and concept based on the *Philosophical Transactions of the Royal Society*. *Medical Transactions* was amongst the first published medical journals, and showed a promising start to a potentially important publishing venture. Unfortunately, unlike its twin at the Royal Society, the journal did not flourish. The second volume was published four years later and the third only in 1785, after which the journal petered out, with publication ceasing in 1820 after the sixth volume. Had it survived, it might have matched the success of *The Lancet*, which started publishing in 1823, and remains the earliest medical journal still in existence.

During this period, the College also continued to update the *Pharmacopoeia Londinensis*, and a new edition was published in 1788 (replacing the previous edition of 1746) and again in 1809. This too became more scientific and less empirical, thus gaining in stature.

Below left and right: Title page
and medicinal recipes of the 1788
edition of the *Pharmacopoeia
Londinensis*.

1784

The President is granted the
right to nominate licentiates to
the Fellowship. By 1800, eight
licentiates had been promoted
in this way, including several
Scottish graduates.

1788

Revision of the *Pharmacopoeia
Londinensis* is published.

1799

The College first announces
its intention to move from Warwick
Lane, and over the next 25 years
searches for new premises.

1800

The creation of the Royal College
of Surgeons marks the beginning of
reform of medical affairs over the
next five decades. This removes
many of the powers of the College
over medical practice.

PHARMACOPOEIA

COLLEGII REGALIS

MEDICORUM

LONDINENSIS.

LONDINI:
APUD JOSEPHUM JOHNSON.

---

108   MELLITA.

OXYMEL ÆRUGINIS.

℞ Æruginis præparatæ ꜰ. unciam unam,
    Aceti ᴍ. uncias septem,
    Mellis despumati ꜰ. uncias quatuordecim.

Solve æruginem aceto, et cola per linteum;
dein adde mel, et misturam decoque ad ido-
neam crassitudinem.

OXYMEL COLCHICI.

℞ Colchici recentis in laminas tenues secti
    ꜰ. unciam unam,
    Aceti distillati ᴍ. libram unam,
    Mellis despumati ꜰ. libras duas.

Macera colchicum cum aceto in vase vitreo
leni calore per horas octo et quadraginta.
Liquorem radice fortiter expressum cola, et
adde mel. Denique misturam, cochleari
ligneo sæpe agitans, decoque ad syrupi crassitudinem.

OXYMEL SCILLÆ.

℞ Mellis despumati ꜰ. libras tres,
    Aceti scillæ ᴍ. libras duas.

Decoque in vase vitreo lento igne ad syrupi
crassitudinem.

TRITA

TRITA in PULVEREM.   109

TRITA in PULVEREM.

PULVIS ALOES CUM CANELLA.

℞ Aloës socotorinæ ꜰ. libram unam,
    Canellæ albæ ꜰ. uncias tres.

Separatim in pulverem tere, dein misce.

PULVIS ALOES CUM GUAIACO.

℞ Aloës socotorinæ ꜰ. unciam unam cum
    semisse,
    Guaiaci gummi-resinæ ꜰ. unciam unam,
    Pulveris aromatici ꜰ. unciam dimidiam.

Aloën et guaiaci gummi-resinam separatim
in pulverem tere; dein cum pulvere aroma-
tico misce.

PULVIS ALOES CUM FERRO.

℞ Aloës socotorinæ ꜰ. unciam unam cum
    semisse,
    Myrrhæ ꜰ. uncias duas,
    Extracti gentianæ exsiccati,
    Ferri vitriolati, singulorum ꜰ. unciam
    unam.

Separatim in pulverem tere, et misce.

PULVIS

Below: This famous print, *The Reward of Cruelty, or an Anatomy*, is from a series of four which William Hogarth produced in February 1751. The series depicts the life of the fictional Tom Nero, who was executed for a string of violent crimes. The print shows the anatomy theatre, where Nero's body is being dissected. On either side are skeletons labelled 'Gentn: Harry' and 'Macleane', after two recently hanged criminals.

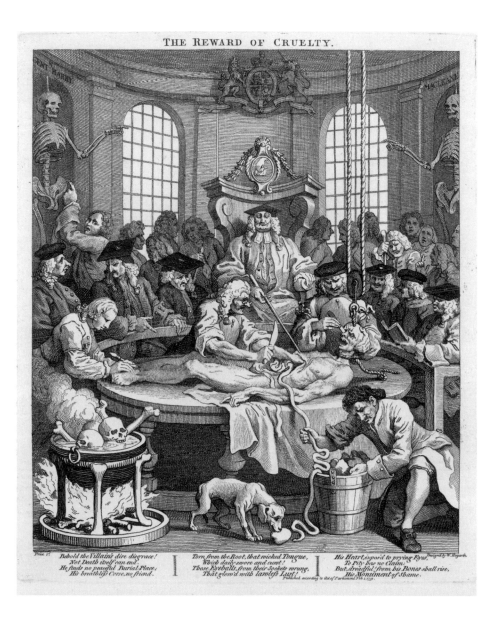

THE REWARD OF CRUELTY.

William Heberden 1710–1801

Heberden was an intellectual, 'a Physician in the Age of Reason', who helped move the College into modern times. He dismissed the Doctrine of Signatures and ridiculed certain ancient herbal remedies in his writing. In 1749 he was elected to the Royal Society, where he became an enthusiastic advocate of the new concepts of Natural Philosophy. There he contributed papers on rainfall, the effects of lightning and on astronomical subjects, and at the College of Physicians he delivered the Goulstonian Lectures on the history, nature and cure of poisons. He was the driving force behind the publication of the College's *Medical Transactions*, and contributed 16 papers in the first volumes of the journal, including his important description of angina pectoris (an 'Account of a disorder of the breast'), which was not then a recognised condition, and also papers on rheumatism, measles, chickenpox and the hazards of London pump water. His major book *Commentaries on the History and Cure of Diseases* was published in English shortly after his death. His patients included Dr Johnson, who called him the '*ultimus Romanorum,* the last of our learned physicians', and King George III. His friend Dr Wells wrote in 1799, 'No other person, I believe, either in this or any other country, has ever exercised the art of medicine with the same dignity or has contributed so much to raise it in the estimation of mankind' – this was no overstatement of his high reputation.

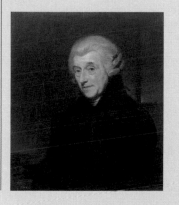

Baillie was related to William Hunter, and was his supporter and student. On Hunter's death, he inherited his house and estates and became trustee custodian of his museum. His book *The Morbid Anatomy of Some of the Most Important Parts of the Human Body* (1793) was immensely popular and published in nine British editions, as well as one Russian, three American, two French, four German and three Italian editions, over the next three decades. It provided descriptions of the pathology of disease, and he was the first to link alcoholism to hepatic cirrhosis, hardening of the arteries to angina and rheumatism to cardiac valve disease. He also had an enormous and lucrative practice (said at its height to exceed £10,000 per year), attending amongst others George III and Princesses Amelia and Charlotte, although the latter's care ended in catastrophe when, with Baillie in charge of her confinement, a 50-hour labour resulted in the death of the child and the mother. Other patients included Lord Byron, Sir Walter Scott, Edward Gibbon and (post-mortem) Samuel Johnson. In spite of his success and wealth, he was a modest man, said to have hated having his portrait copied and having 'a particular dislike to the idea of seeing his face in the window of a print shop!'. He is commemorated with a bust and inscription in Westminster Abbey, and he bequeathed to the College his medical books and papers, along with his famous collection of anatomical specimens, which were transferred to the Royal College of Surgeons of England in 1938 and then sadly destroyed in the Blitz of 1941.

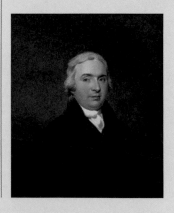

Below: The passing on of a gold-headed cane, from an older to younger physician, was a traditional practice in the 18th century as a sign of regard, and a passing of the baton. This tradition was the basis of the famous book by William MacMichael which is a fictionalised 'autobiography' of the gold-headed cane which was bought by Radcliffe and then passed to Mead to Askew to David Pitcairn and to Baillie, and then given on Baillie's death by his widow to the College. The book recounts the lives of these well-heeled physicians from the cane's point of view, including amusing descriptions of their royal consultations. The arms of Radcliffe, Mead, Askew, Pitcairn and Baillie are inscribed on the top and sides, and the stick is of malacca and about one metre long.

'After listening, with torture, to a prosing account from a lady, who ailed so little that she was going to the opera that evening, he had happily escaped from the room, when he was urgently requested to step upstairs again; it was to ask him whether on her return from the opera, she might eat oysters. "Yes, Ma'am," said Baillie, "shells and all."'

The gold-headed cane describing one of Matthew Baillie's consultations

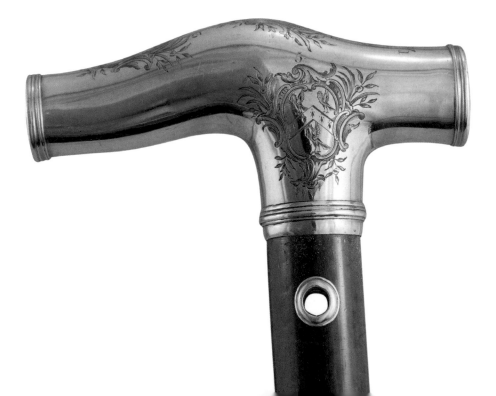

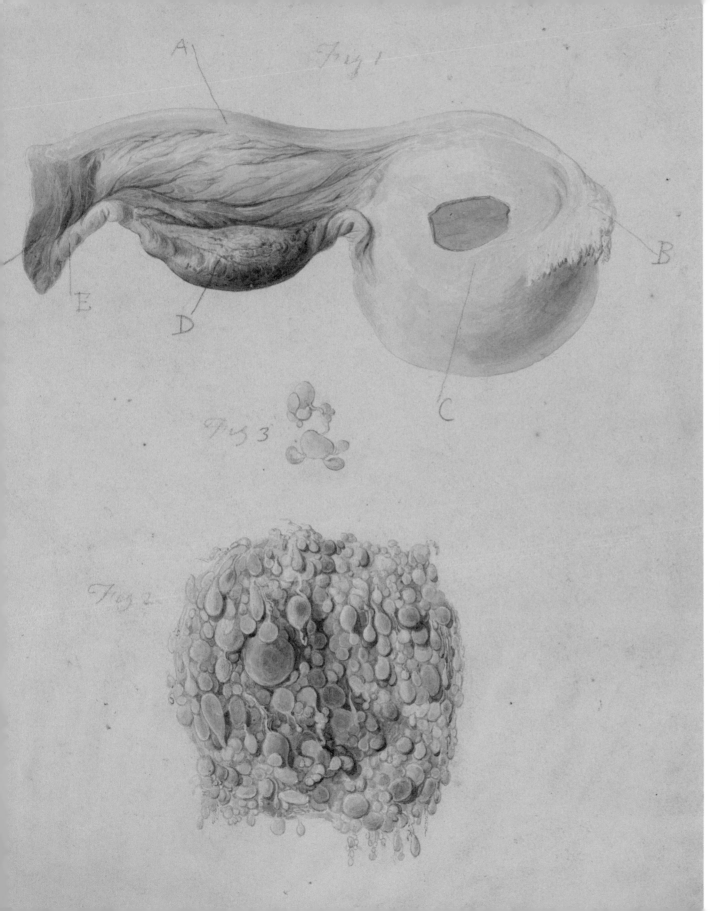

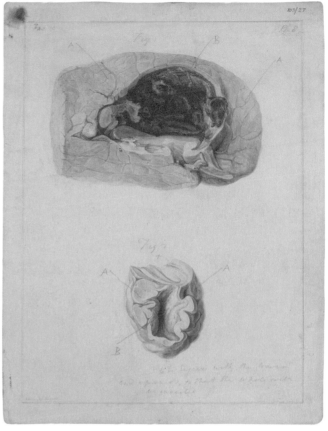

Left and above: William Clift's renowned drawings for Matthew Baillie's book, *The Morbid Anatomy of Some of the Most Important Parts of the Human Body* (1793). In the 10th Fasciculus he concentrated on the cranium, the brain and its membranes, and the 'morbid changes of structure to which the brain is subject [and] which possess a great deal of variety'. These plates deal with venereal disease, hydrocephalus, tumours, tuberculosis and hydatid disease of the brain. These were made to accompany the book.

Great Chatham with his sabre drawn
Stood waiting for Sir Richard Strachan;
Sir Richard, longing to be at 'em
Stood waiting for the Earl of Chatham.

Regarding the Walcheren expedition – attributed to Joseph Jekyll

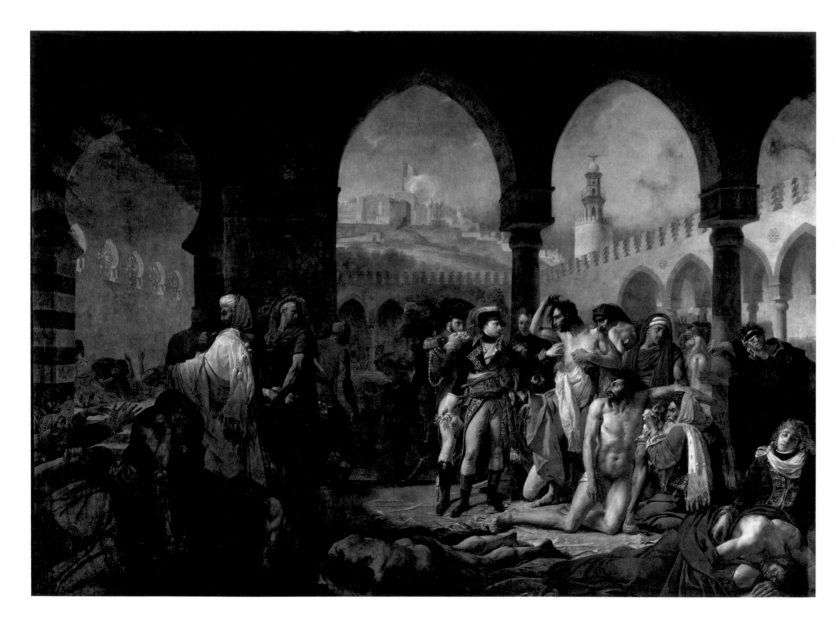

Left: This piece of propaganda was a commission by Napoleon from the artist Antoine-Jean Gros in 1804. It shows Bonaparte visiting his sick soldiers on 11 March 1799, and was an attempt to quell rumours that he had ordered the poisoning of 50 plague victims in Jaffa during the retreat from his Syrian expedition.

Opposite: Detail from the cartoon of *The Meeting of Wellington and Blücher after the Battle of Waterloo* by Daniel Maclise, showing the doctor on the field of Waterloo taking the pulse of an expiring soldier. This sums up the impotence of medicine in war at the time.

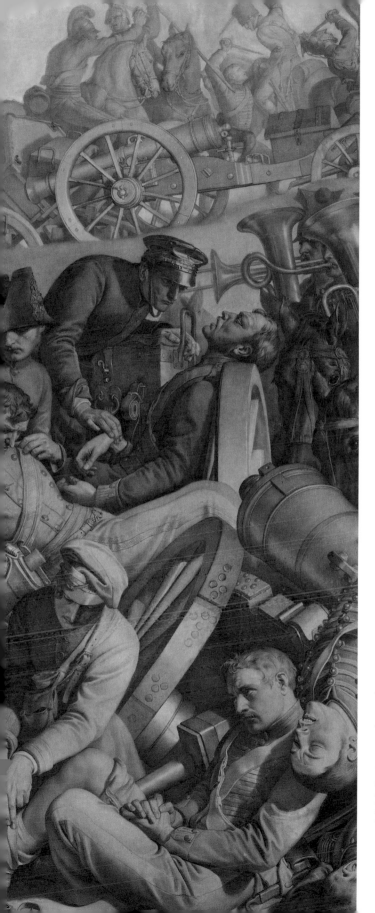

Between 1793 and 1815, Britain was at war with France. This became a tussle between two military geniuses, Napoleon Bonaparte and the Duke of Wellington, and culminated in British victory at the Battle of Waterloo in June 1815. There was a great deal of bloodshed, but physicians had little to contribute on the battlefield. It was only the actions of surgeons amputating and debriding that really influenced survival and recovery, with surgery carried out in improvised settings with a dollop of rum as the only anaesthetic. Instruments were blunt and unsterilised and transportation of injured soldiers was often by wagon cart. The physicians were criticised as being 'too fine for common use ... and able to read Hippocrates in original Greek ... but never to have touched a bleeding wound'.

Sir Lucas Pepys (1742–1830) was President of the College between 1804 and 1811, and was also President of the Army Medical Board for 15 years. His incompetence in this post was matched only by his arrogance. In 1809 he presided over the Walcheren catastrophe in which a large British expeditionary force, under the command of the Earl of Chatham, was sent to this small Dutch island to confront the French army. Before any engagement could start, the British forces were decimated by an epidemic of Walcheren fever, for which the medical services were totally unprepared. The condition affected 40 per cent of the troops and 60 officers, and 3,900 soldiers died. A Parliamentary enquiry was later held, and Pepys appeared before the committee but performed dismally. When asked why he did not personally visit Walcheren he retorted that he was not personally acquainted with diseases of the

camp. He was thereafter quickly retired. The reputation of physicians was somewhat salvaged, however, by the appointment of Sir James McGrigor (1771–1858) to head the Army Medical Board. In contrast to Pepys, McGrigor was practical and effective, introduced numerous improvements in standards of hygiene and medicine and also in its organisation and was in large responsible for the creation of the Royal Army Medical Corps (RAMC).

Casualty figures in the military during the Napoleonic Wars were high. Between 1793 and 1815, the British army lost 240,000 men. Of these deaths only 30,000 or so were due to wounds during battle; the majority of the rest were caused by epidemic infectious disease, such as malaria, smallpox and yellow fever in India and the West Indies, plague and dysentery in Egypt and the Middle East, and typhus, malaria and dysentery in Europe. Ophthalmia was an incurable purulent disease of the eye and alcohol was another potent cause of ill health, as was syphilis (le gros lot) and gonorrhoea (le petit lot), both of which spread through the ranks at various times (as was said, 'an hour with Venus and a lifetime with Mercury').

'[The French soldiers were] as active as ever, and as merry as a beggar under a hedge ... [the afflicted English] pined, drooped, and die ... listless, prone to yawning, suffering from intense thirst, from shivering and burning fits, and finally falling into complete prostration.'

Regarding Walcheren fever

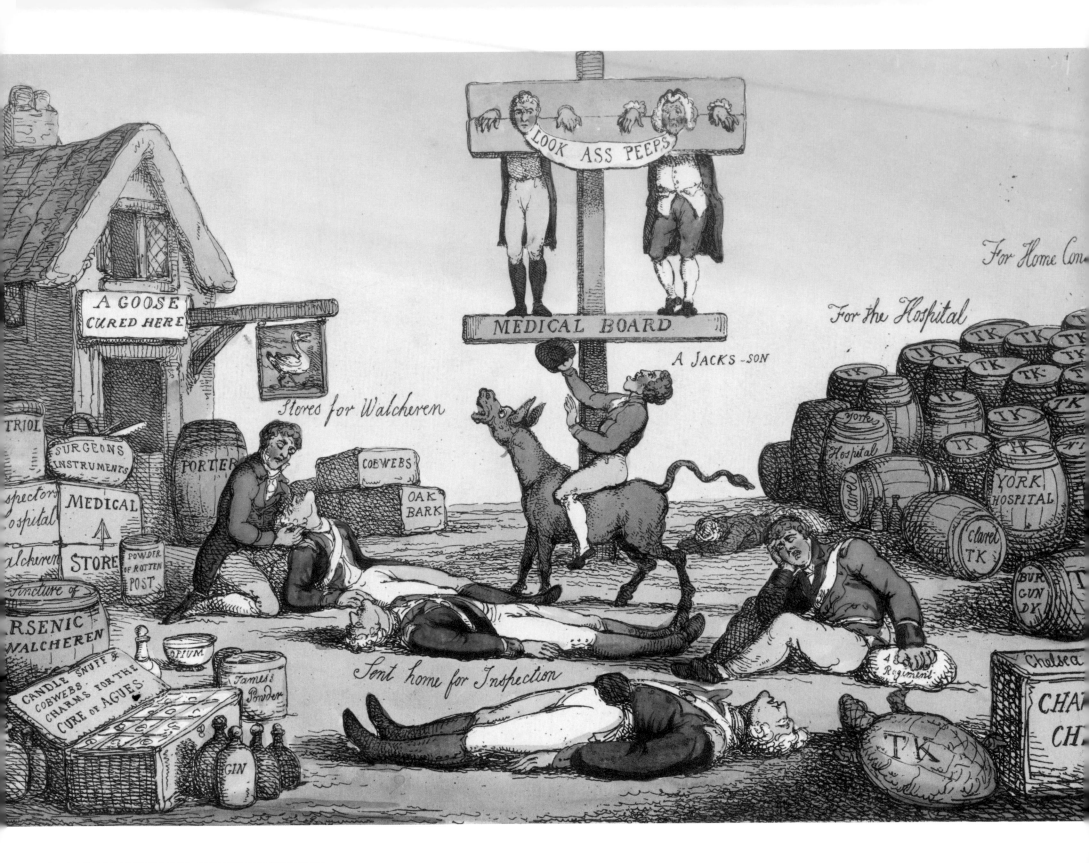

Sir Lucas Pepys elected President
and presides over the catastrophic
Walcheren affair in 1809, resulting
in his condemnation by Parliament.

Between 1806 and 1813, the
College advises the government
on vaccination policy, and is
considered to have performed
great public service.

'Had you the knowledge of Sydenham
or of Radcliffe, you are the surgeon of a
regiment, and the surgeon of a regiment
can never be allowed to be a physician
to His Majesty's army.'

Sir Lucas Pepys (PRCP) to Dr Jackson (the Jack-Ass in the cartoon)

**Opposite: Lucas Pepys, College
President, was responsible for
gross mismanagement of the
army medical services. This
came to a head in 1809, when
the largest British expeditionary
force ever assembled was sent
to the island of Walcheren.
The expedition was a complete
disaster, with an epidemic
of disease (Walcheren fever)
largely destroying the army,
along with Pepys's reputation.
A Parliamentary enquiry was
subsequently held, which
Rowlandson satirises in this
cartoon, *The winding up of
the medical report on the
Walcheren expedition.***

**Right: George Cruickshank's
cartoon of 1809, *The Grand
Expedition,* pokes fun at the
prelude to the Walcheren fiasco.**

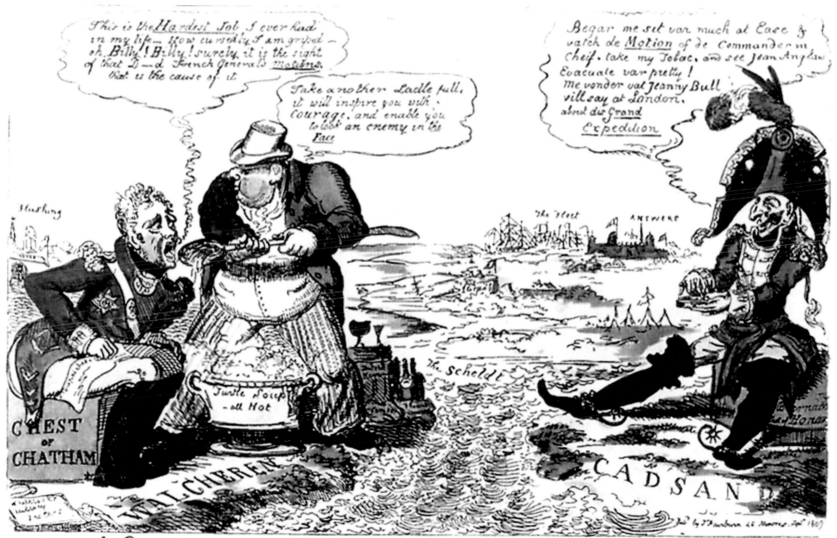

There were significant advances made in both diagnosis and therapy in medicine in this period, and the fellows of the College played their part. Two examples can be given here. From the 16th century, sailors with inadequate diets on long voyages died miserably in great numbers from scurvy – until 1797, when Dr Gilbert Blane persuaded the navy to take lemon juice on their ships. Although not the discoverer of the value of citrus fruit, it was Blane who was instrumental in persuading the sceptical naval high command of its value. At the time, the commonly accepted theory, proposed by Surgeon General and President of the Royal Society Sir John Pringle, among others, was that scurvy was due to putrefaction and a lack of 'fixed air' in body tissue, which could be prevented by drinking infusions of malt and wort, whose fermentation in the body would replace the missing air. James Lind carried out the first scientific clinical trial, dividing 12 scorbutic sailors into six groups of two sailors each. All received the same diet but, in addition, group one was given cider, group two sulphuric acid, group three vinegar, group four sea water, group five two oranges and a lemon, and group six barley water. Only the sailors from group five recovered.

Another important medical landmark was the discovery of the value of digitalis in heart failure. This was first employed by Dr William Withering, who observed that a patient dying of heart failure ('dropsy') was cured by a herbal mixture containing the leaves of foxglove, *Digitalis purpurea*, and this marked a new phase in the scientific study of medicines and their effects. For a dozen years he experimented with the dried leaf on his charity patients, recording the effects and publishing his results in *An Account of the Foxglove* in 1785. The extraction of digoxin, primarily from the woolly foxglove *D. lanata*, continues, using cell cultures of the leaf. An incredibly powerful drug, it constitutes 62.5mcg of a tablet – a grain of sugar weighs five times as much.

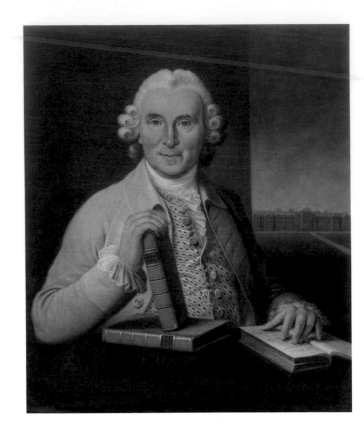

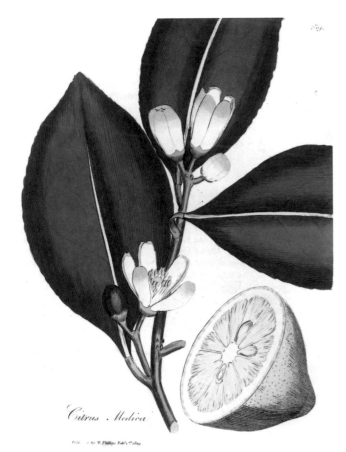

Citrus Medica

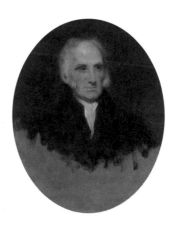

1809

Standing committee formed to oversee the *Pharmacopoeia Londinensis*.

1811

College statutes completely rewritten (although in Latin).

1812

Pressure for medical reform increases outside the College with the application of the Medical and Chirurgical Society for a charter of incorporation, and the formation of the London Committee of Associated Apothecaries and Surgeon-Apothecaries of England and Wales.

1815

Defeat of Napoleon at the Battle of Waterloo, and the end of a somewhat ignominious war for the College and for physicians.

1815

The Apothecaries Act creates an examination in medicine, surgery and later midwifery, and is the first British qualification to cover the whole of medicine (LSA).

1816

The College decides to move to Pall Mall East as part of John Nash's development of the area.

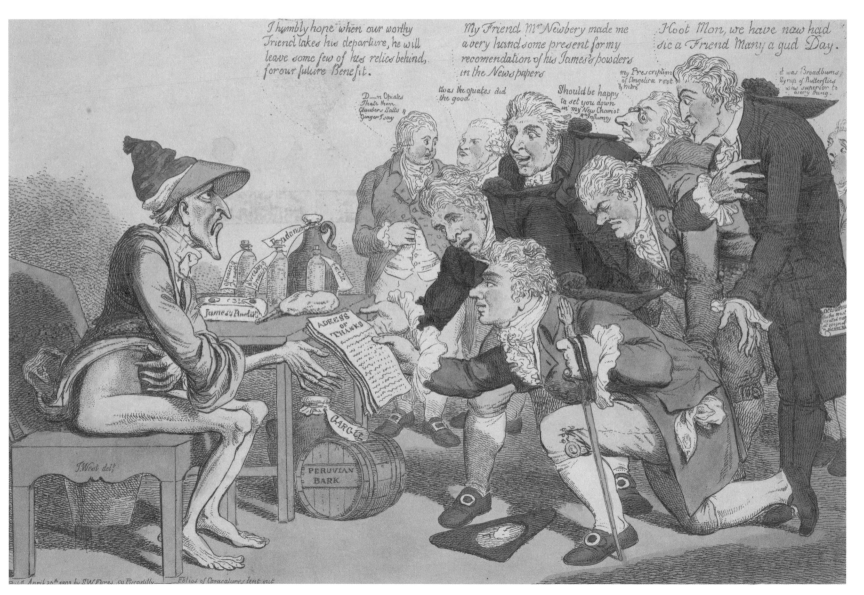

Left: Influenza is a long-recognised disease. The first clear description of what was probably influenza was by Hippocrates, and the first time the word was used was in 1703. It is possible that the 'sweating sickness' was in fact influenza. Pandemics have been recorded since 1580, and the pandemics of 1830–33 were particularly severe. This cartoon by Temple West identifies the visitor as French – another 'French disease' – at a time of intense hostilities between the two countries.

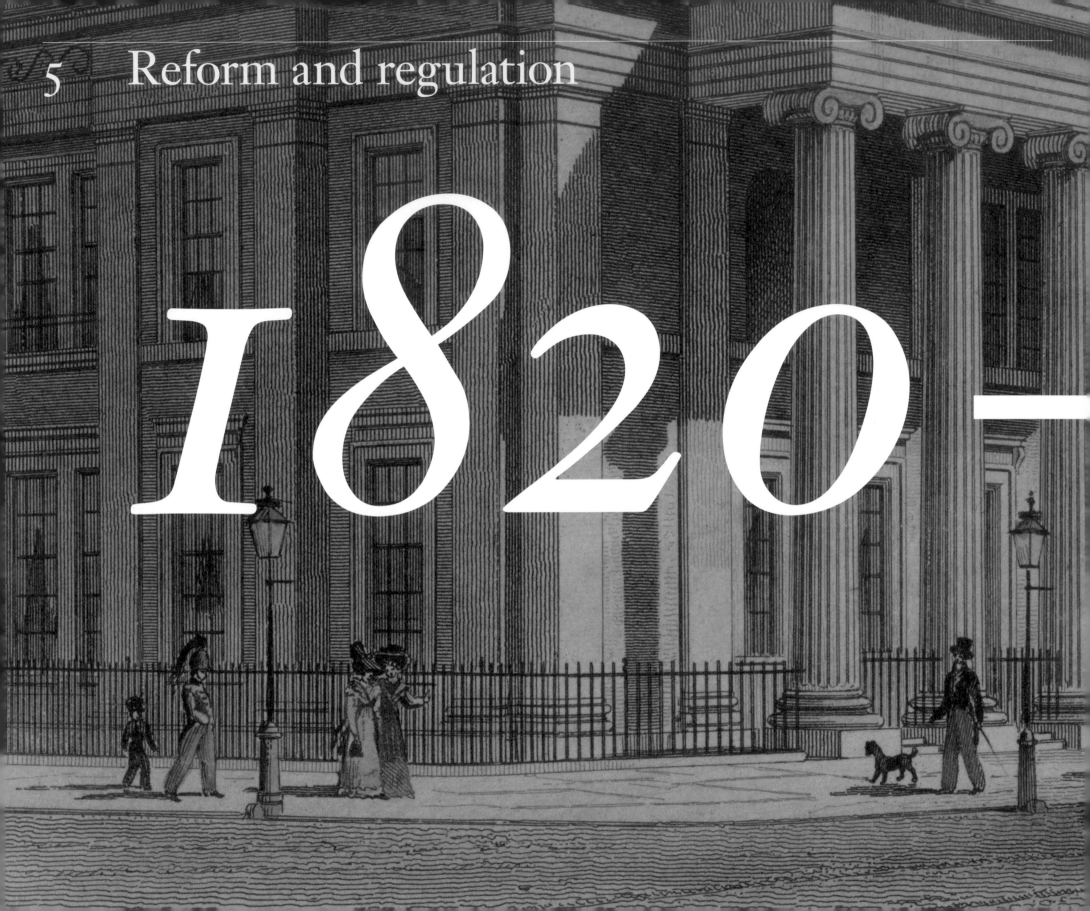

1820–

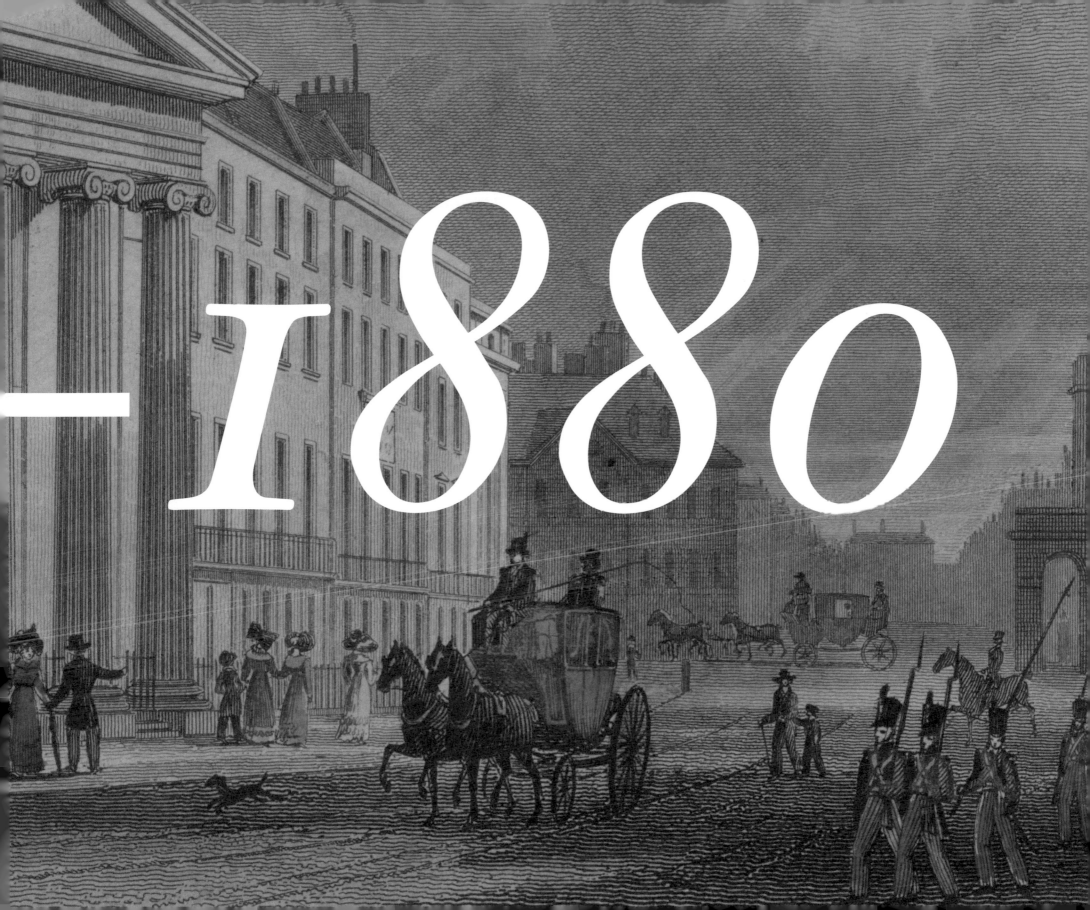

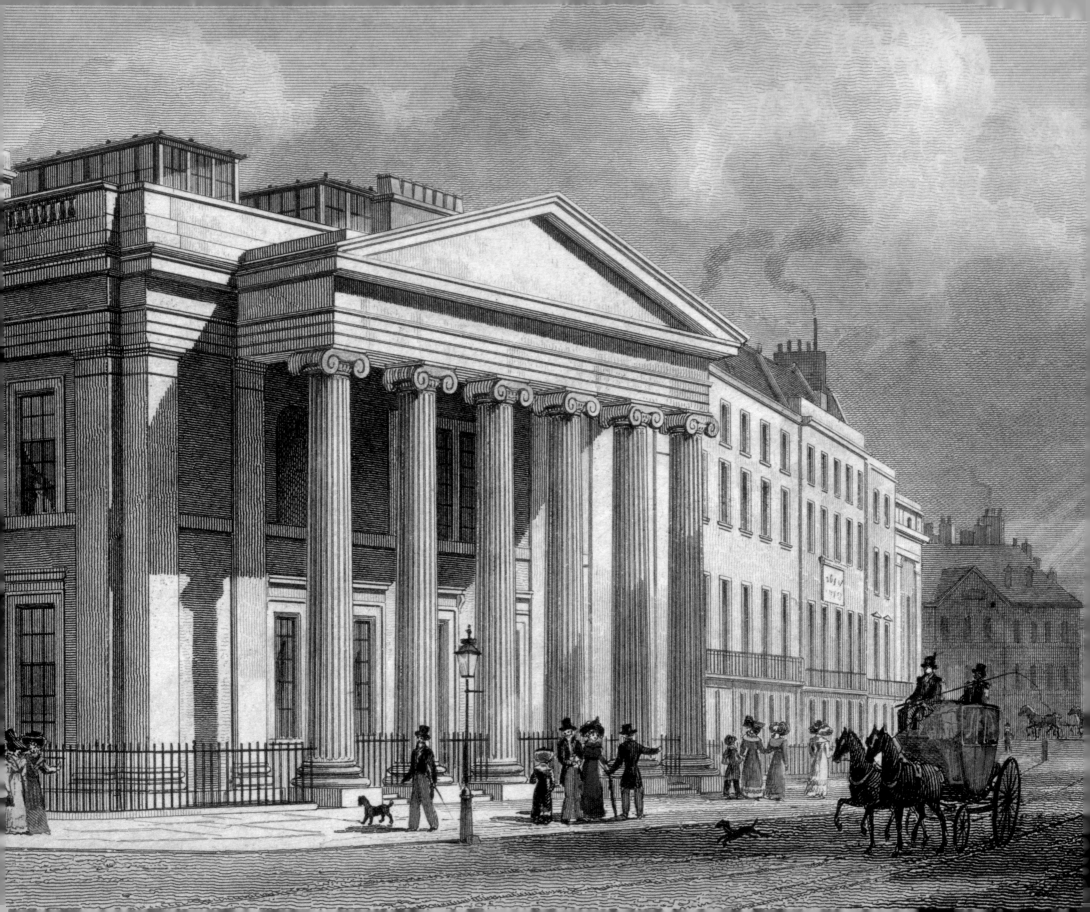

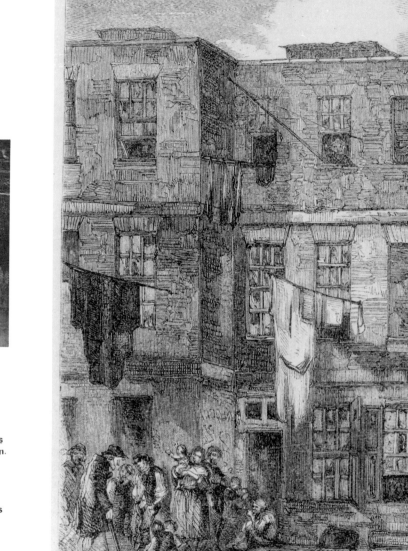

Left: The new College of Physicians in Pall Mall East, now Canada House.

Above: *Street Life in London* was written by radical journalist Adolphe Smith with photographs 'taken from life' by John Thomson. The image shows a destitute woman called a 'crawler of St Giles', whose only means of earning a living was babysitting neighbours' children on the steps of the workhouse.

Right: Wild Court, off Great Wild Street, Drury Lane, 1855. This illustration first appeared in a magazine published by the Labourer's Friend Society, which in 1844 became the Society for Improving the Condition of the Labouring Classes. After an outbreak of typhoid fever, this area was demolished in the Improvement Scheme of 1877.

1820

Sir Henry Halford Bt (1766–1844) elected President annually until his death. He was the longest-serving President in the history of the College.

1823

The Lancet founded by Thomas Wakley (1795–1862). It was a radical journal that attacked the oligarchy of the medical colleges and their resistance to change.

In 1800, overall life expectancy in the United Kingdom was just under 40 years, though a ten-year-old could expect to live to age 56. London's population was about 1 million, with many living in extreme poverty. The 1800 London Bill of Mortality documents 19,374 burials, over a quarter being of children aged less than two. Attributed causes of death were 'age' in 1,562 cases, consumption (TB) in 4,695, convulsions in 3,931, fevers in 2,908 and smallpox in 1,461; other infections – 'cough', 'hooping cough' and measles – were also prominent. Strikingly, modern 21st-century killers were miniscule in number: dropsy (congestive heart failure) 165, cancer 57 and diabetes 1. Epidemic outbreaks of smallpox, scarlatina, measles, influenza and typhus are well documented in the early 1800s, although the major 19th-century epidemic of the UK – 'King Cholera' – did not arrive until 1831. Some estimates blame TB for as many as one third of all deaths at the beginning of the 19th-century. Despite some advance, most therapies remained empiric, and were often bizarre, including bleeding, cupping, scarification and purging. Although many diseases, and particularly the high infant mortality, were those that were common amongst the poor, there were some diseases of affluence – most notably gout, associated with high living and drinking port. Unsurprisingly, being affluent and expensive, but generally ineffective, the medical profession was not held in high public esteem.

The epitome of a fashionable physician, Halford was elegant, oleaginous and the ultimate establishment figure. He served as President of the College for 24 years, longer than any before or since, and physician to several generations of British royalty. Whether he was an effective doctor is arguable, as he was against innovation, did not carry out physical examination of his patients and was ignorant of pathology. Amongst his recorded counsels, no doubt gleefully received, was the advice 'Never read by candlelight anything smaller than the Ace of Clubs'. He obtained a crown lease for a site on Pall Mall East, which enabled the College to move in 1825 to Trafalgar Square. There he presided over the grand opening of Robert Smirke's building, on which day the King decorated him with the Knight Grand Cross of the Royal Guelphic Order.

The Lancet, which had a long feud with Halford, was less kind: 'He is all tact and nothing else. He is ignorant of the modern discoveries in pathology and never employs the modern instruments of diagnosis; he has never written a line that is worthy of perusal on any scientific subject.' Calling the College 'The sanctum of the old dowagers', it teased Halford for starting an 'eating and drinking club' in a scene which was, as it sarcastically put it, 'highly creditable to the dignity and high mindedness of that august body'. Halford sensibly married a baronet's daughter and was himself ennobled in 1809, being known in *The Lancet* thereafter as 'the eel-backed baronet', due to his habit of making frequent bows.

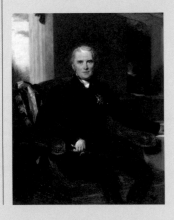

'*… so suave was his bedside manner that aristocratic women were said to prefer dying with Sir Henry than living with lesser physicians.*'

Roy Porter on Henry Halford

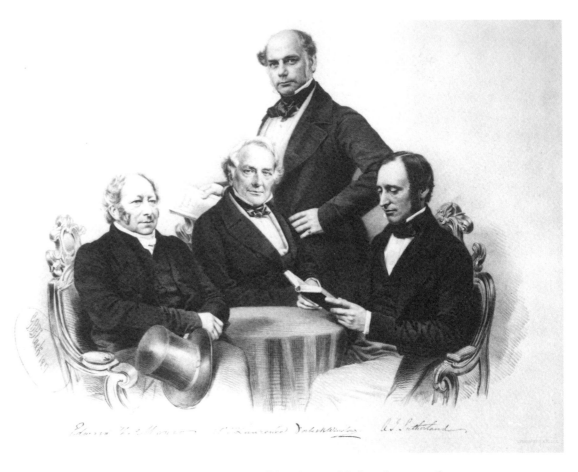

Above: Portrait of doctors Edward Monro, William Lawrence, Forbes Winslow and A. J. Sutherland. Dr Edward Thomas Monro (1789–1856) was Principal Physician at Bethlem Hospital from 1816; Sir William Lawrence (1783–1867) was an English surgeon who became President of the Royal College of Surgeons of London and Serjeant Surgeon to the Queen; Dr Forbes B. Winslow was a psychiatrist and the proprietor of a private psychiatric hospital; Dr A. J. Sutherland was Physician to St Luke's Hospital in London.

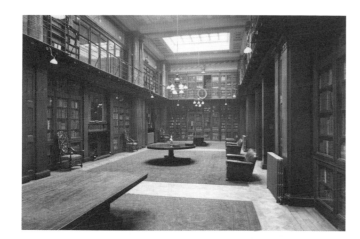

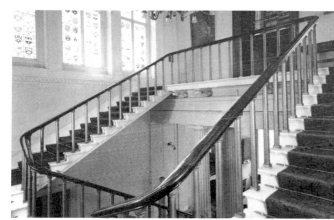

The centre of gravity of London had for at least a century been moving west, and increasingly the fellows found their College in Warwick Lane inconveniently sited in a part of London that was deteriorating and becoming unfashionable, not least because of its proximity to Newgate Prison, which had been rebuilt and extended after the Great Fire. The College had searched for sites further west on several occasions, but it was the President, Henry Halford, with his connections to royalty, who finally obtained a crown lease on a site in Pall Mall East. Here the architect Robert Smirke designed the College's fourth home, overlooking John Nash's Trafalgar Square and conveniently placed in the fashionable West End, close to government offices and gentlemen's clubs. Smirke's Greek revival building, with a grand staircase and ionic columns, indeed had a club-like atmosphere, and is reminiscent of Smirke's other large London buildings, such as the Covent Garden Theatre, the British Museum and the Charlton Club. A bill was required to allow the College to leave the City, and the College sold its building in Warwick Lane and raised the necessary finances. The new building was opened in 1825 by Halford in the presence of a glittering assemblage, the Annals simply recording: 'Die Juni 25th, 1825. On this day the new College was opened.' The building contained the Censors' Room, panelled with the Spanish oak donated by Baldwin Hamey, Jr and removed from Warwick Lane, and the Dorchester Library, dining room, small lecture theatre and museum.

In the early years of the century, the younger reformists and older conservatives among the fellows frequently debated in Comitia alterations to the statutes, and in particular the exclusion from the Fellowship of all but medical graduates from Oxford and Cambridge. However, although a blind eye was increasingly taken to the interpretation of the rules, there was little change until the Parliamentary Select Committee on Medical Education of 1834 suggested that the general governance of the College would be better delegated from Comitia. As part of a general revision of the statutes, in 1835 an elected council was formed to advise, but not overrule, Comitia. This arrangement continues to this day.

Its first 12 fellows were elected in 1836, and for the first time the council started to propose licentiates for election to the Fellowship. It seems a small change, but it ended 300 years of restrictive practice, and slowly the College inched towards its more modern form.

Left above: The Dorchester Library in the Pall Mall building; the portrait of William Harvey (1578–1657) hangs on the left. Meetings of Comitia were held in the library, and Denys Lasdun modelled the 1964 library on that of 1824.

Left below: The fine double staircase and late 19th-century coats of arms of presidents and fellows in stained glass at the College in Pall Mall. The staircase was demolished when the Canadian government took over the building.

1832

The contentious Anatomy Act is passed, requiring all teachers of anatomy to obtain a licence to use bodies for dissection.

1834

The College statutes were modernised between 1834 and 1839, and an elected standing committee of Council was set up to advise Comitia. Rules on admitting non-Oxbridge graduates were formally abolished in 1835.

There was increasing interest in dissection for the teaching of anatomy in the early 19th century. This, and the growth of the numbers of students and the number of private anatomical schools catering for their instruction, caused a shortage of bodies. The public in the capital became fearful of the grave robbers (resurrectionists), who illegally acquired and sold disinterred bodies to the schools. Prominent surgeons set up an Anatomical Society, partly to regularise this supply of cadavers, but against some opposition from the profession, the government passed the Anatomy Act of 1832, by which all anatomy departments and schools had to obtain a licence to dissect a limited number of bodies, after seeking the permission of the relatives of the deceased. Independent inspectors of the schools were appointed, but many of the poor still felt that bodies of paupers would be unfairly selected.

Right: Engraving of the widespread clandestine exhumation of corpses by grave robbers or resurrectionists in London to sell them for anatomical studies, particularly in private schools. This was finally regularised by the 1832 Anatomy Act.

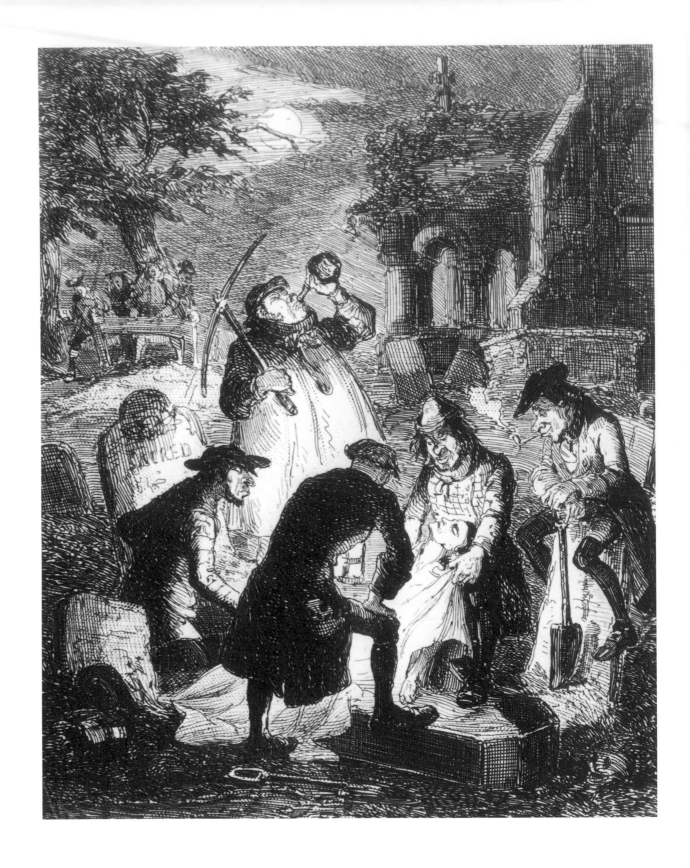

Right: James Gillray, *The Gout*, 1799. Gout, unlike most disorders (prior to the current obesity epidemic) was deemed to be consequent upon indulgence, affecting mainly men, who could afford a lavish lifestyle. The sufferers were easy targets for cartoonists. Gillray, the acid-penned caricaturist, took delight in lampooning King George III, one of history's many eminent sufferers.

Below: A coloured etching illustrating the low public regard in which physicians were held, as a group of physicians wrongly diagnose the case of a pregnant woman (by Isaac Cruikshank, 1803).

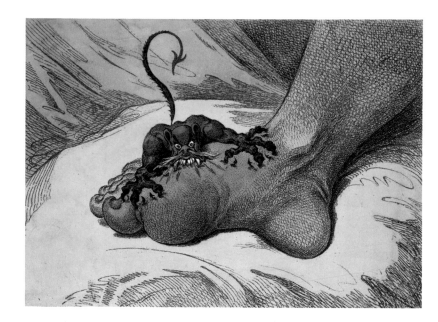

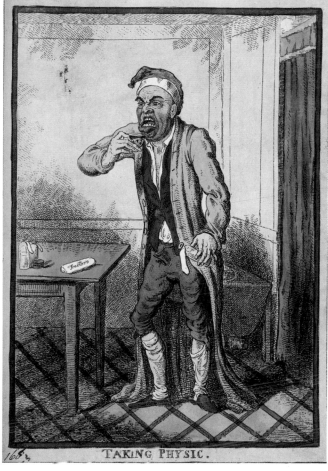

Above: *Taking Physic* (1801), a coloured etching by Cruikshank, after Gillray. It shows an ill-kempt invalid, in a nightcap and wearing a dressing-gown, grimacing with disgust at a cup of medicine. There are medicine bottles, a pill-box, and a small case inscribed 'Tractors' on the table.

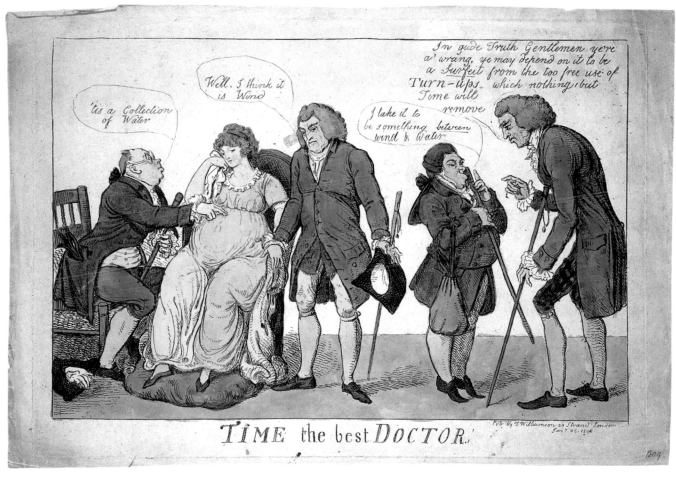

The 19th century was a time when public health measures were taken to prevent disease, medical advances started to make real inroads in the treatment of disease and the great London medical institutions assumed new power and influence.

Vaccination was another development of great importance. Edward Jenner (1749–1823) coined the term in his famous report *An Inquiry into the Causes and Effects of the Variolae Vaccinae* and distinguished between 'true' and 'spurious' cowpox. He also developed an arm-to-arm method of propagating the vaccine from the vaccinated individual's pustule. Despite considerable controversy within the medical profession, and public and Church opposition to the use of animal material, his method was widely adopted, and his report was translated into six languages. By 1801, over 100,000 people had been vaccinated.

Gavin Milroy (1805–1886), another pioneer of public health, examined the spread of leprosy and contributed to the College report on the topic in 1867. He left a bequest of £2,000 to found the Milroy Lectureship on state medicine and public health.

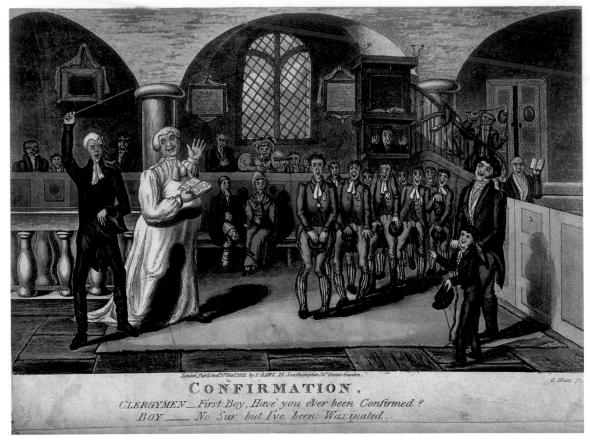

CONFIRMATION.

CLERGYMEN — First Boy, Have you ever been Confirmed?
BOY — No Sur but I've been Waxinated.

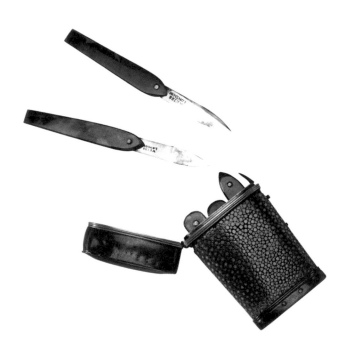

Above: An 1831 satire on the debate over the safety of smallpox vaccination. The College had supported vaccination since the work of Edward Jenner in the 1790s, and pressed the government to legislate, but it was not until 1853 that it became mandatory for infants, and for children in 1867, resulting in a fall in the number of recorded cases.

Left: Made from steel with tortoiseshell protectors, these lancets were owned by Edward Jenner, the pioneer of smallpox vaccination. Lancets were primarily used for bloodletting, but could also be used to apply vaccines.

Right: *The District Vaccinator – A Sketch at the East End.* Engraving by Edwin Buckman (1841–1930). From *The Graphic*, 8 April 1871.

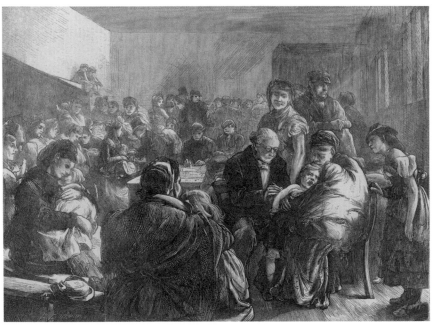

1840

The first Vaccination Act, based on an 1807 College report, bans unsafe and unreliable inoculation or variolation, and offers free vaccination, later made compulsory for infants.

1841

James Hope, an early cardiologist, dies young from consumption (tuberculosis).

1848

An Act to Improve Public Health provided central and local Boards of Health, improved drainage and sewers, refuse removal, clean drinking water and town medical officers.

1848

At the request of the government the College sets up a cholera committee to recommend precautions.

1849

By the will of Dr George Swiney an alternating quinquennial prize for jurisprudence and medical jurisprudence is created.

1849

Dr Elizabeth Blackwell (1821–1910) travels to America and qualifies in medicine at Geneva College, New York, the first English woman to become a doctor. She was ineligible for entry to the College.

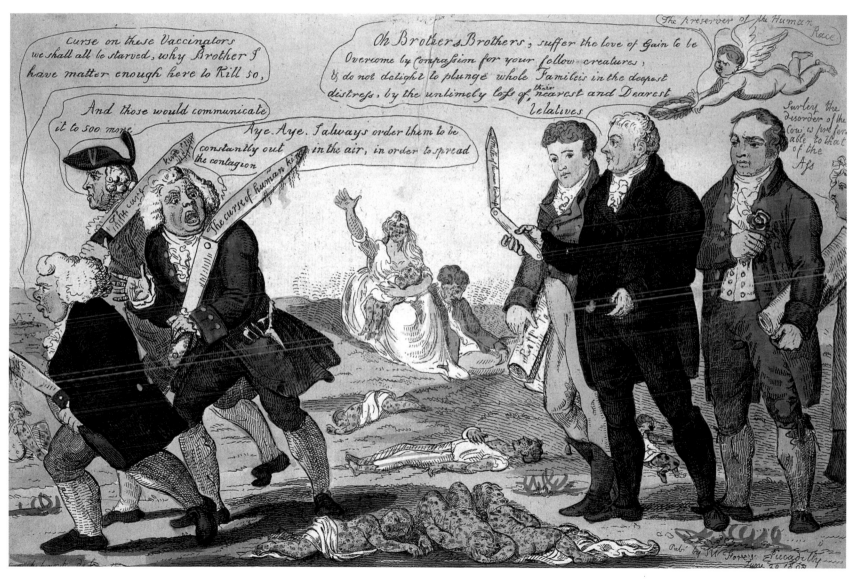

Left: In 1808, half of the people who caught smallpox died – about 400,000 Europeans per year. Smallpox was ubiquitous, but milkmaids did not succumb to the disease. In an eight-year-old boy, Jenner bravely, if somewhat recklessly, demonstrated that inoculation with cowpox prevented smallpox. In this cartoon by Isaac Cruikshank, Edward Jenner and colleagues are shown driving out mercenary physicians from the old school, who denied the value of vaccination, allowing the spread of smallpox and death.

In 1831, the fearful Asiatic cholera reached England from Russia. The previous year the government had consulted Sir Henry Halford to advise on its prevention, and a board of health, including five College fellows, recommended precautions. How effective these were is unclear, but when a second board was later set up the College was not included. Epidemics returned in 1848 and 1854.

A College licentiate, John Snow (1813–1858), who would become famous for his early use of ether, thought cholera was waterborne, and in the 1854 outbreak he meticulously plotted the houses in Soho in which residents were afflicted. He showed that they had drawn water from the municipal pump of a well in Broad Street, and subsequently that one water company supplied water piped from the Thames downstream from discharged sewage. He surmised this to be the cause of the disease. It was pioneering epidemiological research, and although the authorities were sceptical they did agree to remove the handle from the Broad Street pump. Snow was unable with the microscopes then available to see the bacteria, and it was not until Robert Koch in 1884 found the *Vibrio bacillus* in water that the cause was completely understood. From the 1850s, magazines had urged better water quality, and several Parliamentary acts forced the private water companies to improve the piped public water supplies.

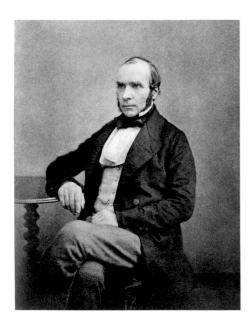

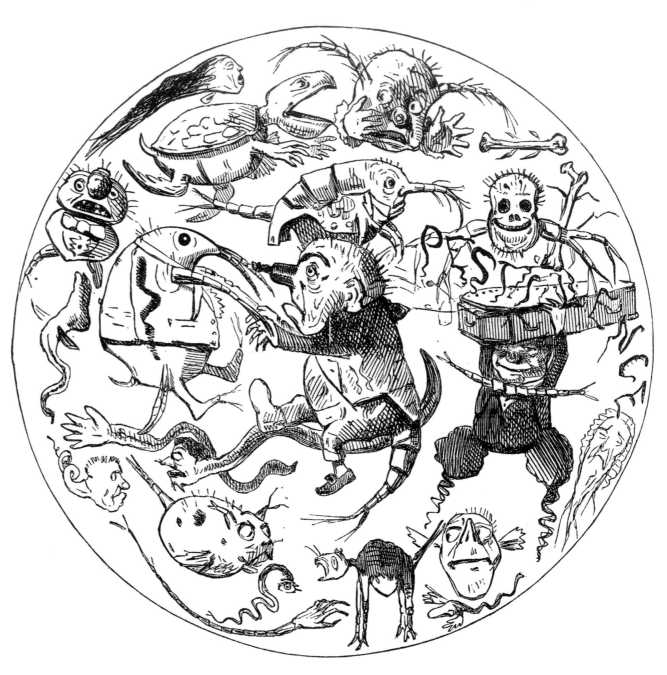

Below: *A Drop of London Water*, 1850. A cartoon from *Punch* satirising what might be found with the microscope in a drop of the Thames water that was supplied by private water companies to London households.

Below left: In addition to authoring *On the mode of communication of cholera* in 1849, John Snow was a pioneer in the field of anaesthetics. He gave chloroform to Queen Victoria at the birth of her son Leopold and her daughter Beatrice, in 1853 and 1857 respectively.

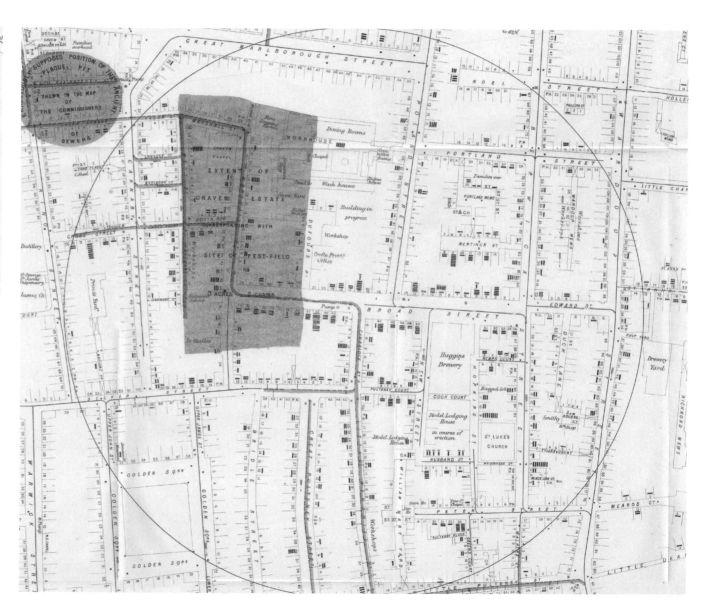

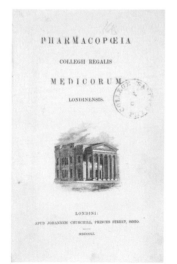

Above and right: Detail from John Snow's map charting deaths from cholera in 1854. The detail (right) shows the area around the contaminated Broad Street pump.

Left: The tenth and last edition of the College's *London Pharmacopoeia*, 232 years after the first edition appeared.

William Jenner 1815–1898

William Jenner trained at University College London and was an ambitious workaholic, but a difficult colleague, although he was adored by children. By 1849, he had acquired an international reputation by defining typhus and typhoid fever as two separate disorders. Public health officials were then able to concentrate on eradicating typhus, by controlling the human flea population, and purify the water supply to prevent typhoid fever.

He was appointed professor of both pathological anatomy and medicine at University College London and joined the Hospital for Sick Children at its inception, adding greatly to its reputation. He wrote papers on rickets and diphtheria – a major cause of childhood mortality.

In 1862, he was appointed Physician Extraordinary to Queen Victoria and cared for both Prince Albert in his final illness and, some ten years later, the Prince of Wales when he too contracted typhoid fever. In gratitude, Queen Victoria made him a baronet and professionally he became the foremost clinician of his day, partly based on his clinical skills and broad experience and partly on his outstanding teaching ability. Nonetheless, he was strongly opposed to admitting women to the profession – a view vehemently upheld by his monarch. He received a plethora of public and professional honours both at home and abroad, including presidency of the Royal College of Physicians. Not surprisingly, Sir William's medical opinion was sought by the wealthiest and most influential members of society, evidenced by the fortune of £325,000 that he amassed during his life.

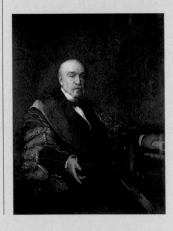

'The great aim of the physician is to prevent disease; failing that, to cure; failing that, to alleviate suffering and prolong life.'

Sir William Jenner

Below: Queen Victoria and Prince Albert visiting invalided soldiers from the Crimean War at the Fort Pitt Military Hospital, Chatham, 3 March 1855, by John Tenniel (1820–1914).

Right: Silver cup and cover, hallmarked 1871, presented to the College by Lady (Adele) Jenner in 1902. It was given to her husband in 1875 by HRH Prince Leopold, who suffered from haemophilia, 'in grateful remembrance of repeated kindnesses', while he was at Oxford University.

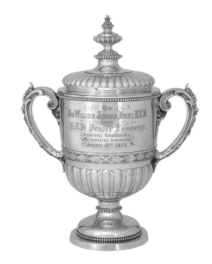

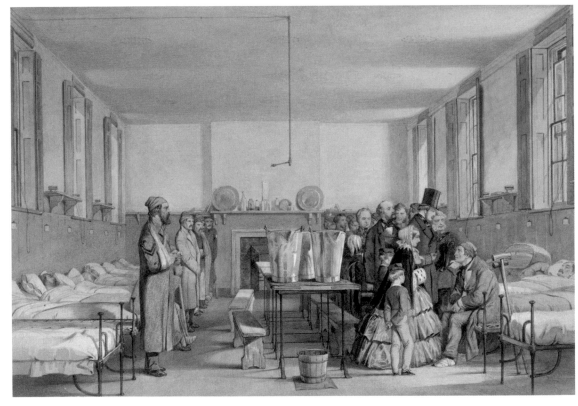

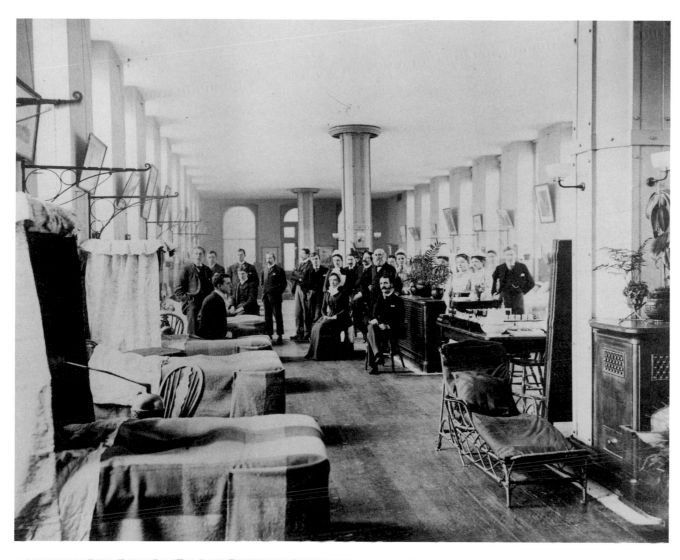

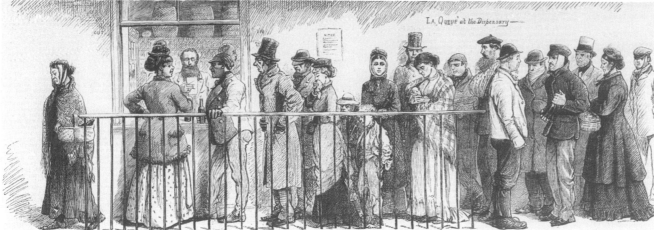

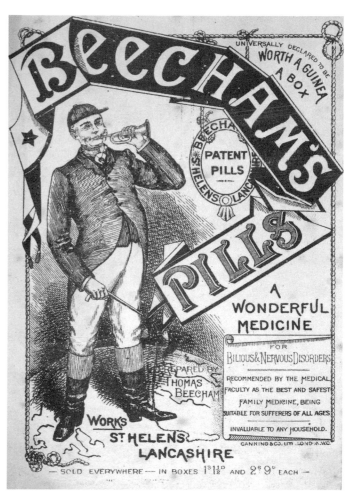

Left: A Nightingale ward at St Thomas' Hospital, *c.*1890.

Below left: Outpatient queue at the dispensary of a London hospital published in *The Graphic,* 18 December 1879.

Below right: An advertisement for an early Victorian remedy of doubtful efficacy.

1855

Dr Thomas Addison of Guy's Hospital describes Addison's disease in *On the Constitutional and Local Effects of Disease of the Supra-Renal Capsule.*

1857

Dr Thomas Mayo is elected President, the last President to be chosen by the College elects. He presided during a critical time when the College was undergoing constitutional change.

Below: Richard Bright, Thomas Hodgkin and Thomas Addison were contemporaries and became known as 'the three great men of Guy's Hospital'. Each correlated pathology with clinical findings and had a disease named after them. Jenner was also an eminent physician and pathologist, practising at University College Hospital, while James Hope practised at St George's Hospital, studied heart murmurs and is recognised as the 'first modern cardiologist'.

As medicine advanced, so many of its great institutions arose. The University of London was founded in 1835 from the nonconformist (dissenter) institution of University College in Gower Street (1828), combined with the staunchly Anglican King's College in the Strand (1829), plus other smaller affiliated colleges. Classes in medicine had opened in 1828, and later the medical schools of the London hospitals were added. In 1854, by statute the right of awarding the London degree of Bachelor of Medicine was given to the university, thus breaking the English monopoly of Oxford and Cambridge. This was opposed by the College, but unsuccessfully. A series of celebrated physicians practised at the great London hospitals. Sir William Jenner (1815–1898), the leading figure in medicine in London in the late 19th century, was a fine clinician and teacher at University College Hospital. At Guy's were Richard Bright (1789–1858), best known for his observation linking protein in the urine and dropsy (oedema) to chronic renal disease, soon known as Bright's disease; Thomas Addison (1793–1860), who described his eponymous disease in 1855; and Thomas Hodgkin (1798–1866), who described Hodgkin's disease and was a vigorous reformer and supporter of indigenous people, dying in Palestine from dysentery. James Hope (1801–1841), from St George's, was perhaps the first cardiologist, for he described the familiar diastolic murmur in mitral stenosis (Hope's murmur), and carefully studied the appearances of the heart post-mortem, correlating his findings with the clinical diagnosis.

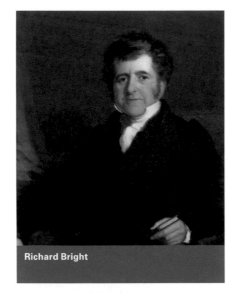

Richard Bright

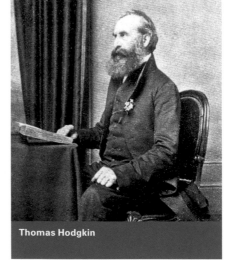

Thomas Hodgkin

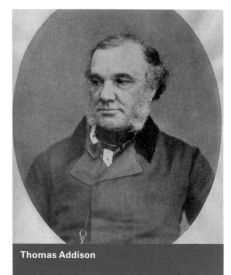

Thomas Addison

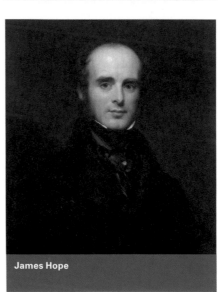

William Jenner

James Hope

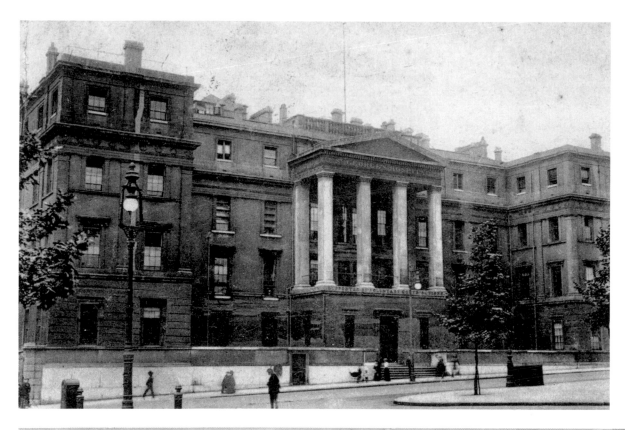

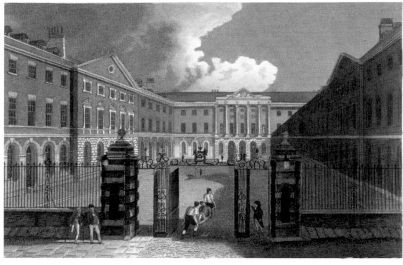

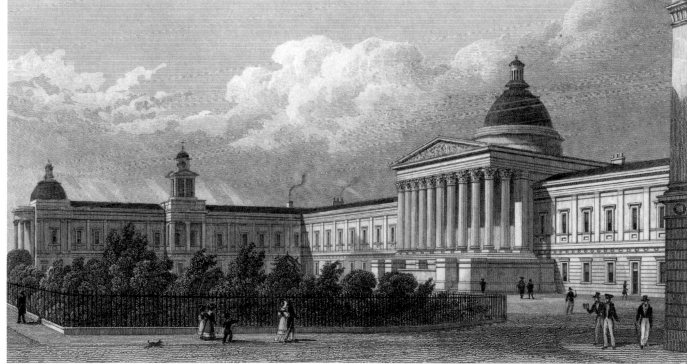

Above: Sketch of Guy's Hospital, 1820, where Richard Bright, Thomas Addison and Thomas Hodgkin worked.

Above left: St George's Hospital at Hyde Park Corner, where James Hope worked. He was a protagonist for the new clinical skill of auscultation, particularly applying this to cardiac murmurs.

Left: University College London, c.1835. The university was founded in 1826 as a secular alternative to the religious universities of Oxford and Cambridge. Initially, there was strong opposition and it did not receive a royal charter allowing the award of university degrees until 1838. The University College Hospital was the 'home' of Sir William Jenner, Holme Professor of Clinical Medicine and, subsequently, Professor of the Principles and Practice of Medicine.

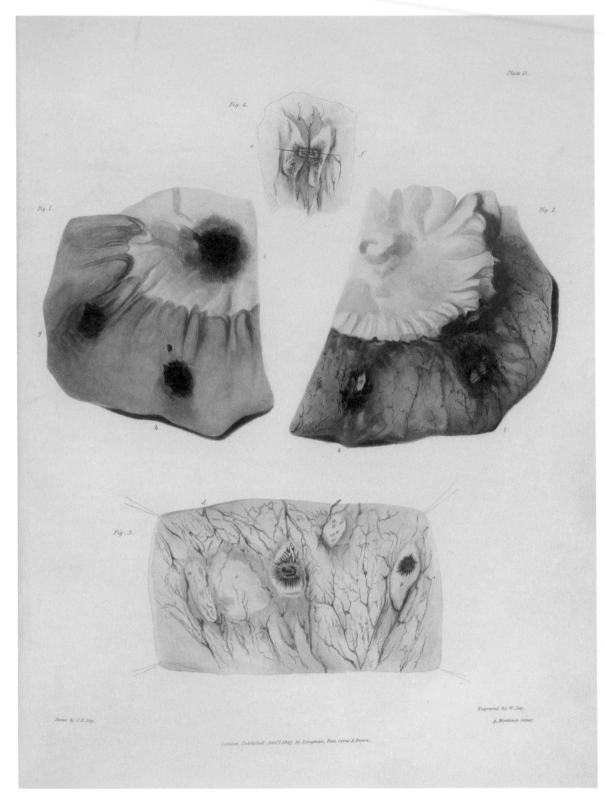

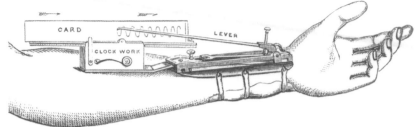

Above: The sphygmograph was developed in 1854 by German physiologist Karl von Vierordt (1818–1884). It is considered the first external, non-intrusive device used to estimate blood pressure.

Left: An illustration by Richard Bright of a gross anatomical specimen and histological section of chronic renal disease.

Below: Acute atrophy of the liver, from *Atlas of the Pathological Anatomy Illustrative of Diseases of the Liver* by Friedrich Theodor von Frerichs (1862).

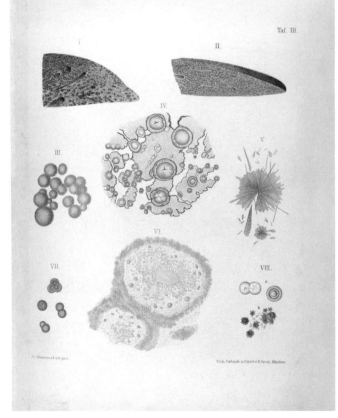

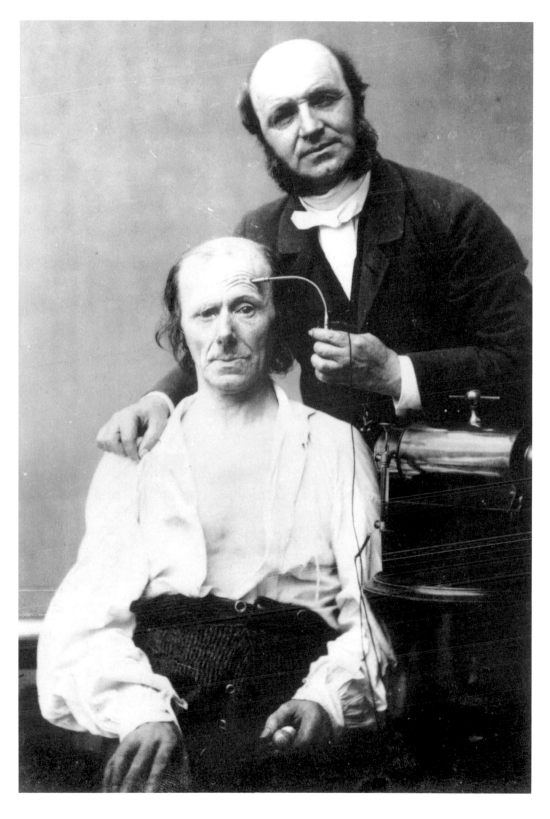

Left: 'Galvanic stimulation of the left frontal muscle'. Photograph by Guillaume Duchenne de Boulogne (1806–1875), pioneer in neurology and photography. In 1856, he advocated the use of an AC as opposed to a DC current for electrotherapeutic stimulation of muscles.

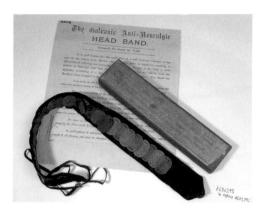

Right above: Galvanic anti-neuralgic headband made up of a series of 24 alternate zinc and copper discs mounted onto a felt and ribbon band. It was used for the treatment of headache and migraine.

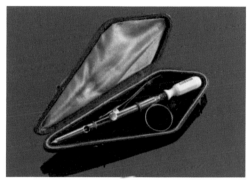

Right below: In 1844, the Irish physician Francis Rynd developed the first syringe with a hollow needle to allow drugs to be introduced under the skin.

Below: TB remained a scourge, with treatment ranging from none to a prolonged stay in a sanatorium, and in rare cases collapsing a lung by injecting air inside the chest but outside the lung itself.

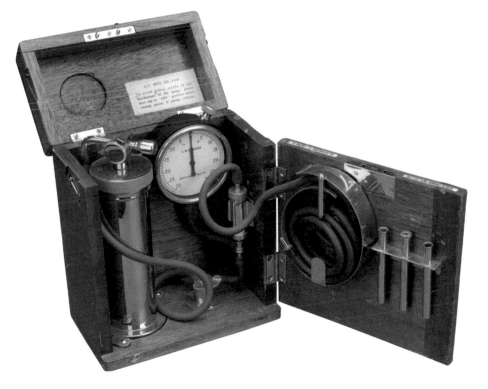

1857

William Munk appointed as the Harveian Librarian, and starts his work on producing *Munk's Roll*, one of the College's most valued publications.

EXPECTATION OF LIFE (in Years).

Age.	PERSONS.			MALES.			FEMALES.		
	Surrey.	Liver-pool.	Metro-polis.	Surrey.	Liver-pool.	Metro-polis.	Surrey.	Liver-pool.	Metro-polis.
0	45	26	37	44	25	35	46	27	38
1	50	33	43	50	33	41	50	34	44
2	51	38	46	51	37	45	52	39	48
3	52	41	47	52	40	46	52	42	49
4	52	42	48	52	41	46	52	43	50
5	52	43	48	51	42	46	52	43	50
10	49	41	45	49	41	44	49	42	47
15	45	37	41	45	37	40	45	38	43
20	42	34	38	42	33	36	42	34	35
25	38	30	34	38	30	32	38	31	35
30	35	27	30	35	27	29	35	27	32
35	31	24	27	31	23	25	31	24	28
40	28	21	24	28	21	22	28	22	25
45	24	18	20	24	18	19	24	18	22
50	21	16	18	21	16	17	21	17	18

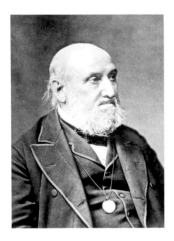

Left and above: William Farr was hired by the General Register Office and became responsible for the collection of official medical statistics in England and Wales. Importantly, he devised a system for recording the cause of death, enabling mortality rates across different occupations to be compared for the first time. The table above, compiled by Farr, is from *Vital Statistics*, published in 1843.

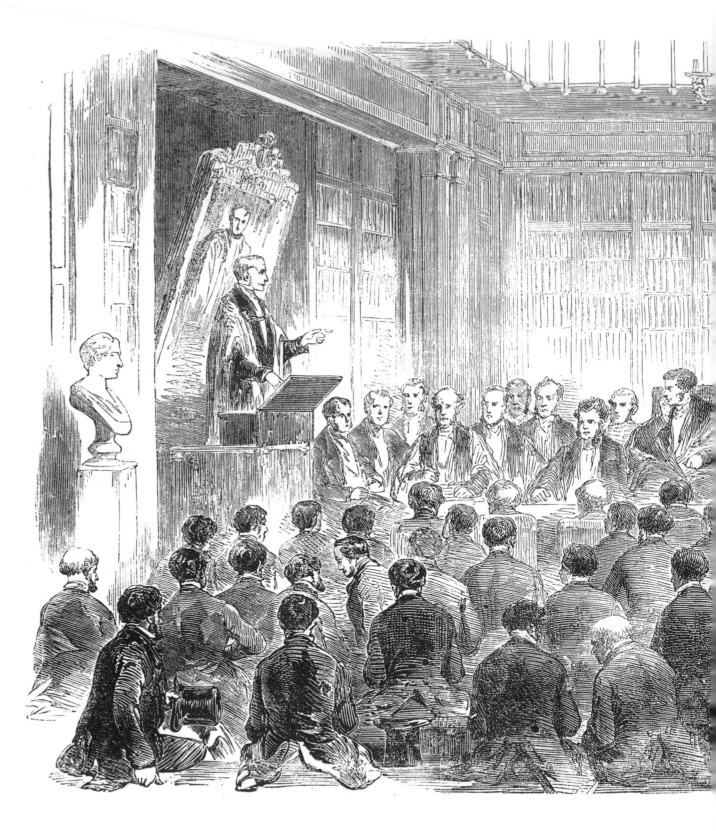

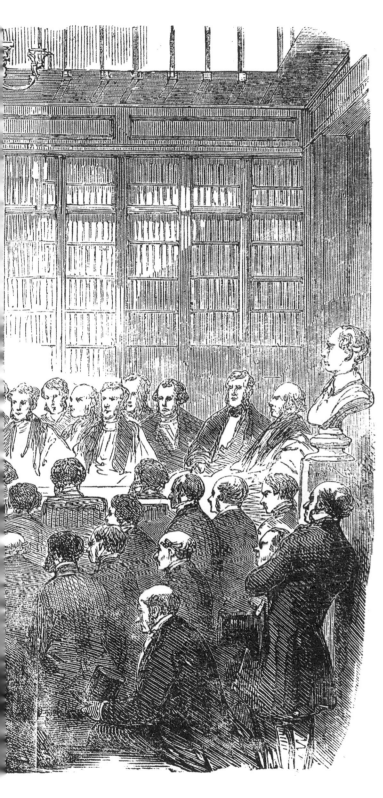

It was in the 19th century that medicine, and the College, began to assume a form which would be recognisable today. It was a torrid period for the College, during which its roles and responsibilities were altered by acts of Parliament, and the state became increasingly involved in regulation and control – much to the disapproval of many doctors.

In 1837, the General Register Office was set up, which, as part of the collection of national statistics, recorded the dates of deaths. Francis Bisset Hawkins (1796–1894), whose College posts included Censor and Lumleian and Goulstonian lecturer, suggested adding the causes of death. In 1858, his namesake Francis Hawkins (1794–1877) resigned after 29 years, as the longest-serving College Registrar, and he became the first Registrar of the General Council of Medical Education and Registration of the United Kingdom (now the General Medical Council). The epidemiologist Dr William Farr (1807–1883), the Registrar General's Compiler of Abstracts, drew up an excellent simple classification of the causes of death, and in 1857 the College set up a large committee of fellows and external experts, with Francis Sibson (1814–1876) as its energetic secretary. It worked intermittently until the first *Nomenclature of Diseases* was published in 1869 in five languages. The *Nomenclature* was well received and the College persuaded the Treasury to distribute 20,000 copies to all medical practitioners and the armed services to make the completion of death certificates more informative. In 1869, the College presented Sibson with a silver cup and cover, which were given to the College museum by his widow, Sarah, in 1876. Since then, there have been seven revisions and editions, the last in 1961. The *Nomenclature* has been an important instrument in both the United Kingdom and the USA for clarifying and classifying the causes of diseases, as knowledge has increased.

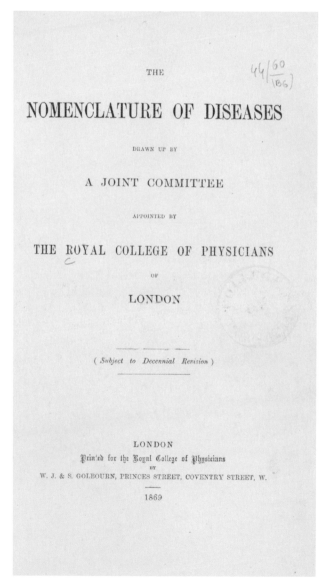

THE

NOMENCLATURE OF DISEASES

DRAWN UP BY

A JOINT COMMITTEE

APPOINTED BY

THE ROYAL COLLEGE OF PHYSICIANS

OF

LONDON

(*Subject to Decennial Revision*)

LONDON
Printed for the Royal College of Physicians
BY
W. J. & S. GOLBOURN, PRINCES STREET, COVENTRY STREET, W.

1869

Left: *The Nomenclature of Diseases* 1869 produced by a joint committee appointed by the Royal College of Physicians enabled more accurate recording of the cause of death.

1858

The momentous Medical Act to help the public distinguish qualified from unqualified medical practitioners radically changes the role of the College in medical regulation.

1858

In response to the Medical Act, the College quickly introduces a written and oral Membership (MRCP) examination. A member is then eligible to be elected to the Fellowship.

1859

The first national Medical Register of practitioners is published. Elizabeth Blackwell joins the register, the first woman to do so.

1861

Munk's Roll first published in two volumes, containing biographies of all the fellows of the College since its foundation in 1518.

Below: *Medical Student at Guy's,* *c.*1880: Medical students at Guy's Hospital in London having some fun playing pranks.

Moves to regulate the practice of medicine had been made at various times in the early 19th century, and this culminated in the Parliamentary Bill to Regulate the Qualifications of Practitioners in Medicine and Surgery (the 'Medical Act'), which was passed after a tortuous course in 1858. The act set up the General Medical Council (GMC), on which all the colleges and other institutions were represented, to control entry into the profession. Medical education was reformed, and examinations and the awarding of qualifying degrees by colleges and universities were regulated by the GMC. Many of the powers previously held by the College were reduced and, although the act took away the College's supervisory powers over apothecary shops and quacks, this was probably not regretted. The College was given the role of conducting the much-improved qualifying examination (LRCP) for the whole of England and Wales for both general practitioners and physicians, which led to the first Conjoint examination with the Royal College of Surgeons in 1884. After 250 years, the College had also lost its pharmacopoeia, replaced with the national *British Pharmacopoeia.* It did however gain the new title of Royal College of Physicians of England.

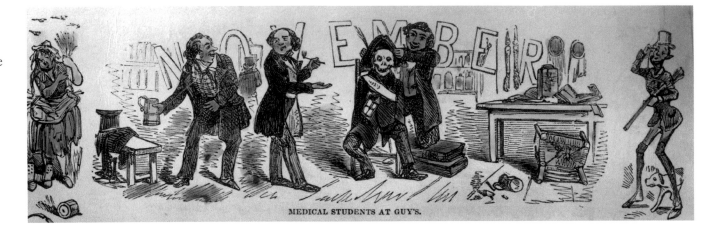

MEDICAL STUDENTS AT GUY'S.

One far-reaching effect of the 1858 Medical Act was the establishment, for the first time, of a national register of medical practitioners, listing the qualifications that were recognised by the new General Medical Council (GMC), and hence awarding licences to practise. A medical register had previously been published by Samuel Simmons (1750–1813) in three editions, 1779–83 (in which he listed physicians with their universities, surgeons, apothecaries and dentists in London, the provinces and abroad), and there was the *London Medical Directory* from 1845, but these were both commercial enterprises, and entries were not compulsory. Before this, the College had regularly issued a catalogue of its members, and in the 1783 edition extra-licentiates practising outside of London were included.

'The hospital is the only proper College in which to rear a true disciple of Aesculapius.'

John Abernethy, 1764–1831

Far left: The 1858 Medical Act regulating the qualifications of practitioners of medicine and surgery, resulting in reform of medical education. The act also set up the General Medical Council, which regulated the award of medical degrees.

Left: The first *Medical Register* of 1859, authorised by the new General Medical Council.

Left below: Questions from papers of the October 1867 membership (MRCP) examination on the Principles and Practice of Medicine, Psychological Medicine, Public Health and Medical Anatomy, including a translation from Greek into Latin or English and Latin into French or English.

Below: *In Propria Persona* (Charles Samuel Keene, 1875) – a cartoon from *Punch* depicting medical students bemoaning the severity of College examinations, which they had to face alone.

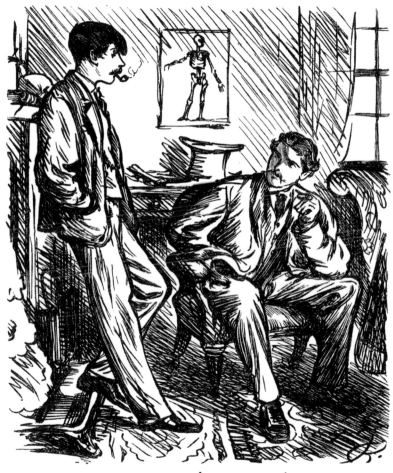

IN PROPRIÂ PERSONÂ.

First Medical Student. "THE BRITISH MEDICAL ASSOCIATION APPEARS TO COUNTENANCE VIVISECTION!"

Second Ditto. "I SHOULD THINK SO, AFTER THE WAY THEY CUT ME UP AT THE COLLEGE!"

Thermometers had been used since the 17th century, but were heavy, a foot long and very slow to record. Working with a glassblower in Leeds, in 1867, Thomas Clifford Allbutt, Censor and Harveian Orator, designed a smaller version. The mercury was expanded by heat and forced from the bulb into a narrow tube, which made the response much faster and more sensitive. It remained there until the column was shaken down and became known as 'Dr Clifford Allbutt's self-registering, short clinical thermometer'. It was rapidly popularised as it could be carried in the pocket, and detailed, earlier research in Germany, on thousands of fever charts, had stimulated interest in recording the temperature of patients. This thermometer stands, with the stethoscope from France and percussion from Germany, as a major advance in the clinical examination of patients in the 19th century. Allbutt was also interested in neurology and, having listened to Trousseau and Duchenne in Paris, published a monograph *On the Use of the Ophthalmoscope in Diseases of the Nervous System and of the Kidneys*, in 1871. He hoped that the use of the ophthalmoscope would end the 'metaphysical or transcendental habit of thought' and bring a more rigorous and philosophical mode of investigation to disorders of the brain. After working in Leeds General Infirmary for 28 years and a Commissioner for Lunacy in England and Wales, Allbutt became Regius Professor of Physic at Cambridge in 1892, and edited the popular *A System of Medicine*, 1896–9, in eight volumes. He was knighted in 1907.

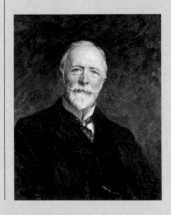

'Nothing seems more natural than that women should be physicians.'

Albert Stille, 1813–1920

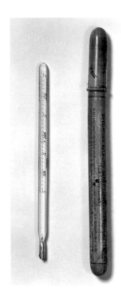

Above: The short self-registering clinical mercury thermometer designed by Sir Clifford Allbutt in Leeds, the use of which revolutionised the clinical management of fevers.

Right: Image of the building of the Metropolitan Railway in 1862, showing the great destruction of the dwellings of the poor that it caused, which the College felt worsened the slums and hence the health of their inhabitants.

Francis Anstie (1833–1874), physician to the now decommissioned Westminster Hospital, liberal contributor to *The Lancet* and first Dean of the London Medical College for Women, was another reforming fellow of the College. In his short life he carried out celebrated work on various aspects of public health. He wrote about the abuse of alcohol, proposing 'Anstie's Limit', that 75ml of ethanol was safe to drink daily (equivalent today to about four units of alcohol). He campaigned for the reform of Poor Law medicine, observing 'that for the state to decline to enquire about such matters as the bodily habits and health of its members was not in favour of liberty but in favour of immorality, dirt, disease, and death'. In 1874, he proposed in Comitia that the College should send to the Prime Minister, Benjamin Disraeli, a *Memorial on the Dwellings of the Poor* to draw attention to the deleterious effects that the Railway and Improvement Acts were having on the already bad housing conditions of the poor. As their tenements were destroyed, the inhabitants were crowded into even worse conditions, which were immortalised by Charles Dickens. The College pointed out that 'overcrowding, especially in unwholesome and ill constructed habitations, originates disease, leads to drunkenness and immorality'. This helped lead to the 1875 Act for Facilitating the Improvement of the Dwellings of the Working Classes in Large Towns.

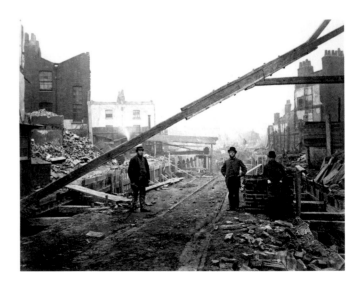

1862

At the request of the Colonial Office, the College sets up a long-lived and sclerotic committee to consider the management of leprosy. In 1868, the College awards its secretary Gavin Milroy (1805–1886) 25 guineas with which he purchased a silver Egyptian inkstand; later he endowed the Milroy lecture.

1864

Elizabeth Garrett Anderson challenges the College to allow her to sit its licensing examination. The request is refused. *British Pharmacopoeia* published, which after 200 years replaces the College's *Pharmacopoeia*.

1865

Elizabeth Garrett Anderson sits and passes the Licence in Medicine and Surgery of the Society of Apothercaries examinations (the first woman in England to do so), and comes on to the Medical Register. First Harveian Oration delivered completely in English.

1867

Survey of leprosy in colonies and dominions published by the College. First visitation of College examinations by Medical Council inspectors.

1869

The first *Nomenclature of Disease* is published by the College, with the final edition in 1961.

1874

The College sends a *Memorial on the Dwellings of the Poor* to the Prime Minister decrying the detrimental effects on public health of the destruction of buildings by the railways.

Left: Registrar of the Royal College of Physicians Sir Henry Pitman's response to Elizabeth Garrett following her request for a licence to practise. May 1864.

Below: *A Court for King Cholera*, 1853. A cartoon from *Punch* illustrating the overcrowding and filth that predisposed London to the epidemics of cholera that were so frequent in the 19th century.

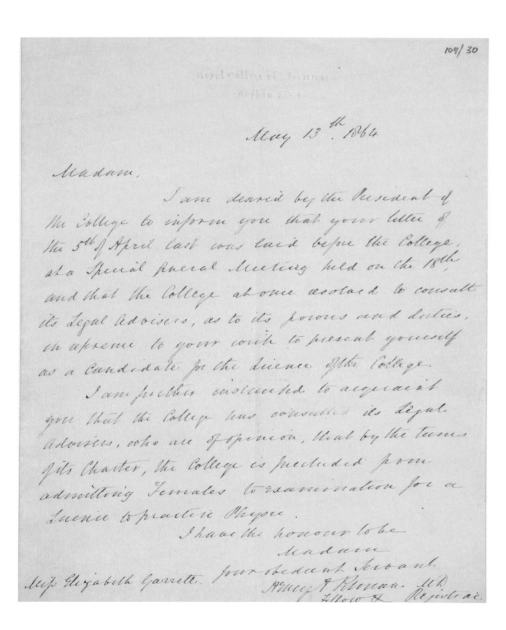

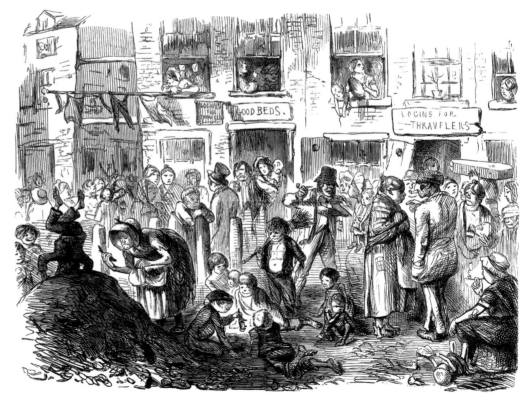

Although Sir John Simon was a towering figure in the important advances made in the regulation of public health in the 19th century, he was first a meticulous and scientific surgeon at St Thomas' Hospital, and an early proponent of asepsis, before the introduction of antisepsis. He was also interested in sanitary science (public health) and the spread of diseases. With the widespread fear of another cholera epidemic in 1855, he was appointed chief medical officer to the General Board of Health, and later to the Privy Council. In this position, following the pioneer work of the civil servant Sir Edwin Chadwick (1800–1890), he wrote a series of hard-hitting annual reports that forced the adoption of extensive legislation in the 1870s to improve public health through central and local regulation, vaccination, clean water supplies, housing, sewage and drainage, clearance of rubbish and better paving of streets. However, he appears not to have been a proponent of the provision of services by the state.

Simon knew John Snow and his work on the spread of cholera through water, and he gradually accepted the 'germ theory' of communicable diseases, which was proved a few years later when the causative agents were demonstrated by microscopy.

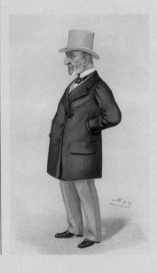

Below: The health of Londoners was hugely improved by the public engineering works masterminded by Joseph Bazalgette, confining the Thames within its embankments and developing the London sewers.

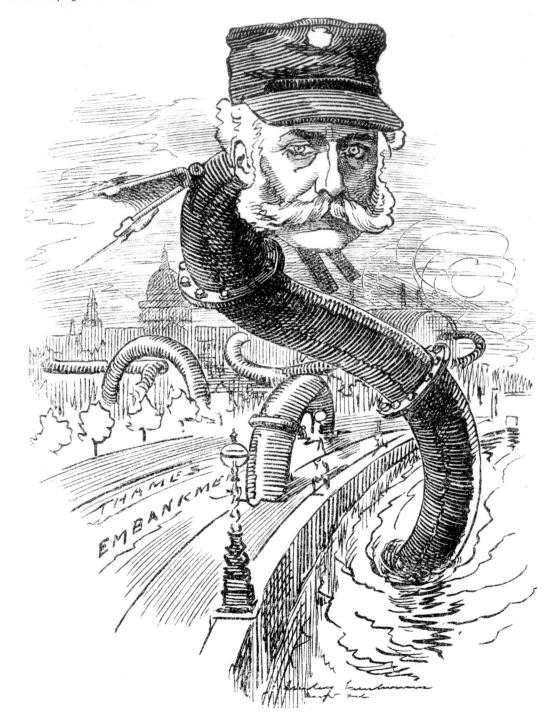

1875

Sir William Jenner (1815–1898)
is presented with a silver cup
and cover by HRH Prince Leopold,
who suffered from haemophilia.

1875

A public health act (Act for
Facilitating the Improvement of the
Dwellings of the Working Classes
in Large Towns) is passed by
Parliament, partly as a result of the
lobbying of Francis Anstie.

1878

The second edition of *Munk's Roll*,
in three volumes, is published.

1878

Fifty-five of the 315 fellows of
the College present to the Fellows'
Club a silver cup and cover, with
shields on the plinth engraved with
their names. From 1857 the Comitia
Club had met after the quarterly
meetings, and was renamed the
Fellows' Club in 1872. It ceased
in 1936.

1879

Louis Pasteur demonstrates the
value of vaccine to protect sheep
against anthrax.

1880

There were 305 fellows, 433
members and 1,370 new licentiates.
Charles Édouard Brown-Séquard
is awarded the Legion of Honour.

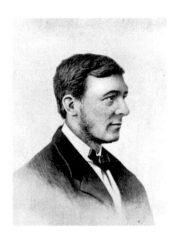

**Above: Daniel Hanbury
(1825–1875), leading British
botanist and pharmacologist.
His *Pharmacographia* (1874,
written with Friedrich Flückiger)
should be the *vade mecum* of
all pharmacognosy students,
as it takes it from the humoural
straitjacket of the previous
millennia into the scientific
age. He died of typhoid in
Clapham aged 50.**

**Right: Colour plate of the
curare vine, *Chondrodendron
tomen* from Bentley and
Trimen's four-volume *Medicinal
Plants* (1880). Robert Bentley
(1821–1893), Professor of Botany
at King's College Hospital,
combined beautiful, hand-
painted botanical images
of 306 plants with scientific
and medical information on all
of them. The illustrations are
a milestone in botanical art.**

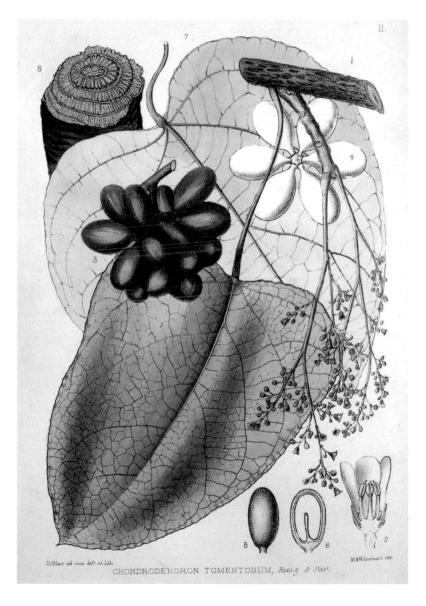

CHONDRODENDRON TOMENTOSUM, *Ruiz & Pav.*

As the 19th century progressed, science began
to underpin the understanding of medicine: Claude
Bernard's work promoted the use of experimental
methodology in medicine, while the miasma theory of
disease transmission of disorders such as cholera and the
black death was replaced by the germ theory based on
the work of Louis Pasteur and Robert Koch. Farr had
introduced epidemiological methodology and the role
of physiology was highlighted by James Carson's work
on the elasticity of the lungs and the role of injecting
air into the plural cavity to aid recovery in tuberculosis.

Scientifically organised books on medicine began
to appear and pharmacy was in the vanguard. Robert
Bentley at King's College produced a structural,
physiologic and systematic account of every plant with
a medicinal use in *Manual of Botany* (1861). With Henry
Trimen, he produced the four-volume *Medicinal Plants*
(1880) with botanical descriptions of hundreds of plants
and 300 hand-coloured plates, along with habitat and
notes on research, medicines produced and uses – in
other words, a modern herbal.

It is the *Pharmacographia: A History of the Principal
Drugs of Vegetable Origin, met with in Great Britain and
British India* (1874) by Friedrich Flückiger and Daniel
Hanbury that is the most famous. The Latin name of
the medicine, with vernacular names in English, French
and German of the plant involved, introduces each
chapter. The following encyclopaedic resource, despite
being unillustrated, contains an outstanding historical
section, followed by the botanical origin, habitat and
description of each plant – essential reading for research.
The microscopic structure, chemical composition and
finally the uses of each drug are given.

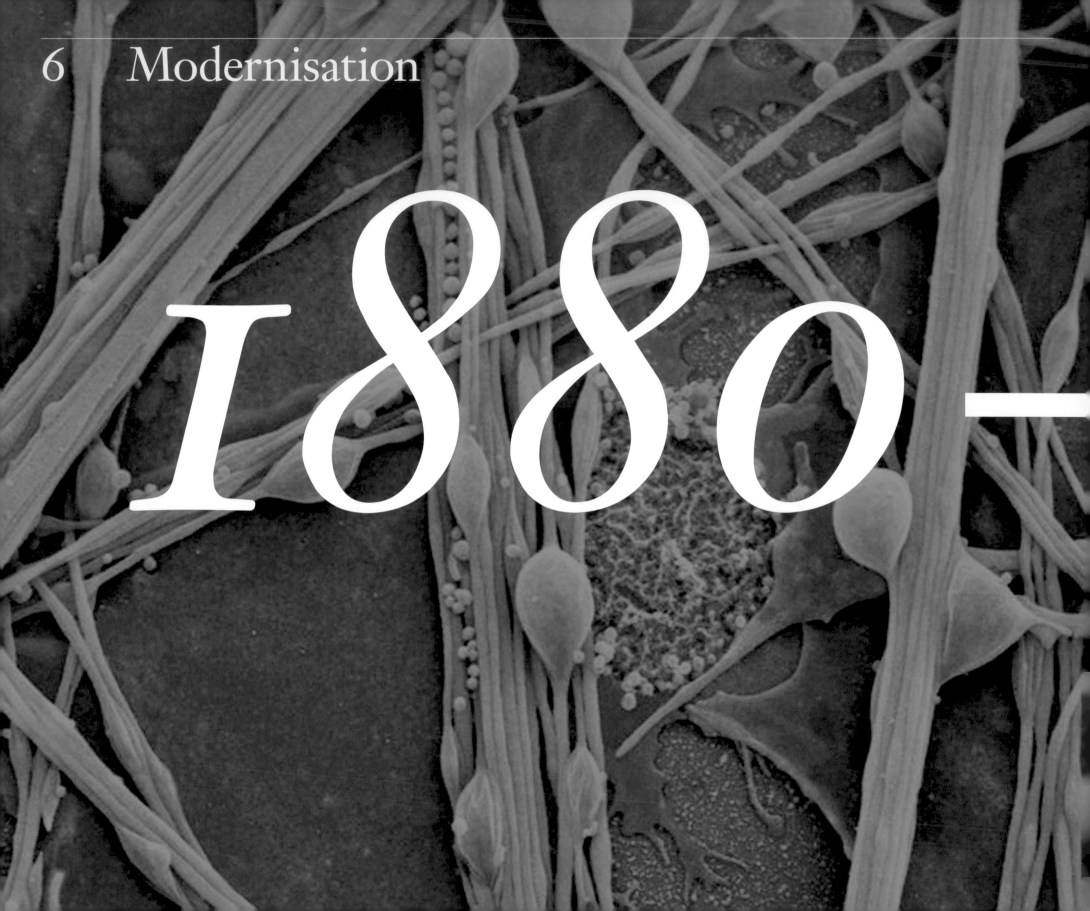

1880–

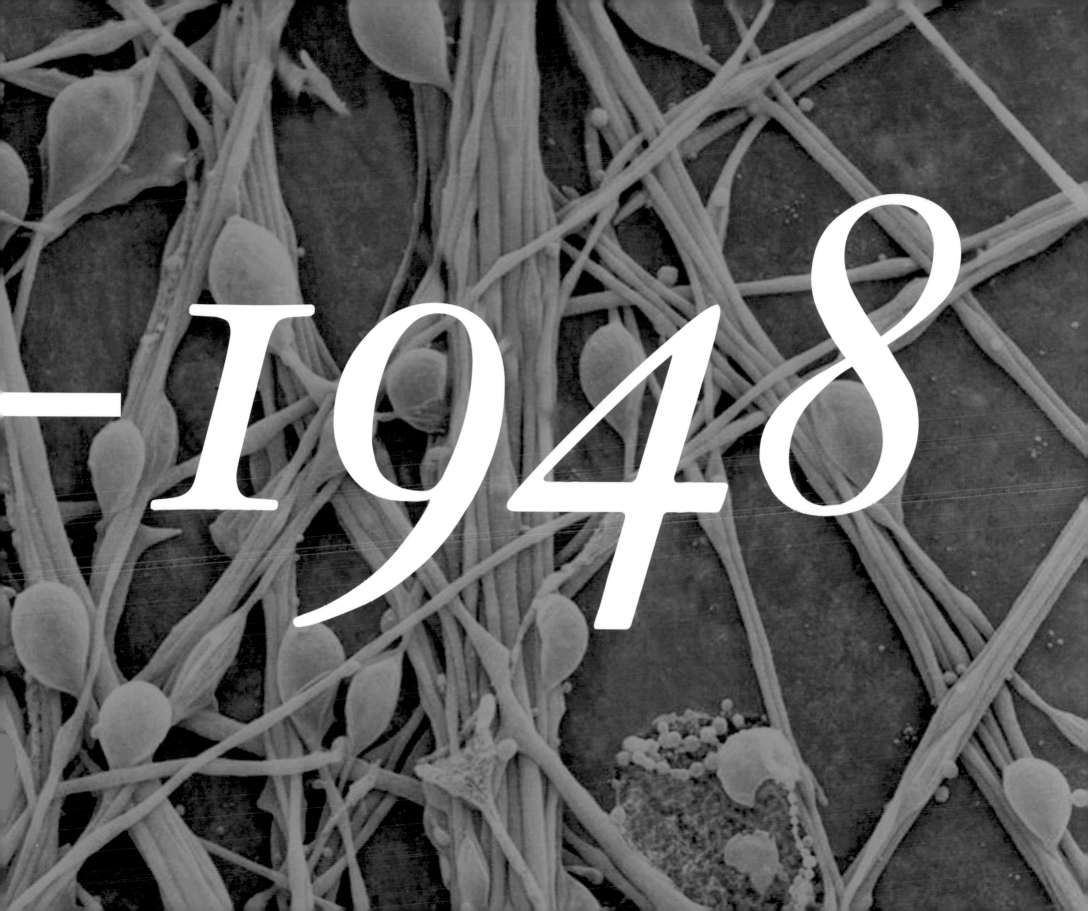

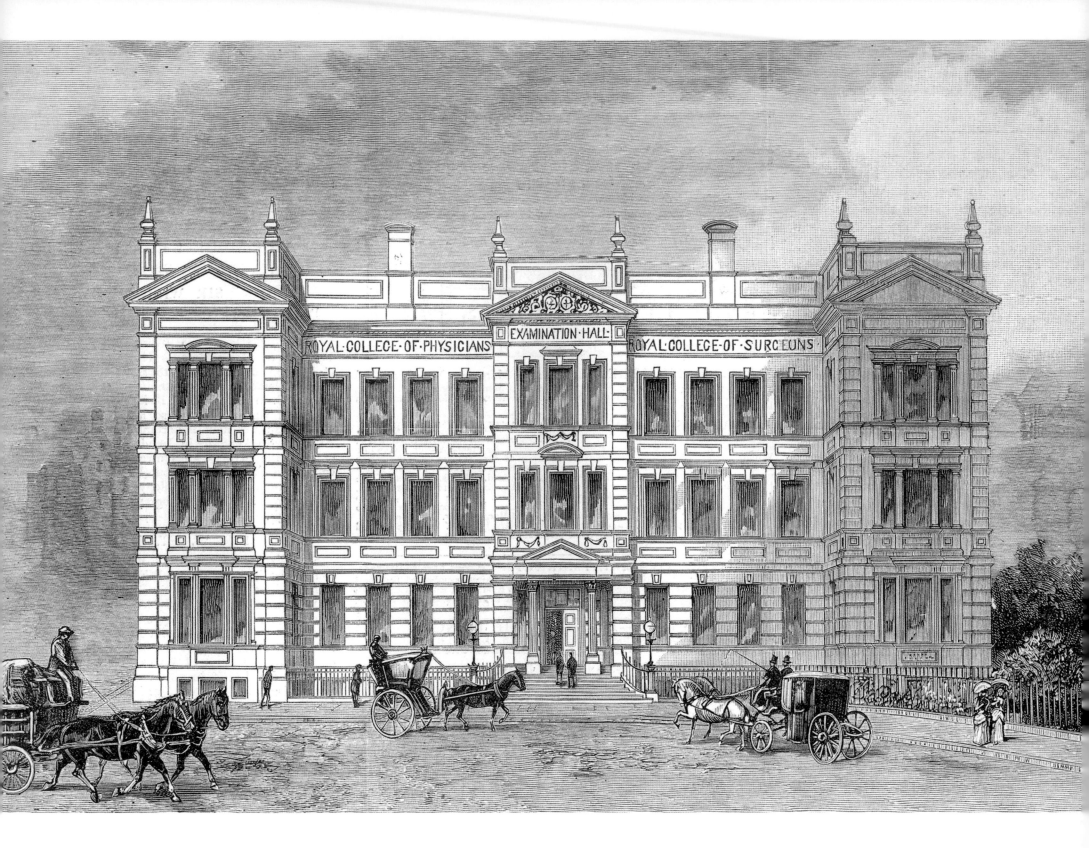

1883

The College begins a campaign to obtain degree-giving powers, reflecting huge dissatisfaction with the University of London, which did not teach medicine but examined in the subject and awarded degrees.

1884

The College building is shaken by an earthquake, sufficient to stop the clocks (though 21st-century readers should be reassured they have been restarted).

1886

Laying of the foundation stone for the Examination Halls – jointly with the Royal College of Surgeons – for the Conjoint licensing exam.

1886

The first specialist diploma of the College is established – the Diploma in Public Health.

Opposite: After the Royal Colleges of Physicians and Surgeons agreed to hold the Conjoint examination, increasing demand required a larger building. Queen Victoria laid the foundation stone in March 1886, and the building was completed in 1889. However finances deteriorated, and the building was sold to the Institute of Electrical Engineers in 1908.

Below: The New Examination Hall was built in Queen Square, and survives today, housing research departments of the Institute of Neurology.

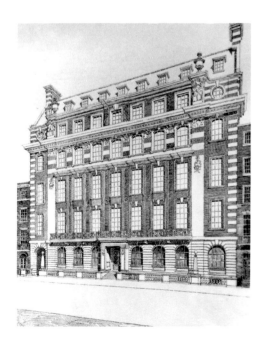

By the beginning of the 1900s the English population had mushroomed – London had a population of over 6 million, six times greater than a century earlier. Life expectancy had climbed to 48 years for a man and 52 years for a woman. During the previous hundred years major strides had been made in the recognition of diseases and understanding of causes. Most fundamentally, Louis Pasteur's proof of the existence of bacteria explained the mysterious phenomenon of contagion and placed microbial infection at the centre of medicine and public health. Recognition of the importance of waterborne epidemic infections had conquered London's cholera epidemics, and improvements such as Bazalgette's sewers and Thames Embankment transformed life for Londoners.

The end of the rigidly class-based Victorian and Edwardian eras and the upheavals of the two world wars wrought major social transformations, which impacted on the College and practice of medicine, as in every area of life. At the end of the 19th century, admission to the College changed to include a membership category based on merit, as judged by theoretical and clinical examinations, initially including Latin and Greek. If successful, this enabled any doctor to enter the College and ultimately be considered for Fellowship, but even more revolutionary, the College had to countenance and finally accept the inclusion of women physicians.

By 1860 at the time of the passing of the Medical Act, there were in the College 220 fellows (physicians in the current meaning of the word, with significant prestige, very much London based, and with involvement in the governance of the College) and about 500 licentiates (essentially general practitioners). Full licentiates had permission to practise within seven miles of the City of London, and extra-licentiates outside that area. In 1860, a new category was created – that of members, open to all medical graduates, but by examination. Members, like fellows, were physicians rather than general practitioners, and membership became the only path to Fellowship; in a vital distinction from licentiates, they were forbidden from practising pharmacy. The membership examination became – and remains – the hurdle that needs to be surmounted by every English physician. In its early form, it covered clinically relevant science, clinical examinations (for participation in which 2s 6d was paid to patients from 1887), oral examinations and a language test. The options for translating from Latin and Greek were not removed until 1936. A very high standard has always been required to pass the various stages of the MRCP examination, and at its most stringent, in 1933, the pass rate was as low as 12 per cent. Currently the qualification MRCP (UK) is jointly administered by the College and the two Scottish medical colleges.

> *'Physicians of the Utmost fame*
> *Were called at once; but when they came*
> *They answered, as they took their Fees,*
> *There is no Cure for this Disease.'*

Hilaire Belloc

1888

A royal commission on the future of London University considers whether the College of Physicians (and the College of Surgeons) should have degree-giving powers.

1889

The College opens its research laboratory, jointly with the College of Surgeons.

1890

The College supports the Midwives Registration Bill in the confidence that 'the majority of medical men in this country are not likely to raise objections to any measure which may conduce to the welfare and comfort of the poor'.

In the mid-19th century a plethora of organisations offered qualifications in medicine, with a race to the bottom to offer the least taxing and cheapest examination. The Medical Act (1858) advocated a more regulated process, but it took over 25 years before a regimented pathway to qualification emerged, in the 1886 Act to Amend the Medical Act. This abolished the option of registering with half-qualifications, requiring doctors to pass examinations in medicine *and* surgery *and* midwifery. In anticipation, the Royal College of Physicians and the Royal College of Surgeons proposed and established their Conjoint Examining Board in 1884, holding its first examination a year later, combining the two independent qualifications of MRCS (Member of the Royal College of Surgeons) and LRCP (Licentiate of the Royal College of Physicians). The two colleges persistently rebuffed the Society of Apothecaries, which wished to participate. 'The Conjoint' was hugely successful; at one point over 80 per cent of registered medical students used it as their pathway to qualification. Foreseeing this demand, the colleges commissioned a large Examination Hall, its foundation stone being laid by Queen Victoria in 1886. The Conjoint examination survived until 1993, when requirements for a university degree for British students rendered it superfluous.

The GMC was given the role of assessing accusations of misconduct by doctors, but despite this, the College Censors' Board also maintained a watchful eye over the behaviour of its fellows, members and licentiates (it still has the remit to do so). One concern was whether physicians were dispensing medication, rather than prescribing it, such behaviour breaching the clear demarcation between physician and apothecary.

Another was canvassing for patients, and a third the tradition that RCP fellows – unlike other medical men – had elected not to be able to sue their patients for unpaid fees. Licentiates were rebuked for using the title 'Doctor' in the absence of a university doctorate. Consorting with spiritual healers, and indeed homeopaths, was strongly discouraged, and one discussion concerned whether Benjamin Disraeli's general practitioner was a homeopath. Self-advertising and the endorsement of commercial products were forbidden, and in 1911 the Censors' Board decided it was undesirable that physicians should be interviewed by the lay press on medical matters. During World War I complaints were made concerning poaching patients from doctors at the front by non-combatants at home, and miscellaneous cases were heard such as of the medical student (undoubtedly patriotic) who impersonated a Royal Army Medical Corps captain and fraudulently passed men as fit for combat.

Right: One doctor who qualified via the Conjoint route, and thus was a licentiate of the College, was William Gilbert (W.G.) Grace. Sometimes known in cricketing circles by the nickname 'The doctor', he was a general practitioner in Bristol, combining his two professions by employing locums during the cricket season.

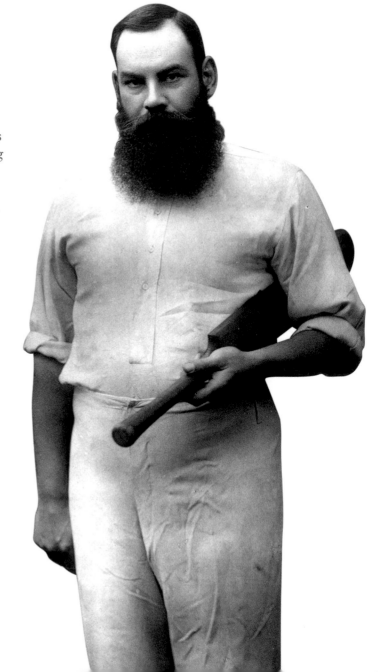

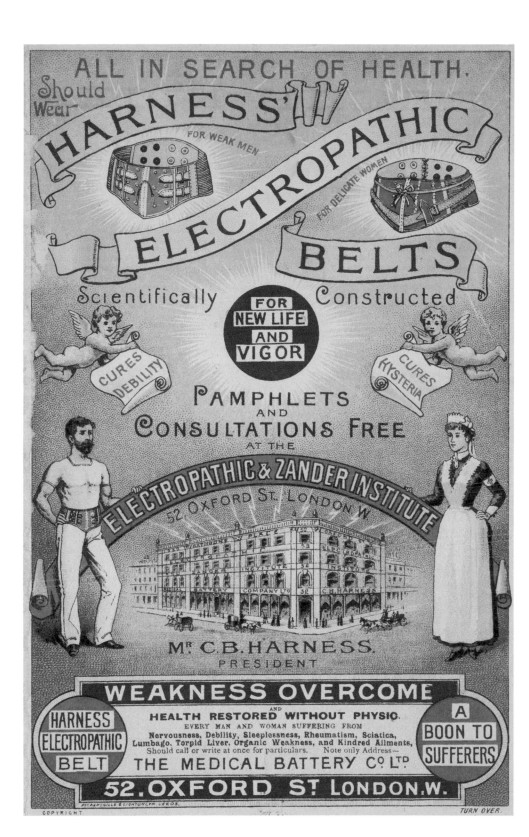

The two colleges jointly ran a research laboratory at the end of the 19th century – established behind the new Examination Hall on the Embankment and fully equipped for the sum of £2,500. A committee approved research projects, controlled publication, and forbade pecuniary remuneration for work done, but enlightenedly its first rule indicated that permission to work there 'shall not be restricted to those whose names are on the medical register'. It has been noted that of the 16 original workers, eight were subsequently knighted. They included Sir Charles Sherrington, neurophysiologist, Nobel laureate and President of the Royal Society, and Sir Almroth Wright, developer of anti-typhoid vaccination, later immortalised as Sir Colenso Ridgeon in Bernard Shaw's play *The Doctor's Dilemma*. The laboratory for several years earned its keep diagnosing diphtheria from throat swabs and preparing diphtheria antitoxin, but soon faced various crises. These included the death of two workers from the enteric fever they were studying, an outbreak of glanders amongst the horses in which antisera were raised, and increasing financial difficulties eventually leading to closure. The buildings became the first laboratories of the Imperial Cancer Research Fund.

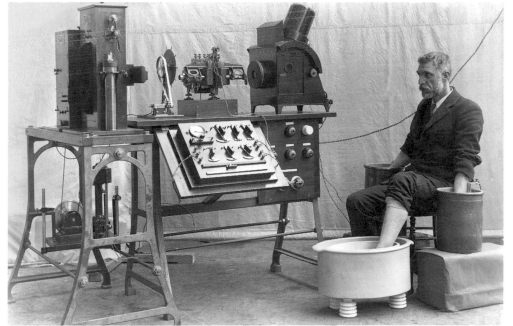

1902

The Midwives Act becomes law, and Sir Francis Champneys becomes its first chairman (he holds the post until 1930).

1909

The College makes women eligible for admission as licentiates and members.

1909–13

Another Royal Commission on the University of London considers the request of the College to share degree-giving powers – but again rejects the request.

1911

Lloyd-George's National Health Insurance Act is passed, despite the widespread opposition of the medical profession including the College.

1912

The College withdraws its objections to licentiates without a university MD degree using the courtesy title 'Doctor'.

1914

Within weeks of the outbreak of World War I, three British women doctors set up a hospital in Claridge's Hotel in Paris.

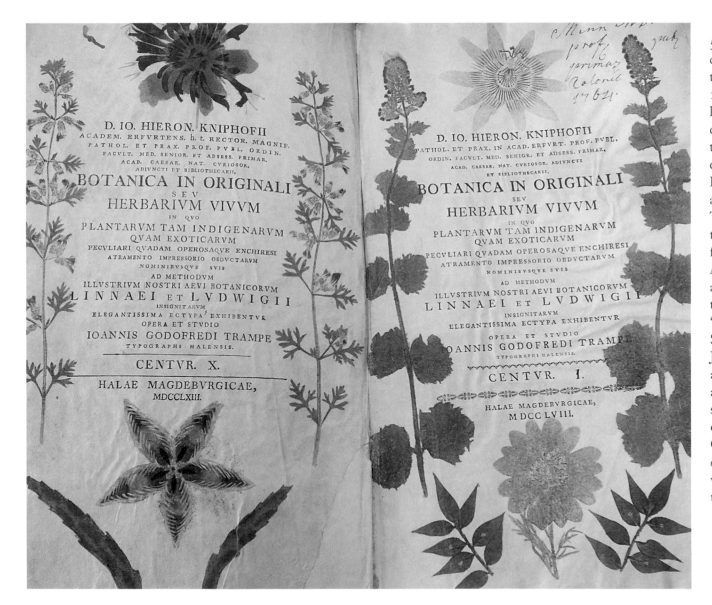

The Pharmaceutical Society Herbarium contains 5,792 herbarium sheets of medicinal plants, pressed, dried, mounted and annotated, which were used for teaching *materia medica* to pharmacy students until 1936, when a knowledge of medicinal plants was no longer required. It is a record of a scientific era now departed. The majority date from 1890 to 1905, though some are much earlier, such as a Cape Colony collection of a thalloid alga in 1795 from Dr William Roxburgh, the 'Father of Indian Botany'. It includes a herbarium from Peking and another from Budapest. The plants were collected from Afghanistan to Chile; the Gold Coast to Australia; Japan to Syria; and even from Sevenoaks in Kent. The collectors include Dr Augustine Henry (1857–1930), the great Irish botanist and physician; Dr John Farrell Easmon (1856–1900), the Sierra Leonean Creole doctor who described 'Blackwater Fever'; Henry Ridley (1855–1956), the first Scientific Director of the Singapore Botanic Gardens; Józef Warszewicz (1812–1866), Lithuanian-born Polish aristocrat, collecting in Central America and Peru; and the pharmacists Hanbury and Martindale. Many sheets are annotated with their indigenous uses. On one of Dr Easmon's collections (Gold Coast – now Ghana – in 1888) of *Brillantasia alata* (now *Brillantaisia owariensis*), with his beautiful pencil drawing, he writes that the 'bruised fresh leaves are applied to ringworm'.

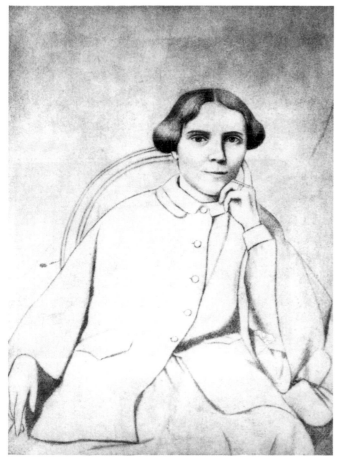

> *'It is not easy to be a pioneer –*
> *but oh, it is fascinating! I would*
> *not trade one moment, even the*
> *worst moment, for all the riches*
> *in the world.'*

Elizabeth Blackwell

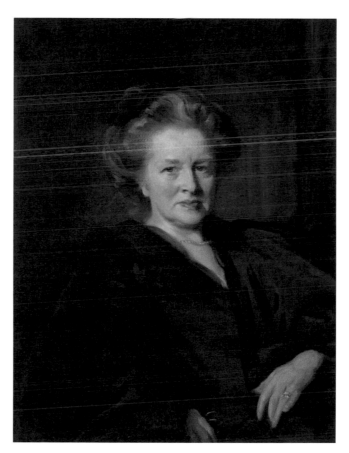

Opposite: A page from *Kniphofi D. Herbarium Vivum* (1757) The prints were made by inking and pressing original plant specimens onto the page.

Above: Dr Elizabeth Blackwell (1821–1910), who went to the USA to gain a medical qualification at Geneva College, New York, and then became the first woman to be admitted to the UK Medical Register in 1859. She worked mainly in the USA, where she set up a medical school for women, subsequently incorporated into Cornell University. She campaigned in London on many aspects of public health.

Right: Dr Elizabeth Garrett (Anderson) (1836–1917), who qualified at the Society of Apothecaries in 1865, which then promptly banned women. The next year she founded the St Mary's Dispensary for Women, later the New Hospital for Women. Her campaign led to the Medical Act of 1876 that eventually allowed women to be licensed to practise medicine.

Even before the suffragette movement of the 1860s, cartoons in the 1850s lampooned the growing idea that women could practise medicine. The universities and the College (and its statutes) were against this, and William Gladstone and Queen Victoria were horrified at the idea. Elizabeth Blackwell went to the USA, and after much difficulty was allowed to study at Geneva (later Hobart) College New York, where the 150 male students voted unanimously to allow her to be admitted. In 1849, she became the first female physician in the USA, where she practised, but on returning to London, she found she could not work in a hospital. She was however included on the first medical register in 1859, even though ineligible as a foreign graduate. It was only in 1876 that Parliament confirmed that women could be admitted to the Register, but the College refused to allow the admission of women to its ranks. In 1909, after considerable debate lasting over 18 months, and 40 years after Elizabeth Garrett's request to sit the LRCP examination had been refused by the College, women were granted the right to take the Conjoint examination and the membership – but with the caveat 'provided always that women shall not be eligible for election as Fellows, or entitled to take any part in the government, management or proceeding of the College'. Miss Ivy Woodward became the first female MRCP in 1909, and the next year Miss Dossibhai Patell the first female LRCP MRCS. It took a further 16 years before the possibility of women being granted Fellowship was conceded, and nine more years before Dr Helen Mackay became the first female FRCP. The risk that 'if girls were encouraged to use their brains the excitement caused thereby would produce insanity' appears not to have materialised. There was one woman, however, who qualified years before any of the others, and this was the cross-dressing Margaret Bulkley, who qualified in 1812 as James Barry and successfully practised as a male army surgeon.

'The awful idea of allowing young girls and young men to enter the dissecting room together, where young girls would have to study things which could not be named before them.'

Queen Victoria

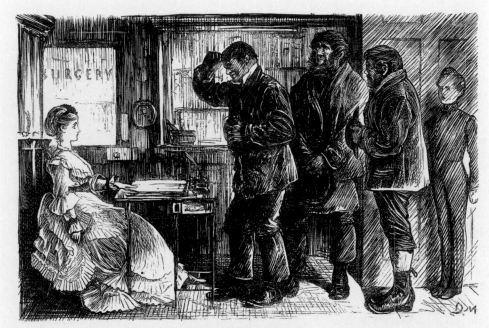

OUR PRETTY DOCTOR.

Dr. Arabella. "WELL, MY GOOD FRIENDS, WHAT CAN I DO FOR YOU?"

Bill. "WELL, MISS, IT'S ALL ALONG O' ME AND MY MATES BEIN' OUT O' WORK, YER SEE, AND WANTIN' TO TURN AN HONEST PENNY HANYWAYS WE CAN; SO, 'AVIN' 'EARD TELL AS *YOU* WAS A RISIN' YOUNG MEDICAL PRACTITIONER, WE THOUGHT AS P'RAPS YOU WOULDN'T MIND JUST A RECOMMENDIN' OF *HUS* AS NURSES."

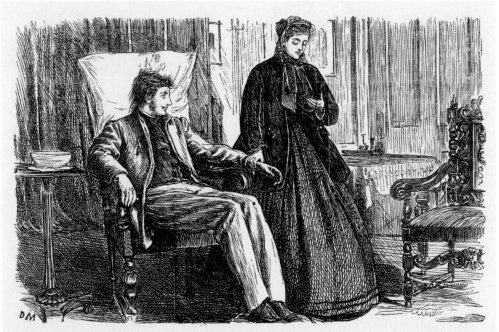

LADY-PHYSICIANS.

WHO IS THIS INTERESTING INVALID? IT IS YOUNG REGINALD DE BRACES, WHO HAS SUCCEEDED IN CATCHING A BAD COLD, IN ORDER THAT HE MIGHT SEND FOR THAT RISING PRACTITIONER, DR. ARABELLA BOLUS!

'But yesterday afternoon my
 reasoning Rivers ran solemnly in,
With peace in the pools of his
 spectacled eyes and a wisely
 omnipotent grin;
And I fished in that steady grey
 stream and decided that I
After all am no longer the
Worm that refuses to die.'

Siegfried Sassoon, in a letter to Robert Graves
on 24 July 1918, about W.H.R. Rivers, the doctor
at Craiglockhart.

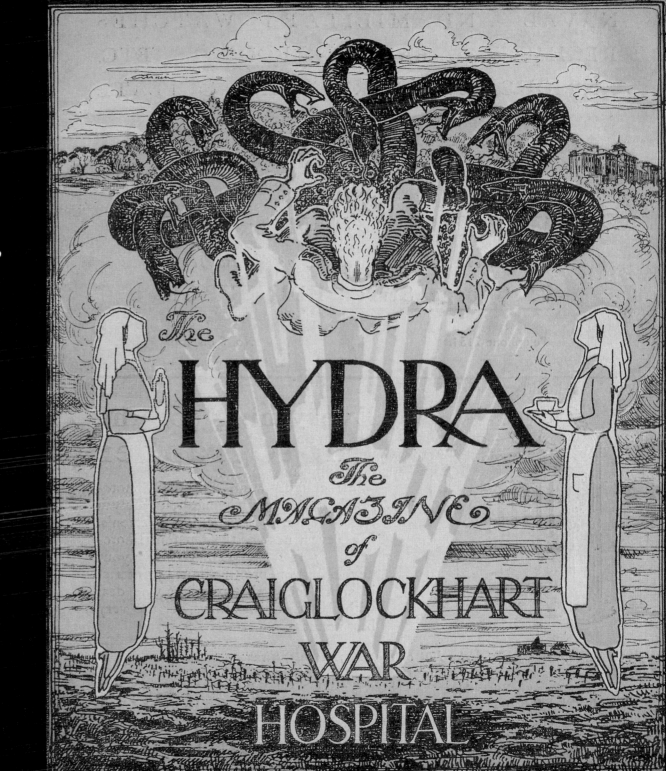

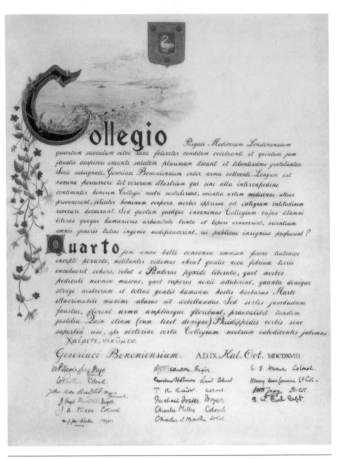

1915

The first zeppelin bombing raid on London. The College's New Examination Hall in Queen Square is damaged.

1915–18

Medical innovations during the war encompass recognition of trench fever, management of shell shock and delineation of neurological consequences of head wounds.

1918

There is no celebration of the 400th anniversary of the College in London, but fellows of the College on active service celebrate with seven courses and fine wines.

1919

As the war ends, the Spanish flu pandemic grips Europe. The College produces guidelines on the management of influenza.

Left: The 16 fellows celebrating the College's 400th anniversary in Boulogne presented the College with a vellum scroll in Latin.

Right: *The Interior of a Hospital Tent*, John Singer Sargent, 1918.

Translation of the vellum scroll celebrating the 400th anniversary of the College

We, the undersigned members, gathered under arms at Boulogne, send heartiest greetings and congratulations to the Royal College of Physicians of London as it celebrates the fourth centenary of its foundation and embarks upon its fifth.

It would be a major task to honour and enumerate so many within our membership who, ceaselessly, have upheld the honour of our College; who have advanced the art of medicine by their learning, and even taught us to restore the bodies of men crushed by disease to full-bodied health. And how rarely does one find a College whose alumni bedeck their learning with both elegance and wit, who have ably built upon knowledge of every kind, who have been of such outstanding benefit to their country. And now

in the fourth year of this war, when all agree that the frenzied German attack has been pierced and halted, in our military duties we see, alas, that a vast cohort of new diseases oppresses the earth, as if from Pandora's box. How many diseases have lice, flies and poisonous gas brought us? And what carnage of our troops and of the whole human race has been required to vanquish the barbarian host, the enemy who has put ruthless war to its foulest forms? But omens are propitious – our side flourished and will flourish further, and in the end justice will prevail. Indeed it is now possible, in the certain hope of victory, to without boasting employ the words of Pheidippes – 'Be of good cheer – victory is ours.'

Boulogne, 23 September 1918

When war was declared on 4 August 1914, the medical services were ill-prepared for the level of military casualties. Of the 8.9 million men enlisted from Britain and its Empire over the next four years, around 1 million men were killed and 2 million wounded. The bloody battles of the Somme claimed 95,000 British and Empire lives and more than 300,000 men were injured. War produced 'new' illnesses and also stimulated medical advance, and challenged the ingenuity of British medicine. Many fellows were involved in wartime medicine and many made great personal and professional contributions. The College as an institution, however, was only peripherally involved in policy decisions. On 9 September 1915, the College examinations halls were bombed in the famous L13 zeppelin raid, but otherwise the buildings escaped quite lightly. It was decided not to celebrate the 400th anniversary of the founding of the College in 1918, as it was felt not appropriate to engage in happy ceremonial, but the President noted that the number of fellows had increased from six to upwards of 300 over the four centuries, and that the College should be congratulated on the fact that no change had taken place in its organisation (not an accolade which would be praised today). Fellows of the College on active service in Normandy had other ideas, celebrating the anniversary in Boulogne with a seven-course dinner and fine wines, and presenting the College with an illuminated Latin address on vellum (left) – although the dinner, it is said, was prematurely curtailed by enemy action.

When the war ended there was a terrible pandemic of Spanish flu, due to the H1N1 influenza virus, infecting more than 500 million persons worldwide and killing 50–100 million (3–5 per cent of the world population).

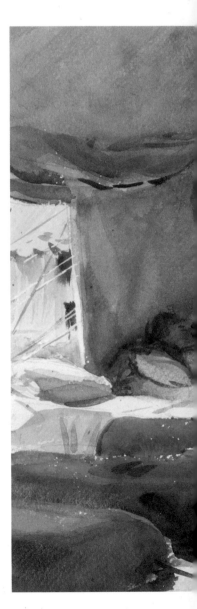

Right: A bomb from the first raid over London, from zeppelin L13, landed in Queen Square and damaged the front of the New Examination Hall, but no injuries were caused. This plaque marks the spot where the bomb landed.

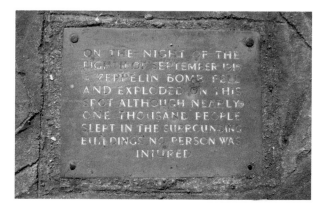

ON THE NIGHT OF THE
EIGHTH OF SEPTEMBER 1915
A ZEPPELIN BOMB FELL
AND EXPLODED ON THIS
SPOT ALTHOUGH NEARLY
ONE THOUSAND PEOPLE
SLEPT IN THE SURROUNDING
BUILDINGS NO PERSON WAS
INJURED

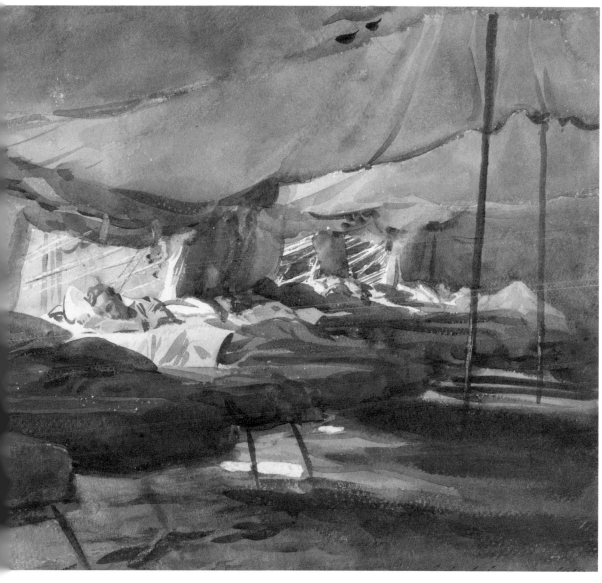

Wilmot Herringham
1855–1936

Wilmot Herringham's biography conjures a medical and military hero: Winchester and Oxford, oarsman, 1st XI, captain of cricket; consultant at Bart's, Senior Censor of the College and Vice-Chancellor of London University until he resigned in 1915 to go to France, as the First Consultant to the British Army, later rising to the rank of major-general. He was involved not only as a practising doctor in the field, but in the investigation of gas warfare from within days of the first attack, and in the organisation of pathology services, such as those that led to the recognition of trench fever as a louse-borne disease. His writings included the official history of the World War I medical services and a discursive and entertaining memoir, *A Physician in France*. In the latter, he reflects on the German and English character, the French way of life, English dentistry, the inelegance of the English (female) ankle contrasted with the neatness of the French, and the quality of war poetry (poor). He received two orders of knighthood, and after the war served on the University Grants Committee, was Chairman of the Old Vic Theatre, and turned down the Oxford Regius Chair of Medicine when Sir William Osler retired.

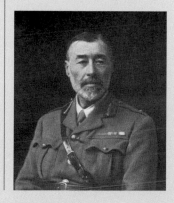

Bertrand Dawson, President of the College 1931–38, was arguably the most influential physician in the UK between the two world wars. He trained at University College London and the London Hospital, joining the consultant staff of the latter in 1906. His very full career was remarkable for its breadth. In 1914, he set up the 2nd London General Hospital, and then served as consultant physician to the British Army in France. Even before the end of the war he had put forward his thoughts on how the nation's medical services should develop. He was instrumental in the setting up of the Ministry of Health, and his 1920 'Dawson Report', commissioned by the new ministry, outlined concepts that eventually led to the NHS.

He was elevated to the peerage in 1920 (Baron Dawson of Penn). In his College role, he broadened the nature of the Fellowship, particularly encouraging younger fellows, and modernised its approach and strategic thinking. In addition, Dawson was twice president of the BMA and, as Royal Physician, he looked after Edward VII and George VI on their death beds, and is credited with the famous bulletin on the latter in 1936, 'that the King's life is drawing peacefully to its close'.

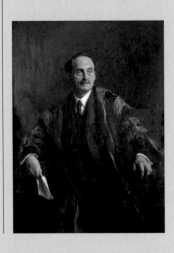

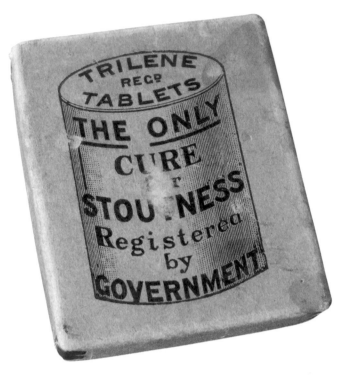

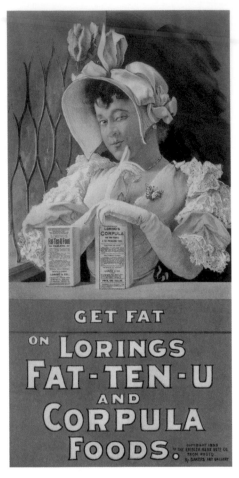

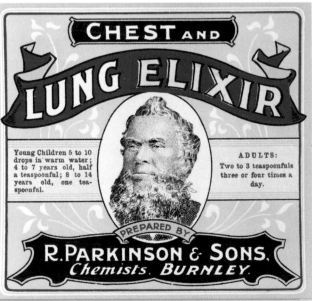

1920

The Dawson Report commissioned
by the Ministry of Health contains
the outline concepts of the future
National Health Service.

1923

The Canadian government offers
£150,000 for the lease of the
College's premises in Pall Mall –
an offer the College refuses.

1925

The College votes to allow women
to be elected FRCP.

1934

The College condemns the
patenting of medical discoveries.

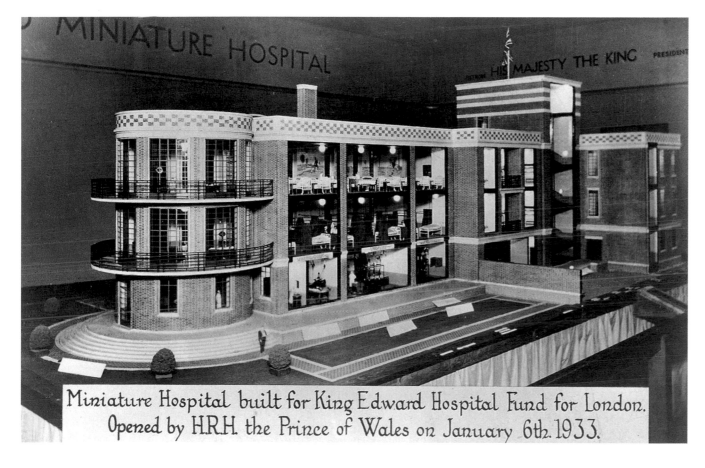

Miniature Hospital built for King Edward Hospital Fund for London.
Opened by H.R.H. the Prince of Wales on January 6th. 1933.

In the early 20th century, the practice of medicine was being transformed. Physiology was emerging as a discipline. Antisepsis and anaesthesia were already established with agreed principles and techniques, changing the practice of surgery. Specific therapies for infections were beginning to emerge, with the production of therapeutic antisera. The era of preventive immunisation, ushered in a hundred years previously by Edward Jenner, had progressed, although there remained a vociferous anti-vaccination lobby which argued against mandatory smallpox immunisation. The ability to culture pathogenic bacteria allowed the preparation of extracts which could be injected to stimulate protective antibodies. Immunisation against typhoid was described in 1896, and proved to be of major benefit in the 20th-century wars to come. One of the most useful drugs of all time – acetylsalicylic acid, aspirin – had just been synthesised by the Bayer company. Specific antimicrobial therapy was still in the future, to be ushered in by the arsenical treatment – Salvarsan – for syphilis in 1908; but the antibiotic era would not start for another 40 years. The physical sciences were beginning to enter the medical arena, most notably with the discovery and very rapid diagnostic application of X-rays. More mundanely, the mercury sphygmomanometer for recording blood pressure was invented in 1902. Psychology was developing – Freud gained his University Chair in 1902. And at the same time the spread of commerce into the medical field was producing a plethora of ingenious machines and attractively packaged medicines and potions directly advertised to the public.

Robert Bridges is unique – the only medical graduate to become Poet Laureate. His medical career was not quite so distinguished: a Bart's student, house physician, then casualty physician, where he personally reviewed over 30,000 patients in one year. He published an outspoken critique describing the system as 'virtually inoperable'. He subsequently held posts at the Great Northern Hospital, Islington – where his swift action is said to have aborted a smallpox outbreak – and Great Ormond Street Hospital for Children. He retired from medicine aged 38 after a bout of pneumonia, but is recorded as having planned from the start to retire at 40 and use his experience as a doctor to enrich his literary output.

He published poems from his student years onwards, being appointed Poet Laureate aged 69; his last work, *The Testament of Beauty* (1929), is considered his greatest achievement. His poem 'On a Dead Child' must reflect his time at Great Ormond Street:

> Thy hand clasps, as 'twas wont,
>   my finger, and holds it:
> But the grasp is the clasp of
>   Death, heartbreaking and stiff.

Perhaps curiously for a recipient of the Order of Merit, he is quoted as saying the distinction by which he set most store was his Fellowship of the RCP.

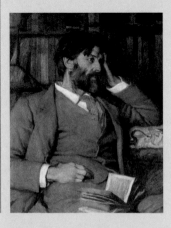

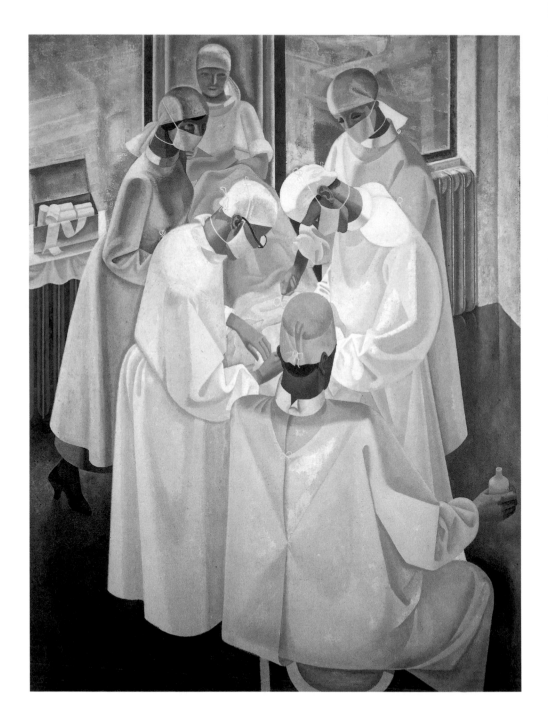

Below: *A Surgical Operation* by Reginald Brill (1934–35), from a series called *The Martyrdom of Man*.

Opposite: London on fire in the Blitz of 1940–41.

World War II

'*Your services will be given with devotion and your voice will be heard with respect.*'

Winston Churchill referring to the Royal College
of Physicians, during lunch on 2 March 1944

World War II was even more devastating than World War I. It was a global conflict, and up to 75 million persons died, including 20 million military personnel. As in World War I, adversity spawned innovation and new diseases were described, organisation of care was transformed, and novel treatments developed, for instance in the fields of antibiotics, vaccines, blood transfusion, kidney disease, trauma and rehabilitation. As in World War I, the College was, as an institution, largely ignored when it came to making medical policy, which was left to the military authorities and central government. The College buildings were hit by bombs in the Blitz attacks of October and November 1940, with serious damage caused. Four fellows, 18 members and 243 licentiates lost their lives in the war (out of over 3,000 fellows, members, and licentiates present in 1945).

A significant outcome of the war, from the College's point of view, was the appetite amongst the British people to set up a state medical service, which took shape in the form of the NHS in 1948. The College initially took up an extremely hostile view to the development of a state-led medical service and to state-salaried doctors, but eventually bowed to the inevitable as it fell in step with the plans of the post-war Labour government. At the same time, plans were also being considered to move out of Pall Mall into more suitable accommodation, and even to be co-housed with both the Royal College of Surgeons and the Royal College of Obstetricians.

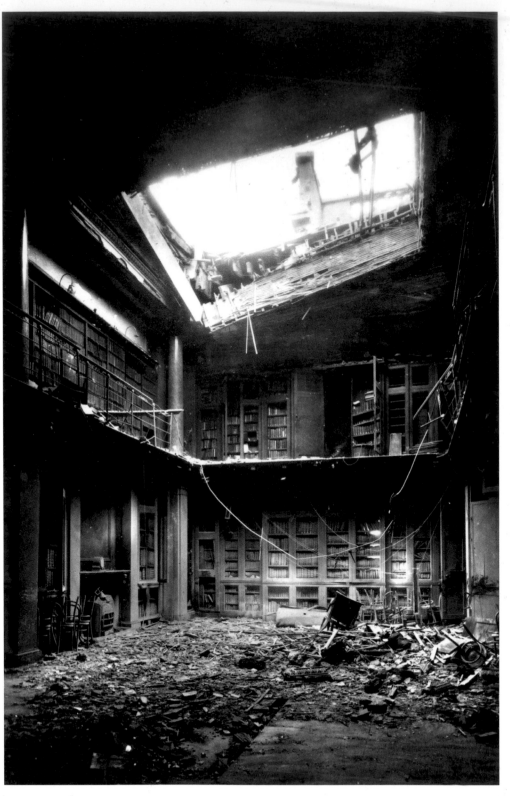

1939

Outbreak of World War II.
A suggestion by the then President to suspend the activities of the College for the duration of hostilities is rebuffed by younger members.

Left: The College library after the bombing in 1940.

Right: Guy's Hospital bomb damage.

Far right above: Proposed building in Lincoln's Inn joining the three colleges – Physicians, Surgeons and Obstetricians. The proposed building had three separate front entrances to emphasise the continuing separate identities of the constituent colleges, surgery, medicine and obstetrics, despite coalescence into an 'Academy of Medicine'. A 21st-century equivalent would require 21 entrances.

Far right below: The roof of the College after the bombing in 1940.

1940

The College building in Pall Mall receives two direct bomb hits, in October and November.

1940

The Emergency Medical Services plan for London is initiated – allowing central control of all hospitals – and offering a practical vision of what a state-controlled health service might deliver.

1941

The Royal College of Surgeons (also severely damaged by bombing) suggests a 'closer association of houses' with the Royal College of Physicians, to bring about 'closer association of thought and action'.

1942

The College begins to debate the shape of a National Health Service.

1944

The College entertains Prime Minister Winston Churchill to luncheon at the Savoy Hotel – 220 fellows attend.

1945

The College considers proposals for an amalgamation of the three royal colleges – physicians, surgeons and obstetricians – on one site.

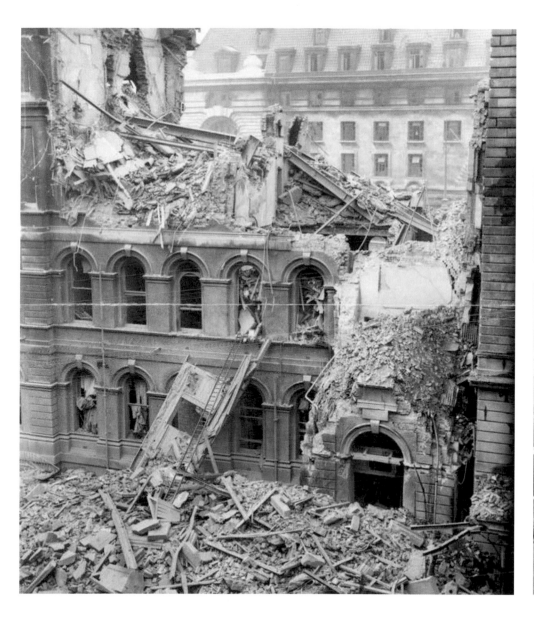

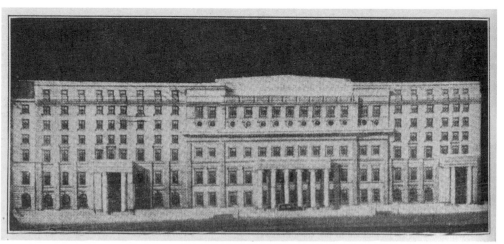

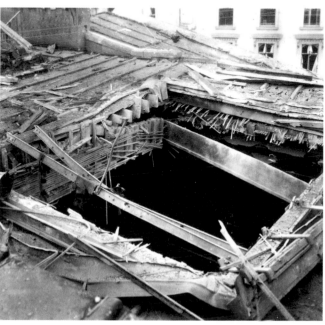

On 2 March 1944, the College entertained Prime Minister Winston Churchill at the Savoy Hotel to a luncheon featuring lobster mousseline, roast turkey and fruit salad. This was a landmark meeting, attended by 222 fellows and 58 guests. Lord Moran gave an address drawing attention to the similarities between the professions of medicine and the military, but stressing the importance of the emphasis on research and independence of thought in medicine, to which Churchill responded:

> Our policy is to create a national health service in order to ensure that everybody in the country, irrespective of means, age, sex or occupation, shall have equal opportunities to benefit from the best and most up-to-date medical and allied services available. The plan that we have put forward is a very large-scale plan, and in ordinary times of peace would rivet and dominate the attention of the whole country; but even during this war it deserves the close study and thought of all who can spare themselves from other duties for that purpose. We welcome constructive criticism; we claim the loyal and active aid of the whole medical profession.

THE
ROYAL COLLEGE OF PHYSICIANS

Savoy Hotel,
March 2nd, 1944.

The Prime Minister hopes to be present at this luncheon, and you are asked to keep secret the date, time and place.

The President and Fellows
of the
Royal College of Physicians of London
request the honour of the company of

at a Luncheon at the Savoy Hotel
on Thursday, March 2nd, 1944, at 1 for 1.30 p.m.

An early reply is requested to the—
Royal College of Physicians,
Pall Mall East,
London, S.W.1.

GUESTS OF THE ROYAL COLLEGE OF PHYSICIANS

Rt. Hon. Winston S. Churchill, C.H.
Dr. H. A. Aksel
Rt. Hon. A. V. Alexander, C.H.
H. E. The American Ambassador
Rt. Hon. Sir John Anderson, G.C.B., G.C.S.I.
Rt. Hon. C. R. Attlee, M.P.
Sir Girling Ball
R. M. Barrington-Ward, Esq., D.S.O., M.C.
Rt. Hon. Ernest Bevin, M.P.
Rt. Hon. Brendan Bracken, M.P.
Rt. Hon. The Lord Cherwell, F.R.S.
Field Marshal Sir Philip Chetwode, G.C.B., O.M.
H. E. She Chinese Ambassador
H. Claughton, Esq.
Air Vice-Marshal Sir Arthur Coningham, C. B., D.S.O.
Rt. Hon. R. Coppock
Rt. Hon. The Lord Cranborne
Admiral Sir Andrew Cunningham, Bart., G.C.B., D.S.O.
Dr. H. Guy Dain
Professor A. Fleming, F.R.S.
Major Sir David Maxwell Fyfe, K.C
Sir William Goodenough D.L., J.P.
Air Marshal Sir Arthur Harris, C.B., O.B.E.
E. Vincent Harris, Esq., O.B.E., R.A.
Brigadier General P. Hawley
Dr. Charles Hill
Lt.-Gen. Sir Alexander Hood, K.C.B., C.B.E.
Professor F. Horton
Sir Richard Hopkins, G.C.B,
Miss F. Horsbrugh, C.B.E.

Rt. Hon. Thomas Johnston, M.P.
Sir Alan Lascelles, K.C.V.O., C.B., C.M.G,
Rt. Hon. Richard Law, M.P.
Rt. Hon. The Lord Leathers, C.H.
Col. The Rt. Hon. J. J. Llewellin, C.B.E., M.C.
Rt. Hon. Oliver Lyttelton, D.S.O., M.C.
Major-General R. M. Luton
Sir John Maude, K.B.E., C.B.
Rt. Hon. Herbert Morrison, M.P.
The Rt. Hon. The Earl of Munster
Dr. D. P. O'Brien
Marshal of The Royal Air Force Sir Charles Portal, K.C.B., D.S.O., M.C.
Rt. Hon. The Lord Portal, D.S.O., M.V.O.
Sir Arthur Rucker K.C.M.G., C.B.; C.B.E
Professor Sarkisov
Rt. Hon. Viscount Simon, G.C.S.I., G.C.V.O., O.B.E.
Rt. Hon. Sir Archibald Sinclair, Bt K.T., C.M.G.
Major-General Bedell Smith
H. S. Souttar, Esq., F.R.C.S.
H. E. The Soviet Ambassador
Dr. B. N. Taskiran
Air Chief Marshal Sir Arthur Tedder, K.C.B.
Professor B. Tugan
Brigadier Harvie Watt
Sir Alfred Webb-Johnson, K.C.V.O., O.B.E., D.S.O.
Rt. Hon. H. U. Willink, M.P.
Rt. Rev. The Lord Bishop of Winchester
Rt. Hon. The Lord Woolton, C.H.

'Just right Moran – makes you look like a medieval poisoner.'

Regarding Moran's portrait – attributed to Winston Churchill

Right: A wartime ward in Guy's Hospital, 1941.

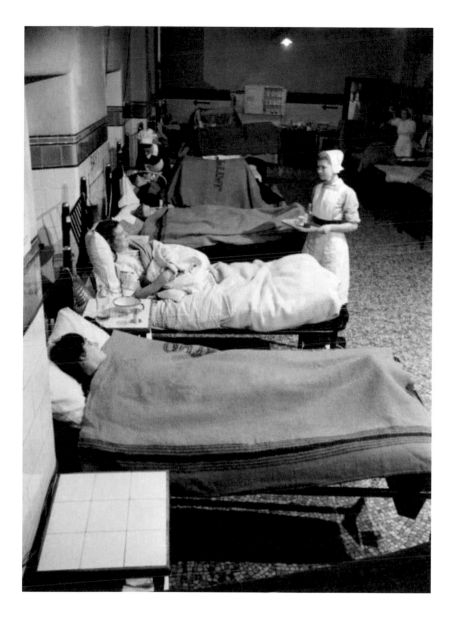

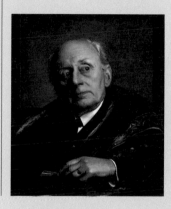

After surviving a headmistress's judgement as 'too stupid to be educated', Janet Vaughan qualified from Oxford and UCLH – where exposure to London's poor made her a socialist (and later, briefly, a communist). In early studies on pernicious anaemia, she prepared raw liver extracts (using her cousin Virginia Woolf's mincer) that made dogs sick, so she self-experimented; she progressed to understanding and classifying anaemia on the basis of red cell morphology, producing the classic text *The Anaemias* in 1934. Before and during World War II, she took a lead in blood transfusion, planning London's Emergency Blood Transfusion Service from her sitting room. She also ran the wartime blood service in Slough, and pioneered the use of blood substitutes for hypovolaemia. As the war ended, she went to Brussels to help malnourished British POWs, and subsequently to Belsen to help determine the best means of treating extreme starvation – 'doing science in Hell' she called it. After the war, she was Principal of Somerville College for 22 years, continuing research into radiation and bones, and becoming a world expert in plutonium. Her wish: 'to be remembered as a scientist. That I have been able to solve, to throw light onto fascinating problems. But as a scientist who had a family. I don't want to be thought of as a scientist who just sat thinking. It's important you have a human life.' She was the first female Councillor of the Royal College of Physicians and the first female named lecturer (Bradshaw Lecture, 1947).

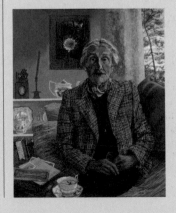

'Start Bleeding.'

Telegram from Medical Research Council to Janet Vaughan, 31 August 1939, three days before the outbreak of World War II

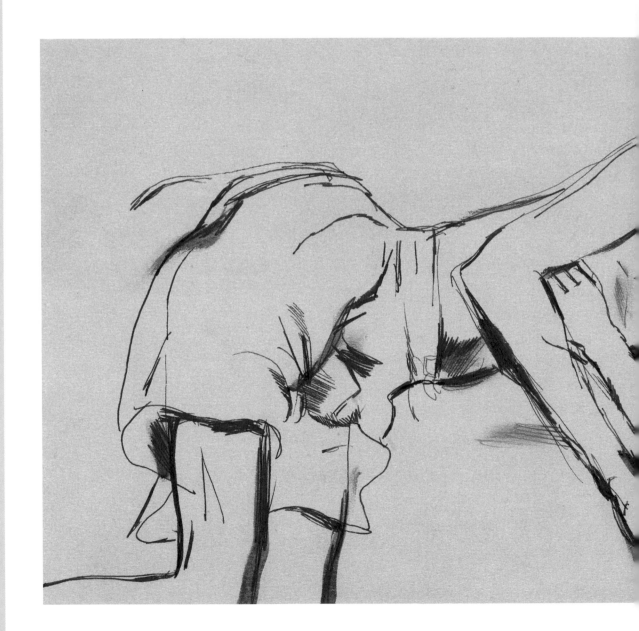

Below: *Prisoner Sleeping after Eighteen Hours Work, Changi Gaol,* 1944.

Right: Sir Almroth Edward Wright, the leading bacteriologist and immunologist in Britain in the two wars. He wrote extensively, and amongst his books was the excellent *Pathology and Treatment of War Wounds* (1942). He was a virulent opponent of female suffrage.

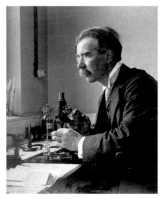

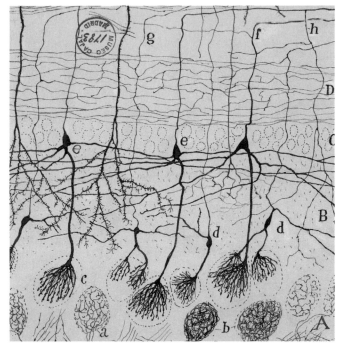

Left: The 20th century witnessed the beginning of a real understanding of the complexity of brain micro-structure. This image published by Ramón y Cajal, using his technique of silver impregnation, illustrates this complexity.

Below left: World War II left its mark on health in many ways. The spread of poliomyelitis was one consequence, and as the incidence of polio gradually increased in the West, the assisted ventilation provided by iron lungs became a lifesaver.

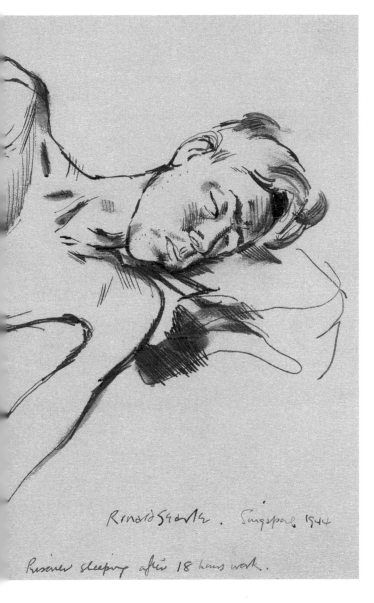

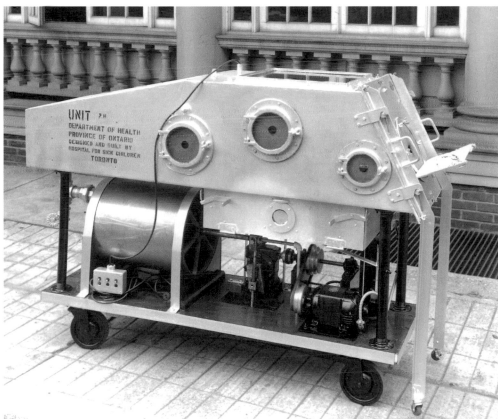

1948-

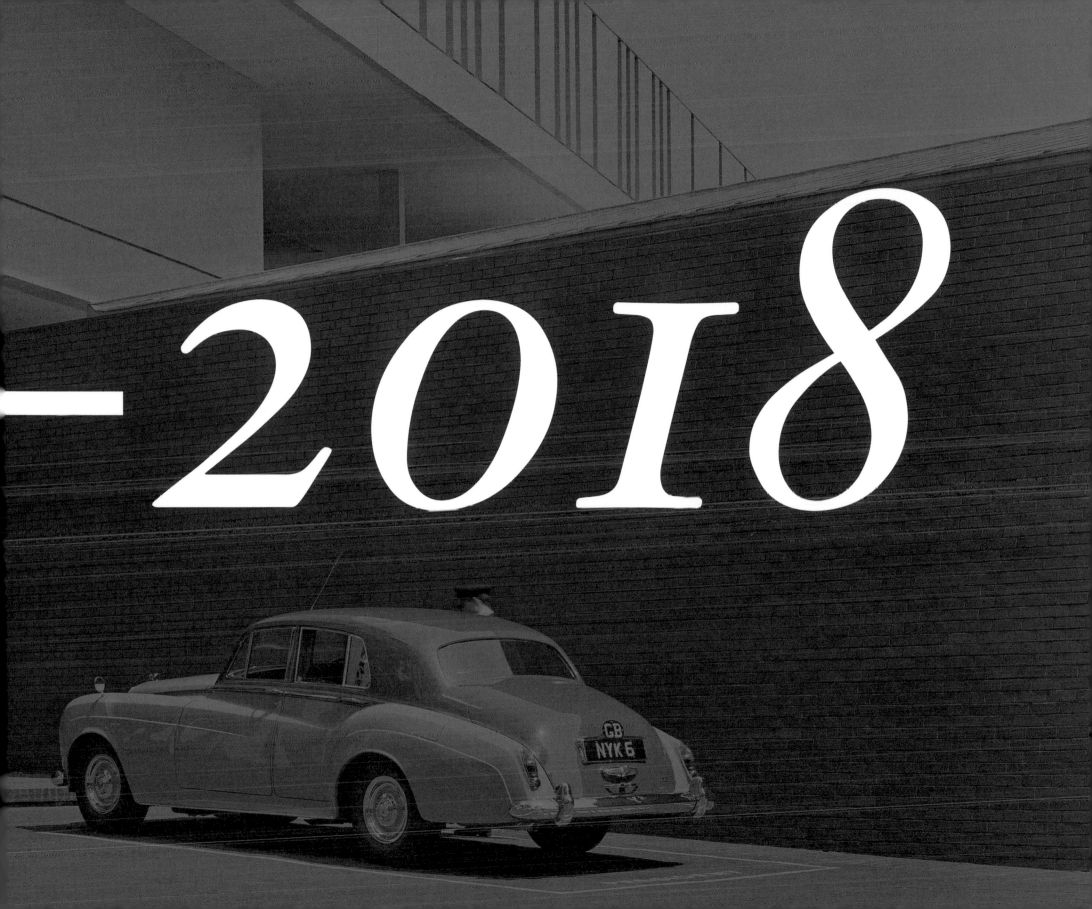

—2018

THURSDAY, MARCH 21, 1946

Evening Standard

37,911

24-HOUR FORECAST:
Bright spells. showers, mild.

MOON: Rises 10.20 p.m.; Sets 8.1 a.m. to-morrow.
LIGHTING-UP TIME: 6.44 p.m.

ONE PENNY

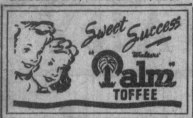
The National Health Bill is out. It will cost £152,000,000 a yea

STATE TAKE OVER DOCTORS HOSPITALS AND DENTISTS

'Free for all'—1948

PRIVATE PRACTICE STAYS, BUT NEW DOCTORS DIRECTED

From WILLIAM ALISON

From 1948 everybody's health will be looked after by the State without fee. That is Mr. Aneurin Bevan's new National Health Service, details of which are published to-day. It is estimated to cost £152,000,000 a year.

It comes under three main heads: the general practitioner service; the facilities to be provided by hospitals which are taken over; and the new Health Centres.

Publication of the plan will begin a great Parliamentary controversy which follows months of discussions outside Parliament. The big Parliamentary battles will be on the taking over of the voluntary hospitals, and the new conditions for the State doctors.

What you get—

Free treatment by doctors and dentists, and you can choose your present doctor or dentist if he takes part in the new scheme.

The relationship between the doctor and any patient on his personal list "will be similar to the ordinary relationship of doctor to patient as it is now known, except that the doctor's remuneration will come from public funds and not from the patient."

Doctors and dentists are to be free to join the new service or not as they choose. Those who join will not be debarred from treating for private fees patients who do not take advantage of the new scheme.

You can have your treatment at the new Health Centres, at the doctor's surgery or in your own home, and hospital treat-

Can they stay outside?

Evening Standard Political Correspondent

Under the new Bevan health plan a doctor who remains outside the scheme will automatically lose the grant made to him for his panel patients and will have to rely on a sufficient number of private patients who wish for medical treatment outside the National Service.

Almost everyone will become compulsorily insurable, and the service is available to everyone—insured or not. This was made clear by the Ministry of Health this afternoon. It was pointed out that doctors will inevitably lose a large proportion of their

FIGURES

As the new health service will not start until 1948 it is impossible to say what the cost will be to the individual, but here are some comparative figures.

In 1938 an expenditure of £152,000,000 would represent about 2s. 6d. in the £ on income tax. Now it would represent roughly 1s. 3d.

The 1946-47 Service estimates are:—

Navy	£255,075,000
Army	£682,000,000
Air	£255,500,000

HAMBURG WITHOUT BREAD

From RICHARD MacMILLAN

HAMBURG, Thursday.—Seventy per cent of the people of Hamburg have no bread.

They have eaten their month's ration in a fortnight, said a British official here to-day, and are not likely to get any more for another fortnight.

In the past 24 hours four more "food incidents" have occurred.

One involved 50 hungry women and children stopping a bread van and trying to make the driver give them bread. They had to be moved on by the police.

Despite these incidents and the fact that last night it was known officially that a crowd of nearly 200, including women, stormed a goods train and plundered a goods truck, ripping off the door of one before they were dispersed by police, a British public safety officer said to-day.

PLANE DIVE ON SCHOOL

200 children at play: All s

Evening Standard Correspondent: Tunbridge Wells, Th

A blazing Mosquito airplane crashed betw two buildings of Rusthall girls and inf schools, near Tunbridge Wells, Kent, du the morning break to-day. Two hun children in the playground escaped se injury.

Mothers rushed to the but after a roll call it wa that every child was saf pilot and co-pilot were

Many children were blo by blast, but neighbou adjoining houses quickly c took them in. The childr later sent home.

Ten-year-old Jean Dipl her hair badly singed, an two other children were tr shock.

Many houses were scorched, as petrol was fl a wide area.

Parts of the airplane w against the wall of the schools.

The N.F.S. were soon scene but it took considera before the flames were put only part of the airpla recognisable was a charred

'Steep dive'

Major Moore, who was witness of the crash, sa

"The airplane was about 600ft. when it sudde into a steep dive to the

Mr. Claude de Bernales

'CIVIL PROCEEDINGS IMPENDING'

Mr. Claude de Bernales, the financier, sent the following statement to the Evening Standard to-day:

"It is to be regretted that the Press should have seized upon certain statements made in the course of proceedings to which I was not a party and in which I accordingly had no opportunity of defending myself, for the purpose of giving publicity to most serious imputations upon myself.

"It is doubly to be regretted that this should have been done at a time when civil proceedings are

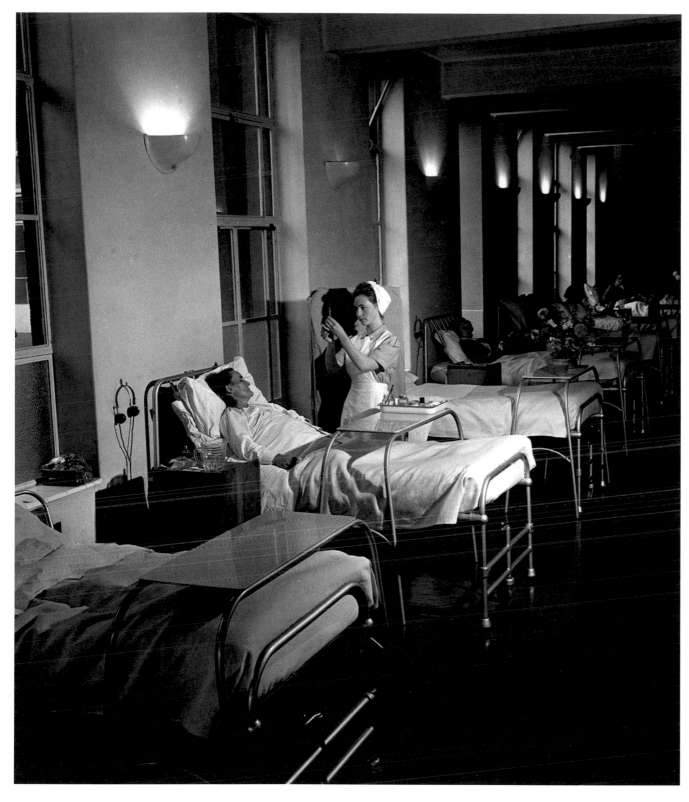

'This is the biggest single experiment in social service that the world has ever seen undertaken.'

Aneurin Bevan

The last 70 years have seen remarkable change in three areas of medicine: the mode of delivery of healthcare, the exponential increase in the cost of good healthcare, and the primacy of research in underpinning the improvements in medical treatment, health and life expectancy around the globe.

The National Health Service (NHS) Act received royal assent on 6 November 1946 and the NHS officially came into being on 5 July 1948, 'the appointed day'. Plans for a comprehensive national health service had gathered pace during World War II with Sir William (later Lord) Beveridge's report for the Conservative-led wartime coalition government, *Social Insurance and Allied Services*. Before the NHS, healthcare was neither comprehensive nor co-ordinated and left many people without access to adequate medical care or impoverished if they fell ill.

Far left: *Evening Standard* headline from 1946 trumpeting the plans for the National Health Service to be launched in 1948.

Left: A typical ward soon after the formation of the NHS in 1949. Nightingale wards had approximately 15 beds on either side of a long ward, with the nursing station in the centre, so that all patients could be observed.

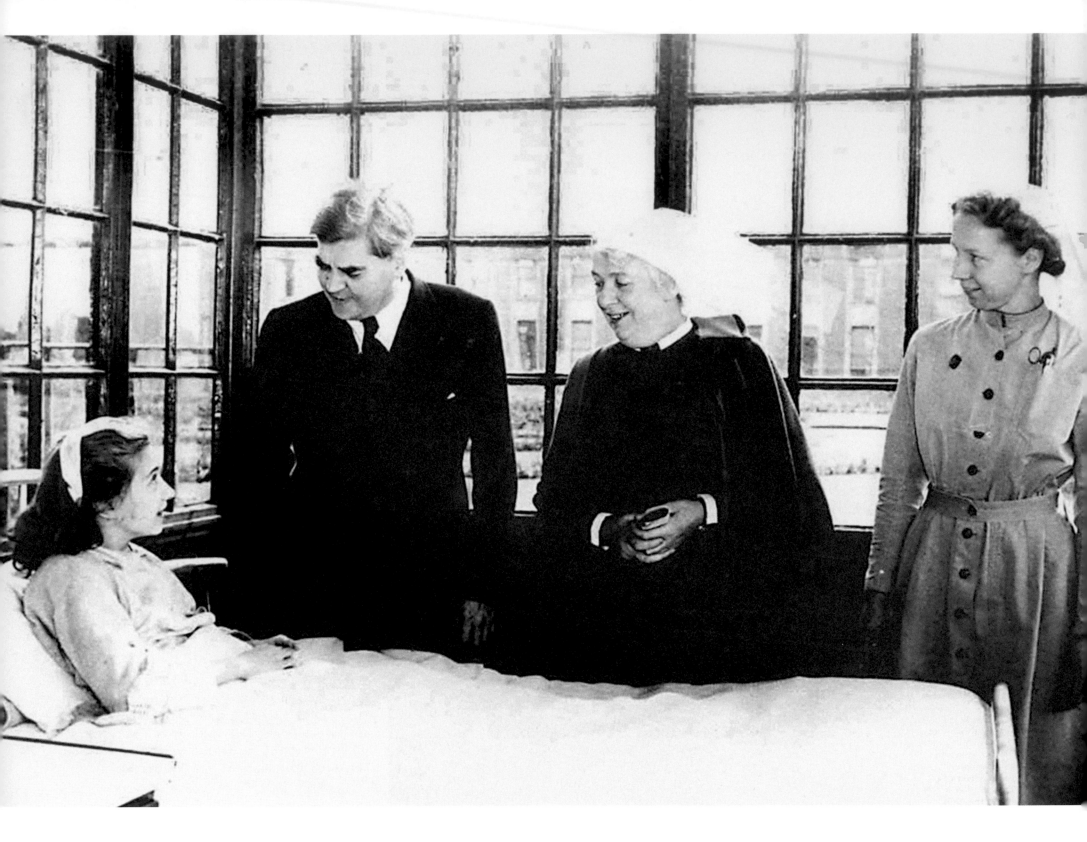

1946
National Health Service (NHS) Act receives royal assent.

1948
5 July: foundation of the NHS – a pivotal moment for healthcare in the UK. Sylvia Diggory, aged 13, becomes 'the first NHS patient'.

1951
Winston Churchill made honorary FRCP.

1953
Watson and Crick publish the structure of deoxyribonucleic acid in *Nature*, based on Rosalind Franklin's crystallography studies.

1956
Parliament passes the Clean Air Act.

1958
Polio and diphtheria vaccination programmes launched.

> *'We shall never have all we need… Expectations will always exceed capacity. The service must always be changing, growing and improving – it must always appear inadequate.'*

Aneurin Bevan

Left: Aneurin Bevan talking to Sylvia Diggory, aged 13, with nursing staff in Trafford General Hospital.

Right above and below: The changing face of nursing, from a predominantly white, female, uniformed profession, providing a primarily caring role on large, single-sex, Nightingale wards in the 1900s to 1970s, to the more casually dressed, ethnically diverse, graduate nurses providing an administrative and medical role, often in four-bedded units in the 2010s.

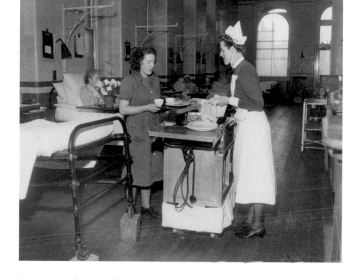

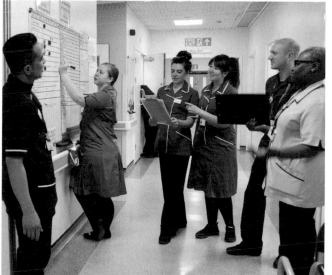

The establishment of the NHS with care for all, 'free at the point of use', in the period of austerity following WWII, was described in the words of Lord Brain (PRCP 1950–1956) as a brave experiment. In the 1950s the NHS made great strides, not least with a new hospital building programme, but since then the service has been the subject of innumerable reports and intense scrutiny. There have been a series of restructurings and reorganisations, notably in 1973, 1977, 1982, 1990 and 1994 with the introduction of the purchaser-provider split and GP fundholding. Most recently, there have been the large-scale changes of the Health and Social Care Act 2012. The need for change and the mismatch between resources and finance had been predicted by Bevan, who at a meeting for nurses in the early 1950s had said prophetically 'It can be argued that the success of medicine under the NHS, after 1948, *itself* led to the need for structural change'. However, every government over the last two decades has felt the need to stamp its imprint on the NHS with continuous change. Sometimes it seems that this has been for largely ideological reasons. The College has given valuable evidence to all of these initiatives by providing advice and leadership on behalf of its members and fellows, putting forth the doctors' position and also advocating for the patient. Indeed, right from the start of the NHS, the RCP has influenced government on issues of health policy and patient care, and developed its own policies and standards to support these efforts. The College's work has been particularly effective in relation to public health and improvements in medical practice.

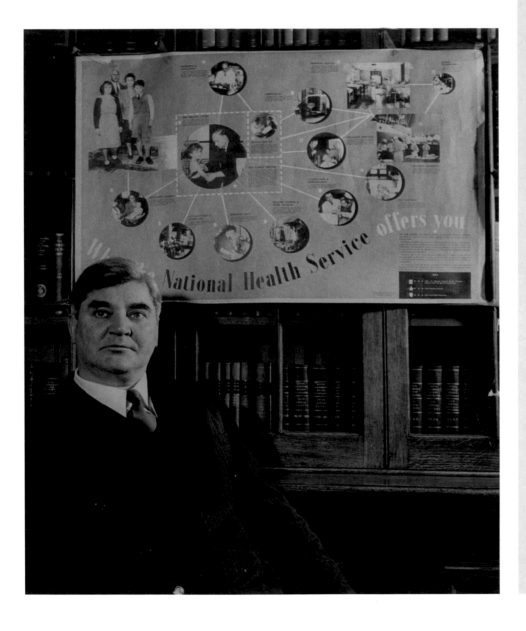

YOUR NEW NATIONAL HEALTH SERVICE

On 5th July the new National Health Service starts

Anyone can use it—men, women and children. There are no age limits, and no fees to pay. You can use any part of it, or all of it, as you wish. Your right to use the National Health Service does not depend upon any weekly payments (the National Insurance contributions are mainly for cash benefits such as pensions, unemployment and sick pay).

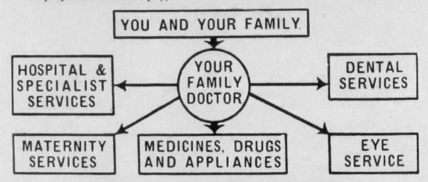

CHOOSE YOUR DOCTOR NOW

The first thing is to link up with a doctor. When you have done this, your doctor can put you in touch with all other parts of the Scheme as you need them. Your relations with him will be as now, *personal and confidential.* The big difference is that the doctor will not charge you fees. He will be paid, out of public funds to which all contribute as taxpayers.

So *choose your doctor now.* If one doctor cannot accept you, ask another, or ask to be put in touch with one by the new "Executive Council" which

has been set up in your area (you can get its address from the Post Office).

If you are already on a doctor's list under the old National Health Insurance Scheme, and do not want to change your doctor, you need *do nothing.* Your name will stay on his list under the new Scheme.

But make arrangements for *your* family now. Get an application form E.C.1 for *each* member of the family either from the doctor you choose, or from any Post Office, Executive Council Office, or Public Library; complete them and give them to the doctor.

There is a lot of work still to be done to get the Service ready. If *you* make *your* arrangements in good time, you will be helping both yourself and your doctor.

Issued by the Department of Health for Scotland

A

This advertisement appears in selected Sunday, Morning and Evening newspapers in Scotland.

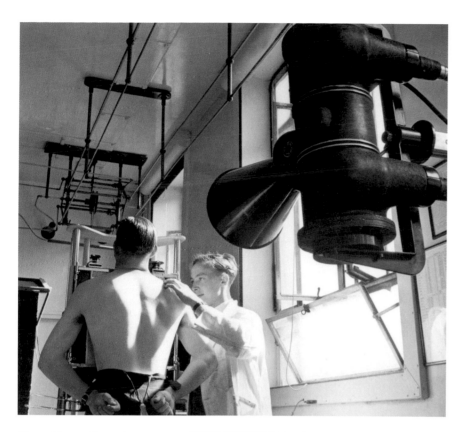

Above: Chest radiography in the 1950s.

Right: Princess Margaret opens a new department of the Queen Alexandra Hospital at Cosham, Portsmouth in 1952. With the princess is the Matron Miss L.C. De La Court and the Lord Mayor Alderman Albert Johnson.

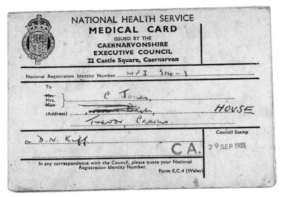

Left: An NHS medical card, with patient and doctor's details and NHS number.

Below: Ward sister and consultant on a female ward at the Montagu Hospital in Mexborough, South Yorkshire in 1952.

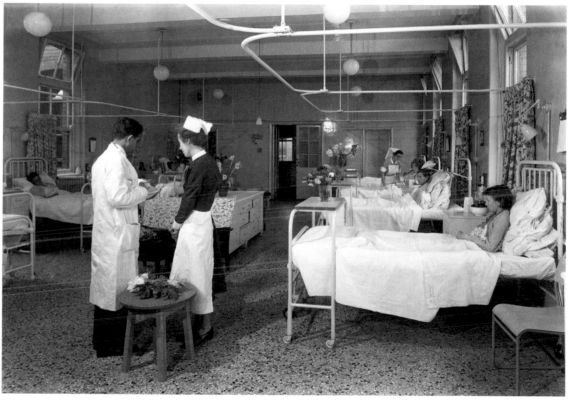

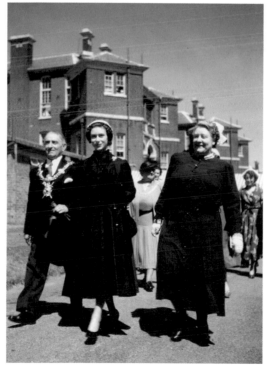

Robert Platt
1900–1978

Robert Platt trained and practised in Sheffield before military service in North Africa, Italy and India during World War II. After the war, he took up the Chair of Medicine in Manchester and then, as President of the RCP between 1957–1962, it was Platt who was largely responsible for the College's move to its current building in Regent's Park and for the choice of Denys Lasdun, as the dynamic and innovative architect. Initial proposals to enlarge the College's existing home in Pall Mall were unrealistic and a site in Harley Street had been first considered. By good fortune, the Canadian High Commissioner then offered to acquire the Pall Mall building, which became part of the renamed Canada House. With a donation of £500,000 from the Wolfson Foundation the College was then able to purchase the 100-year lease from the Crown Estate, on the current site in Regent's Park, giving the opportunity, in Platt's words, to build a new home 'of grace and dignity sufficient for our needs and appropriate to our tradition'.

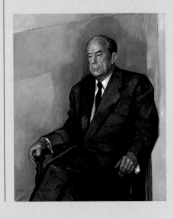

'Our job is to give the client, on time and on cost, not what he wants but what he never dreamed he wanted and, when he gets it, he recognises it as something he wanted all the time.'

Denys Lasdun

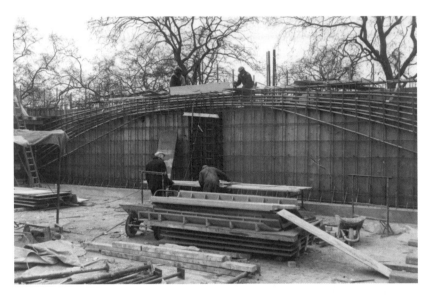

Left and below: Building work at 11 St Andrews Place, erecting the new Lasdun-designed Royal College of Physicians, which replaced the earlier Someries House, designed by Nash.

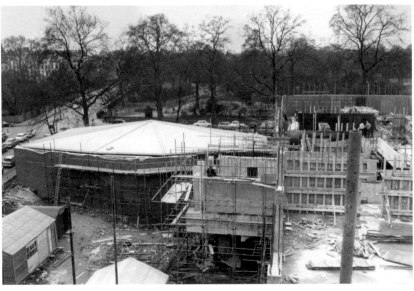

1959

Platt reported that the architect was 'taking the greatest care to study the functions, traditions and ceremonies of this old society'.

1960

Royal College of Physicians of London Act finally ratified officially the name 'Royal College'. Invention of cardiopulmonary resuscitation.

1962

RCP report *Smoking and Health* published.

1962

Enoch Powell's Hospital Plan, which recommends the development of district general hospitals covering populations of around 125,000 persons: 'This plan … will provide for patients … an environment which will challenge comparison with that available anywhere in the world'.

1964

RCP moves to Regent's Park.

1964

Queen Elizabeth II opens the new College in 1964.

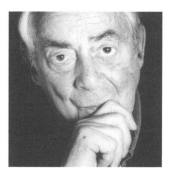

Above: Sir Denys Lasdun (1914–2001) was the architect of the RCP's Regent's Park building. He was influenced by Le Corbusier and Mies van der Rohe and is widely considered one of the most influential British architects of the post-war generation. Other famous buildings designed by Lasdun include London's National Theatre; the Institute of Education; the core buildings of the University of East Anglia in Norwich, and New Court in Christ's College Cambridge.

Right above: Lasdun's model of his proposed design for the new Royal College of Physicians in Regent's Park.

Right: An illustration of the architectural affinity between human anatomy, as represented by Leonardo da Vinci's famous illustration, and a building, represented by Lasdun's innovative design for the RCP, with the Censors' room as the 'heart'.

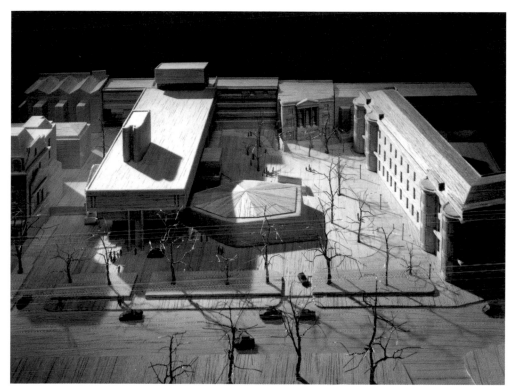

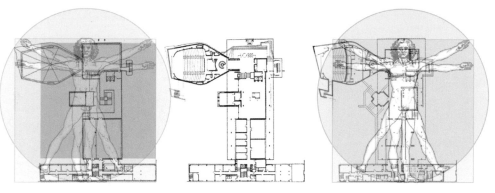

The foundation of the NHS fundamentally altered the practice of medicine in the UK. A tripartite structure was established of: Hospital Services, with non-teaching hospitals supporting the community and teaching hospitals supporting the nation; Primary Care Services, comprising GPs, dentists, opticians and pharmacists as independent contractors; Community Services such as maternity and child welfare clinics, health visitors, midwives, immunisation, health education and ambulance services. This system (and particularly its governance) has since been repeatedly altered in various ways, depending on the political complexion of the government. However, its basic elements remain in place. Since 1948, in order to meet the need for the provision of consultant services in every major discipline across the country, there has been a modernisation of almost every aspect of the work of the RCP, initially under the direction of Robert Platt. This increase in College activity was paralleled by the commissioning and building of an ambitious new headquarters, and the beginning of a revolution in workforce demographics.

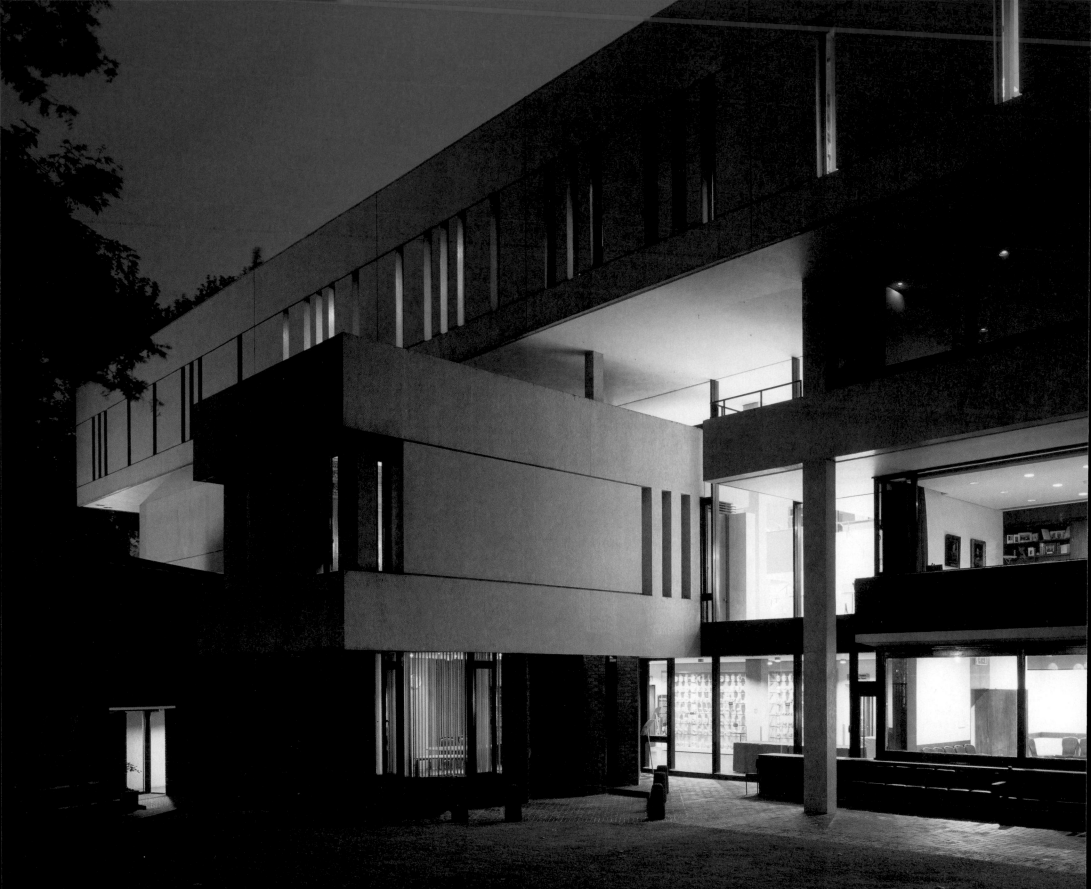

Left: The Royal College of Physicians at night, viewed from the medicinal garden in St Andrews Place. The Victor Hoffbrand collection of apothecary jars, a registered National Treasure, can be seen through the ground-floor windows.

Right: The Lasdun Marble Hall with the magnificent 500-year collection of presidential portraits.

Below: The Censors' Room, which projects from the main building into the medicinal garden and is architecturally conservative in comparison with the rest of the building. It houses the Spanish oak panelling, originally in Robert Hooke's 1675 building in Warwick Lane.

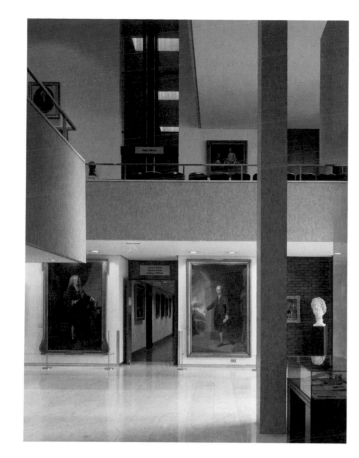

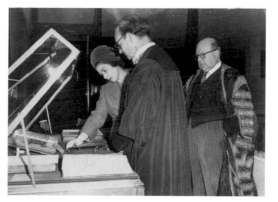

Left: HM Queen Elizabeth II, with Sir Charles Dodds (1899–1973) in presidential robes, and Dr Charles Newman (1900–1989), Harveian Librarian, opening the new Lasdun building in 1964.

Below: The heraldic stained-glass window by Keith New (1925–2012), diffuses multi-coloured light into the entrance of the College.

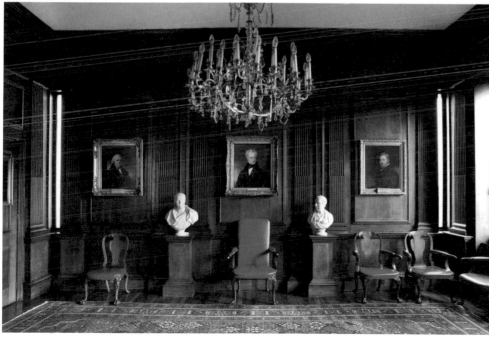

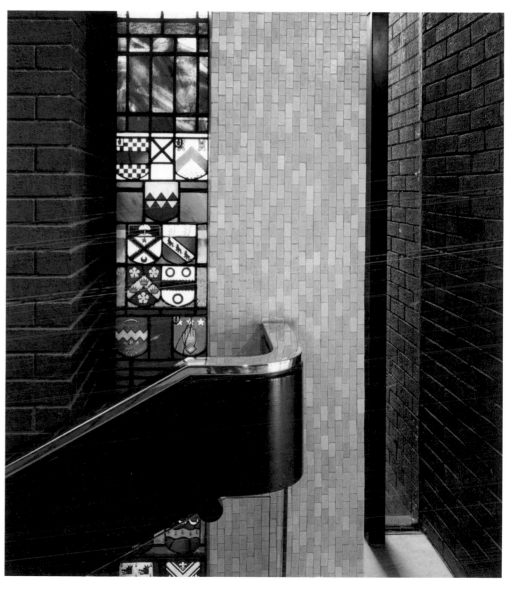

1966
Genetic code deciphered: four bases, 20 amino acids.
The first issue of the *Journal of the Royal College of Physicians of London* is published.

1967
British Association for Emergency Medicine established. A recommendation is made that at least 200 fellows should be elected to the RCP annually.

1967
Dame Albertine Winner appointed first woman Linacre Fellow.
Dame Cicely Saunders founds first modern hospice.

1968
Report of the Royal Commission on Medical Education (the Todd Report) published.
Joint Royal College of Physicians Training Board (JCHMT) established.

1969
Appointment of RCP regional advisors and College tutors.

1970
RCP report on air pollution.
Faculty of Community Medicine (now Faculty of Public Health) established as a joint autonomous faculty by the three Royal Colleges of Physicians of the United Kingdom.

The RCP made a deliberate choice of a modernistic building in Regent's Park for its new home – a new building for a new style of College. Denys Lasdun, a young 'Brutalist' architect, was chosen and spent a year watching the workings of the College to develop the anatomical theme underpinning his building design. His other major works included the University of East Anglia and the National Theatre, but neither demonstrated the mature design detail and variety of materials displayed in the building in Regent's Park. The outside of the building is of horizontal design in the style of Le Corbusier, wider at the top than the bottom and clad in small white tiles. Its broad 'front' actually faces a garden and classical quadrangle of Regency stucco buildings to the side of the road. Inside, the marble-clad three-storey central atrium displays the College exhibitions and portraits. The Wolfson and Seligman lecture theatres (the latter added in 1995–96) support key functions of the building, as a place for education and as a conference centre. The building is constructed with subtle design touches, including the use of 37 types of dark engineering brick, light effects and luxurious imposing materials: bronze, brass, mosaic and marble. The Dorchester Library houses the College's historical book collections and is the location for College ceremonies. The Censors' Room is lined by Spanish oak panelling originally made for the 1675 building in Warwick Lane and transferred first to Pall Mall East and then to Regent's Park.

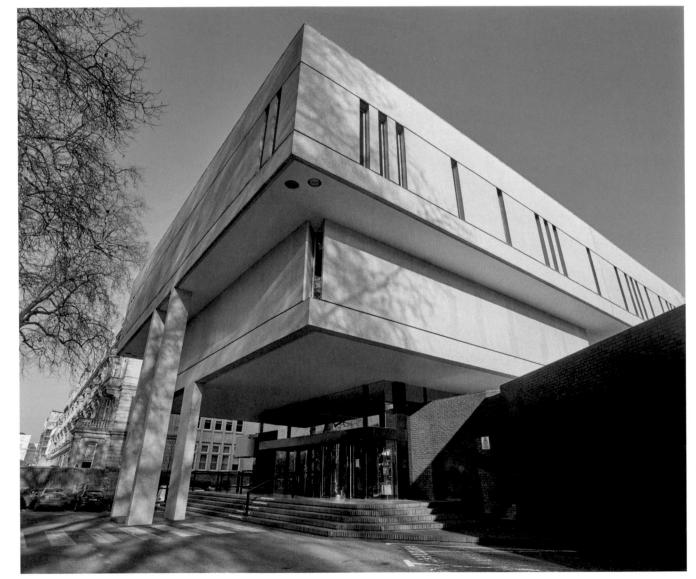

The 'Brutalist' building stands in stark contrast to its Regency surrounds and provides, as Lasdun intended, a magnificent backdrop and exhibition area for the College's collection of historical paintings, archives and artefacts stretching back over 500 years. The collection includes more than 5,000 oil paintings, prints, drawings and sculptures, the Symons collection of medical instruments, the Victor Hoffbrand collection of apothecary jars, listed as a National Treasure and the RCP's silver and medical collections, including a rare set of 17th-century anatomical tables. In recent years, the RCP has presented acclaimed exhibitions including *Reframing Disability: Portraits from the Royal College of Physicians*; *The Mirror of Health: Medicine in the Golden Age of Islam*; and *Scholar, Courtier, Magician: the Lost Library of John Dee*.

Lasdun constructed the building to complement the Regency terrace, and it provides spectacular views of the opposite side of St Andrews Place, through vast plate-glass windows. Since it was built, a fine medicinal garden has been developed, which adds to the beauty of the RCP environment. The garden takes a deliberately historical perspective. Pliny Secundus wrote in 70AD that he knew all the medicinal plants 'except very few' from visiting a distinguished physician, Antonius Castor, 'who had a pretty garden of his own, well stored with simples [medicinal plants] of sundry sorts, which he maintained for his own pleasure and his friends, who used to come and see his plot, and indeed it was worthy of the sight'. The College garden carries on the tradition of Castor's garden, well stored with simples and worthy of the sight. Over 1,100 plants are grown, some 80 named after doctors and about 70 which form the basis of modern medicines; the remainder are the herbal medicines of our predecessors and herbalists worldwide. The eight beds along St Andrews Place have the plants found in the College's *Pharmacopoeia Londinensis* (1618) arranged according to the part of the plant used. Elsewhere they are set out principally by the continent in which they originate. The medicinal garden is, arguably, the largest medicinal plant collection in Europe, and is pedagogic and inspiring.

Left: The front of the Regent's Park building of the RCP, designed by Denys Lasdun and opened in 1964.

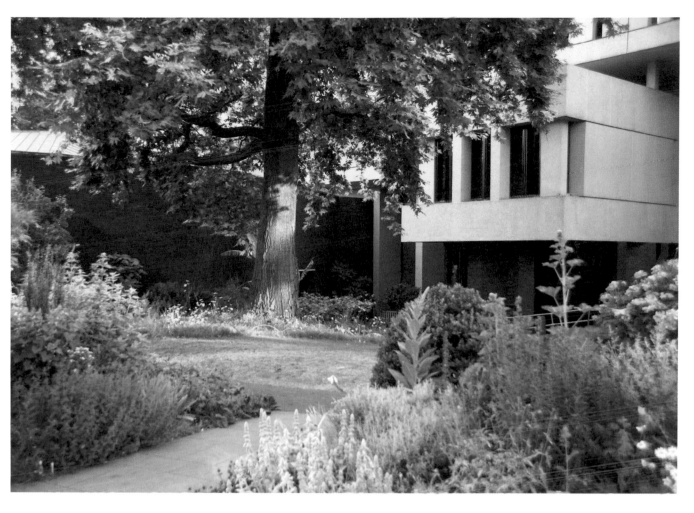

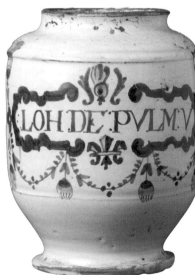

Left: A ceramic apothecary jar from the Victor Hoffbrand collection, *c.*1675. It stored *Lohoch de Pulmones vulpis*, a thick linctus used for coughs, breathing problems and tuberculosis, according to Culpeper (1649). A recipe from Cordus (1546), and attributed to Mesue, listed the ingredients as dried fox lungs, liquorice, fennel, anise, maidenhair and coltsfoot crushed up and mixed with water and sugar.

Above: The medicinal garden of the Royal College of Physicians, with the Hippocratic plane tree which commemorates Hippocrates, the father of medicine. It is a scion of the tree on the Island of Cos under which Hippocrates taught his medical students 2,300 years ago.

Max Leonard Rosenheim 1908–1972

In 1966, Max Rosenheim became President of the College and his presidency marked a decade of change. He enthusiastically picked up the banner of development and modernisation, capturing the mood of national and international collaboration. He had been educated at the University of Cambridge and University College Hospital Medical School and then served in World War II, rising to the rank of brigadier. He spent the rest of his career at University College Hospital, London. Collaboration with the Royal Colleges of Physicians of Edinburgh and Glasgow led to the formation of the common MRCP (UK) examination in 1968, success in which has become a key requirement for career progression for physicians. Another collaborative venture was the establishment of the Faculty of Community Medicine (now the Faculty of Public Health) established in 1972. Lord Rosenheim also pioneered overseas activities of the RCP and, although his focus was on Europe, the principles he established underpin the College's current activities in Africa, Asia and the Middle East. During this period about a thousand new fellows were elected and the College's modern regional structure and outlook were established. Moreover, mirroring the rapid changes in society in this period, more women were entering medicine.

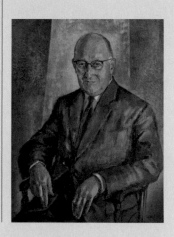

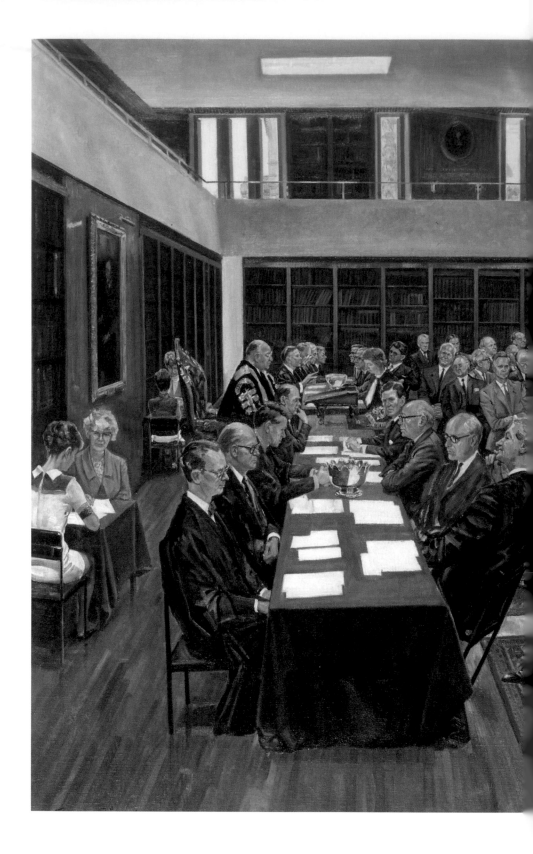

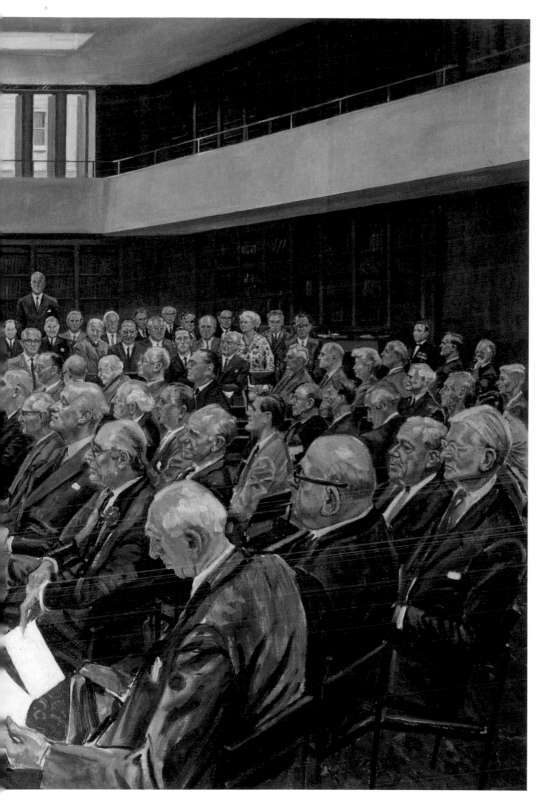

Left: Raymond Piper's painting (1968) of the Comitia in session was in fact painted at several quarterly meetings. The members of the Comitia were asked to sit in the same place each time they attended. The painting is set in the Dorchester Library, where Comitia meetings are still held. Of the 89 persons present (many identifiable today) there were only seven women, including Albertine Winner, Sheila Sherlock and Elizabeth Stokes. Four were administrators and included the stalwart Ina Cook (facing, far left).

1973

NHS Reorganisation Act passed by Parliament after years of debate.

1975

The Merrison Report published. It recommends that the General Medical Council (GMC) should become responsible for regulating postgraduate medical education and training, and that the GMC should hold a list of all registered specialists and GPs.

1979

In its report *Patients First*, a Royal Commission reporting on the NHS raises concerns about the effects on the NHS of an ageing population and the cost of technological developments. However, it concludes that the NHS is in no danger of collapse.

The male dominance of medicine until the mid-20th century and the barriers facing women medical pioneers, such as Elizabeth Blackwell and Elizabeth Garrett Anderson in the late 19th and early 20th century, are described earlier. It was only in the latter part of the 19th century that women started medical training in any numbers and only after the founding of the NHS that all UK medical schools were finally open to women. The changing position of women in the College, since 1948, has mirrored that of the wider medical community and society. The first FRCP was Dame Janet Vaughan, elected in 1943 (see page 140). The first female College officer was Dame Albertine Winner (Linacre Fellow 1967–78), the first woman Senior Censor and Vice-President of the College (1971–77) was Dame Sheila Sherlock, the first woman Treasurer (2010–16) was Professor Linda Luxon and the first woman President (1989–91) was Dame Margaret Turner-Warwick. Since then there have been two further women PRCPs: Dame Carol Black, and the current President, Professor Jane Dacre. According to the 2016 GMC statistics 52 per cent of doctors on the GP Register and 34 per cent on the Specialist Register are women, as are 55 per cent of medical students.

1980

Black Report on health inequalities is published. Flowers Report on London medical education.

1982

Area Health Authorities abolished in NHS reorganisation.

1983

First human disease mapped onto the genome (Huntington's disease to Chromosome 4).

1986

First AIDS Health Campaign.

1987

RCP report on the risks and dangers of alcohol.

1989

Dame Margaret Turner-Warwick elected first woman President. RCP Faculty of Pharmaceutical Medicine created as a joint faculty of the three Royal Colleges of Physicians of the United Kingdom.

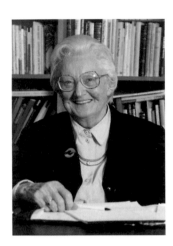

Left: Dame Cicely Saunders was an Anglican nurse, social worker, physician and leader, who insisted that dying people needed dignity, compassion and respect, as well as rigorous scientific methodology in the testing of treatments. She founded the first modern hospice and was responsible for establishing the discipline of palliative care.

Right: Dame Cicely Saunders caring for a patient in St Christopher's hospice.

Below left: The Faculty of Public Health was formed in 1972 as a result of a key recommendation of the Royal Commission on Medical Education (1965–68). Professor Alwyn Smith served twice as President and, as professor at the University of Manchester, developed cervical- and breast-screening programmes. In 1988, he supervised the production of the Nation's Health report, highlighting the impact of social, environmental and economic factors on health, so influencing public policies.

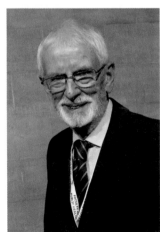

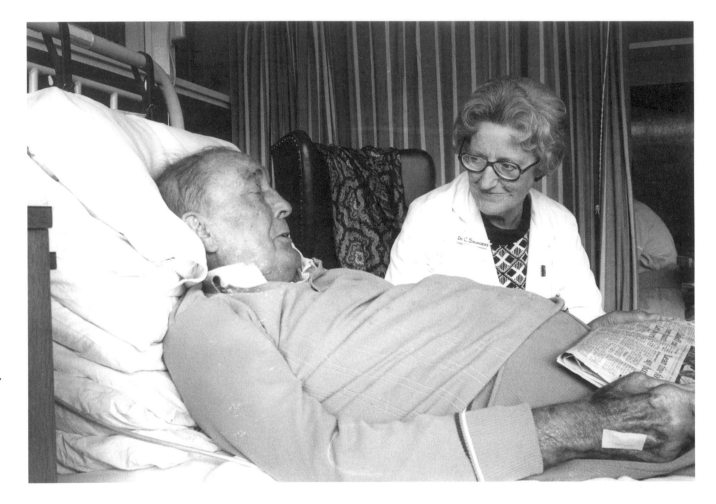

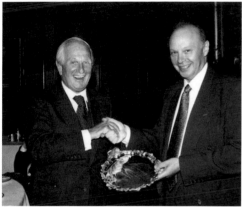

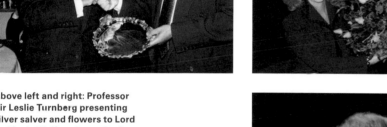

Above left and right: Professor Sir Leslie Turnberg presenting silver salver and flowers to Lord and Lady Wolfson in gratitude for their tireless support of the College.

Right: Dame Albertine Winner (1907–1988) was a remarkable physician and administrator. She served during the war in the RAMC, rising to the rank of lieutenant colonel. She was the first female College officer, when she was appointed Linacre Fellow and was responsible for forming the training posts that were to be recognised by the newly formed JCHMT. She became DBE in 1967.

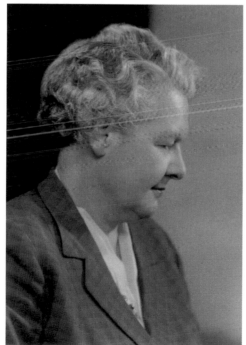

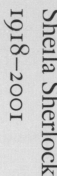

Sheila Sherlock
1918–2001

Dame Sheila Sherlock epitomised the rise of women to senior academic medical positions in the 1960s. Having been turned down by a number of English medical schools, Sheila Sherlock trained in Edinburgh, graduating top of her class. In 1942, at the Hammersmith Hospital, she won the gold medal for her MD thesis on acute hepatitis. After a year in the USA, at Yale on a Rockefeller travelling fellowship, she returned to the Hammersmith Hospital at the age of 30 to set up a liver unit there. Then, in 1959, she moved to the Royal Free Hospital, as the first woman to be appointed to the chair of any British department of medicine. In 1971, she was elected the first woman Vice-President and Senior Censor of the RCP. She was made DBE in 1978 and elected as FRS in 2001. She helped to establish hepatology in Britain and her contributions spanned almost every aspect of the field, including the establishment of the link between the hepatitis B virus and liver cancer. She had a major impact on the Royal Free Hospital and its Medical School, not least through the many fellows and trainees whom she taught and who have practised throughout the world.

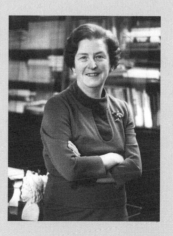

1989

Working for patients (NHS reforms)
proposed to introduce a split
between purchasers and providers
of care, GP fundholders and a state-
financed internal market, in order
to drive service efficiency.

1990

National Health Service and
Community Care Act creates
an 'internal market' in the NHS.

1991

The Patient's Charter stressed
the patient as a customer with
rational expectations.

1992

A white paper, *The Health of the
Nation*, is published. This targets
improvement in five key areas:
coronary heart disease, cancers,
mental health, sexual health and the
prevention of accidents. Tomlinson
Report into London's Health Services.
Private Finance Initiatives (PFIs)
introduced into NHS.

1993

Faculty of Accident and Emergency
Medicine established.

1994

Quarterly Comitia changes to an
AGM on College Day. NHS donor
organ register established.

Since 1948, the College's work has been particularly effective in relation to public health and improvement in medical practice. In 1950, Richard Doll and A. Bradford Hill published a seminal paper in the *British Medical Journal* showing a clear statistical association between smoking and lung cancer, but there was reluctance among politicians to take action to reduce tobacco consumption. In Britain, in the mid-1950s, 12 million men and 6 million women were smoking and tax revenue on cigarettes was greater than that from income tax. When *Smoking and Health* was published by the RCP in 1962 it created a stir. Within six weeks, 50,000 copies of the report were distributed and it contributed to a change in public attitudes. In 1969, the newly created Health Education Council launched the first anti-smoking campaign and in the 1970s anti-smoking advertisements became routine. Further reports in 1971, 1977 and 1983 and more recently have continued to stress the harm from tobacco and the need for continued action.

Other RCP public health initiatives include its reports on air pollution (1970), alcohol (1987) and obesity (2013) and its hosting of the National Clinical Guideline Centre (NCGC), now renamed National Guideline Centre.

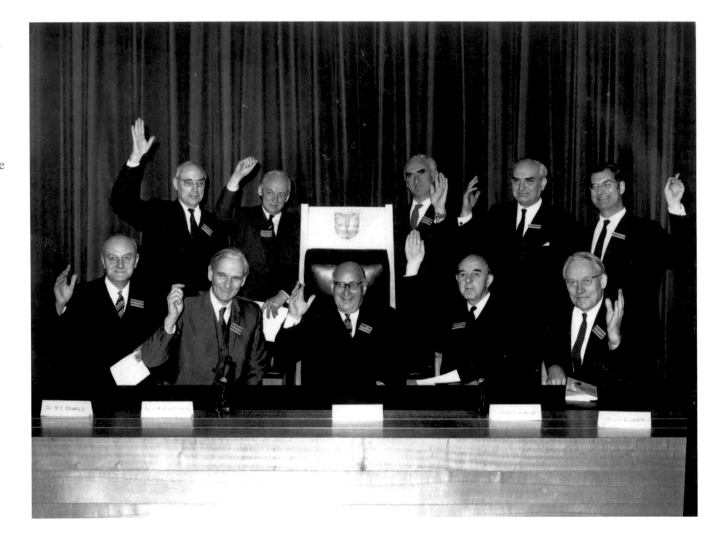

1997

The white paper *The New NHS: Modern, Dependable* is published. It states that 'If you are ill or injured, there will be a National Health Service there to help, and access to it will be based on need and need alone.'

1998

The RCP Education Department and the National Institute for Health and Clinical Excellence (NICE) are established. The Department of Health publishes the Acheson report on *Inequalities in Health*. NHS Direct launched, becoming one of the largest single e-health services in the world, handling more than half a million calls each month.

1999

Department of Health publishes *Saving lives: Our Healthier Nation*. The government plan focuses on the main killers: cancer, coronary heart disease, stroke, accidents and mental illness.

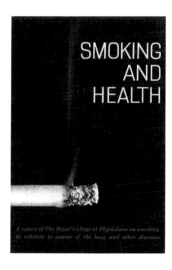

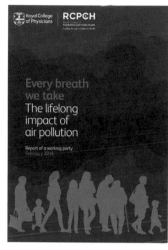

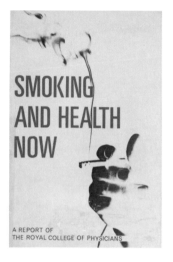

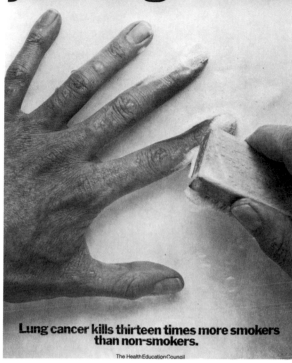

Left: On 1 January 1970, the RCP held a press conference to launch the second RCP smoking report, *Smoking and Health Now*. Following a question about their own smoking habits, all members of the committee raised their hands to confirm that they had given up smoking cigarettes.

(L to R — back row): Dr J.G. Scadding; Sir Francis Avery Jones; Dr P.J. Lawther; Dr D.D. Reid; Dr L.H. Capel (L to R — front row): Dr N.C. Oswald; Dr C.M. Fletcher; Lord Rosenheim; Sir Kenneth Robson and Dr J.C. Gilson.

Above: The BMJ noted that the 1950 report *Smoking and Health* was 'a turning point in the approach to one of the most challenging opportunities for preventative medicine today. A deadly habit.' RCP followed up in 1970 with *Smoking and Health Now* and, with the RCPCH, the seminal air pollution report *Every breath we take* in 2016.

Right above: Anti-smoking campaign poster.

Right below: 1940s advertisement for Piccadilly cigarettes.

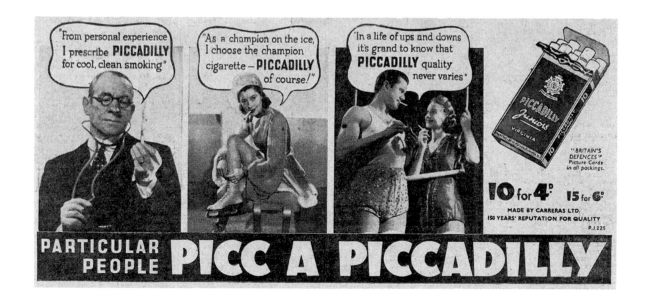

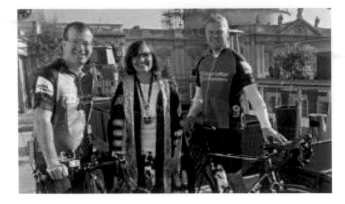

Another key report under the chairmanship of Douglas Black was published in 1980 (the Black Report). It identified the social inequalities in health and set out measures to reduce them. In 1974, Black had been appointed as the first Chief Scientist at the Department of Health, and served as President of the RCP between 1977–1983. He was asked to produce his report by David Ennals, the then Labour Secretary of State for Health, but when the report was finalised, Margaret Thatcher had been installed as Prime Minister and the political landscape had radically changed. The report was out of tune with the prevailing mood, but nevertheless provided convincing data that the poorest in the community had the highest rates of ill-health and death, and the costs of addressing these inequalities would have been significant. Instead of formal publication, 260 stencilled copies were circulated on a Bank Holiday Monday, but, despite this lacklustre launch, the report led to similar initiatives by the World Health Organization and the Organisation for Economic Co-operation and Development (OECD). Black's contribution was recognized by his colleagues and he was elected president of the British Medical Association from 1984–85.

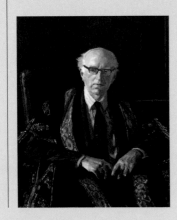

Above: The President, Professor Jane Dacre, the chief executive Ian Bullock (right) and the RCP Registrar, Dr Andrew 'Bod' Goddard (left) promoting physical exercise and cycling around England and Wales to visit as many acute NHS trusts as possible and invite RCP fellows and members to sign the RCP's modern charter and raise money for Physicians for Africa.

Opposite: A recent exhibition, *This bewitching poison*, highlighted the problems of alcohol abuse and the role the College has played in dealing with them. The RCP promotes public awareness of the health harms of alcohol and advocates with government for regulation to limit these dangers. The past President Professor Sir Ian Gilmore is chair of the Alcohol Health Alliance and Special Advisor on alcohol to the Royal College of Physicians.

Since 1948, there have been significant changes in medicine; workforce demographics; the ethos, scope and effectiveness of medicine and multiple, frequent, administrative reorganisations leading to a complex NHS infrastructure. On a professional level, 'patient-focused care' and the democratisation of access to information has made medicine a partnership between doctor and patient that is wholly different from previous, more paternalistic, models of care.

In addition, there have been revolutionary medical advances during this period, some listed in the table opposite. Many other factors have impacted both positively and negatively upon medical care, including public health focusing on illness prevention and self-care; affluence in the developed, and to a lesser extent in the developing world, resulting in epidemics of disorders of excess (obesity and diabetes); and climate change and globalisation. Emergent infectious diseases, some rapidly spreading worldwide – as exemplified by the recent SARS, bird 'flu, Ebola and Zika epidemics – have become major concerns. The importance and value of global cooperation is highlighted by the 145 countries that have ratified their commitment to the Paris Agreement, part of the UN Framework Convention on Climate Change, which will have universal health benefits, especially for vulnerable and disadvantaged populations. Due to multiple and often unnecessary usage, the initial success of antibiotics has been superseded by the rapidly increasing threat of pandemics of antibiotic-resistant infections of previously treatable conditions, such as tuberculosis. These issues require urgent investigation, research and public dissemination, if human health is to remain protected.

2000

New NHS plan published, promising a ten-year modernisation programme of investment and reform.

2002

First successful gene therapy carried out.

2003

New contracts for GPs and hospital consultants are agreed, changing the delivery of services to patients. The Health and Social Care (Community Health and Standards) Act is passed, resulting in a further major reorganisation of the NHS. Full human genome published, showing that there are 20,000–25,000 genes in human DNA and that it is composed of 3 billion base pairs.

2004

The first ten foundation trusts are established, with more control over their budgets and services.

2005

The report *Commissioning a Patient-Led Service* is published.

2006

The white paper *Our Health, Our Care, Our Say* is published. Inaugural meeting of the Faculty of Forensic and Legal Medicine.

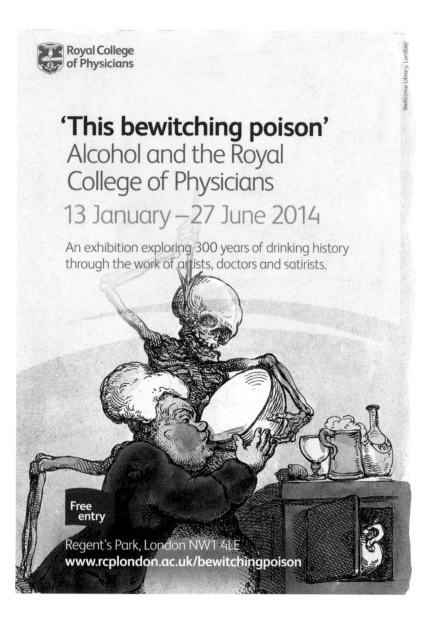

Wellcome Library, London

Royal College of Physicians

'This bewitching poison'
Alcohol and the Royal College of Physicians
13 January – 27 June 2014

An exhibition exploring 300 years of drinking history through the work of artists, doctors and satirists.

Free entry

Regent's Park, London NW1 4LE
www.rcplondon.ac.uk/bewitchingpoison

Advances in Medicine 1948–2018

1940s

First antibiotics (penicillin, streptomycin and Chloromycetin)
Vaccine for influenza
Renal dialysis
Implant of intraocular lens
Chemotherapy
Defibrillator
Mechanical assistor for anaesthesia
Rhesus blood grouping

1950s

Salk polio vaccine
Discovery of stem cells
Cardiac pacemakers
Artificial ventilation
Kidney transplantation
In vitro fertilisation
Cortisone
Ultrasound scanning
Percutaneous angiography

1960s

Oral polio vaccine
Combined oral contraceptive pill
Total hip replacement
Beta blockers
Measles and mumps vaccines
Heart, liver, lung, kidney, pancreas transplantation
Combination chemotherapy
Betablockers
Cardiopulmonary resuscitation
Cochlear implant

1970s

Rubella, pneumonia and meningitis vaccines
Immunosuppressive agents
Cimetidine
IVF + test tube babies
Coronary artery bypass
Endoscopy and laparoscopic surgery
MRI, CT and PET Imaging
Coronary angioplasty
Laser eye surgery
Antiviral drugs
Bone marrow transplantation

1980s

Smallpox eradicated
Vaccine for hepatitis B
Artificial heart implanted
Statins
Helicobacter pylori
Coronary stents
Artificial skin
Human insulin
First surgical robots

1990s

Antiviral therapy for HIV
Vaccine for hepatitis A
Cloning
Stem cell therapy
Targeted therapies e.g. Herceptin
Electroactive polymers (artificial muscle)
Synthetic clotting factors

2000s onwards

Telesurgery
First successful gene therapy
Face and limb transplantation
Kidney and liver grown from stem cells
Cancer immunotherapy
Thrombolysis for stroke
Pharmacogenetics
Proton beam therapy
100,000 Genomes Project

2007

A ban on smoking in nearly all enclosed work places and public places in England is introduced.

2008

Health Minister Lord Darzi publishes *High-Quality Care for All*, a report outlining a ten-year vision for the NHS. 100,000 Genomes Project launched.

2009

National Clinical Guideline Centre established. The Faculty of Pharmaceutical Medicine formed part of the working party that develops the RCP report *Innovating for Health: Patients, Physicians, the Pharmaceutical Industry and the NHS.*

2010

Professor Linda Luxon appointed first woman Treasurer of the College.

2011

The Academy of Medical Royal Colleges establishes a Faculty of Medical Leadership and Management. National Clinical Guideline Centre is opened.

2012

The Health and Social Care Act introduces the most wide-ranging reforms since the NHS was founded in 1948, abolishing both Strategic Health Authorities and Primary Care Trusts. London Olympic Games Opening Ceremony pays tribute to the NHS.

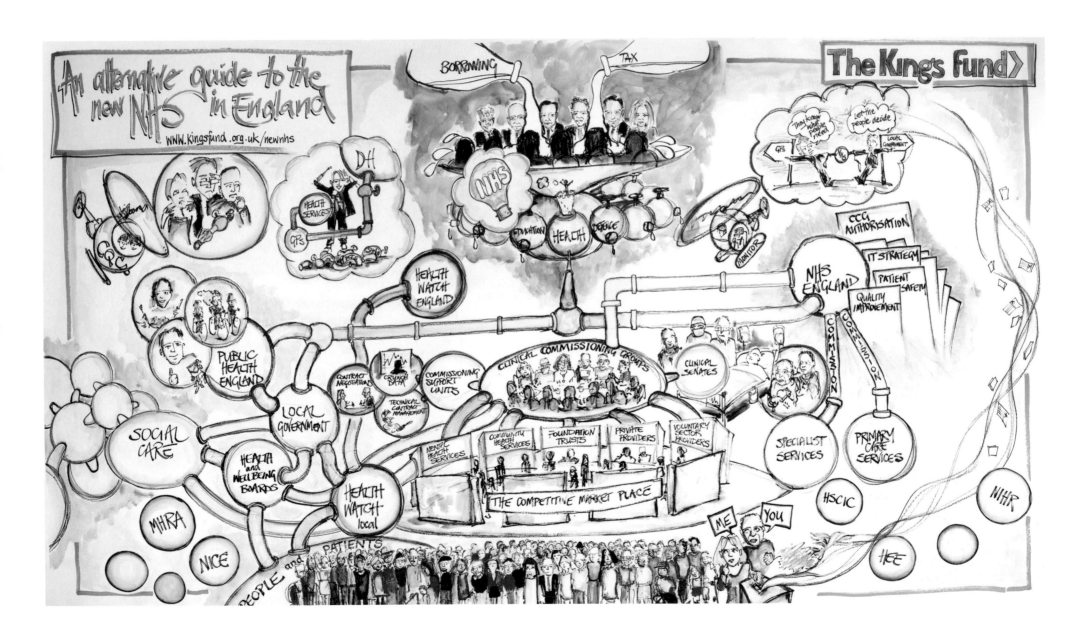

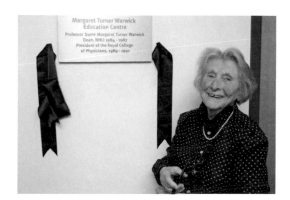

'If they [doctors] can ensure that their professional integrity in the selfless care of patients is sacrosanct then all will be well for the future of medicine. However, if doctors allow their commitment to patients to be pushed into second place by political or managerial diktats, or more personal factors, then medicine will be at risk of losing its soul. In the end, the future of medicine will depend on those who really care for patients.'

Professor Dame Margaret Turner-Warwick

Left: The 2013 King's Fund infographic illustrating the complexity of the NHS following reorganisations, with the Secretary of State for Health, *c.*200 clinical commissioning groups, commissioning support units, clinical senates, NHS England undertaking specialist commissioning and GP services commissioning, Public Health England, Health and Wellbeing Boards, Healthwatch... to name but a few.

Above: Dame Margaret officially opened the Margaret Turner Warwick Education Centre for the National Heart and Lung Institute at the Royal Brompton Campus of Imperial College, on Thursday 16 April 2015.

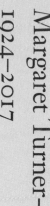
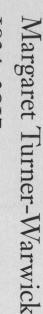

Margaret Turner-Warwick 1924–2017

Professor Dame Margaret Turner-Warwick was an internationally recognised expert in thoracic medicine, the epitome of an excellent clinical academic, a role model for the many young women who were beginning to enter the medical profession and the first female President of the Royal College of Physicians. She demonstrated clinical and academic excellence, while placing great importance upon her family and maintaining great humility and charm. Indeed, despite the prevailing ethos of sexism in her early career, she was emphatic that she did not wish to be seen as a pioneering feminist. From her perspective, gender had no place in medicine. Having trained in Oxford and London, she was appointed Professor of Thoracic Medicine at the Cardiothoracic Institute of London University in 1972 and was elected President of the College in 1989 and served until 1992. She was immediately faced with the difficulties of a major health service reorganisation. She highlighted the clinical, research and educational concerns surrounding Margaret Thatcher's major reforms of the NHS through the introduction of the purchaser/provider split, but met with total intransigence on the part of the government. This was a source of great disappointment to her, but she diverted her very considerable energy and skills to major governance reforms and developments in the College.

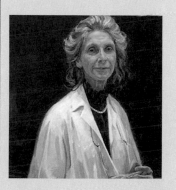

2013

RCP publishes *Action on Obesity: Comprehensive Care for All.*
The Keogh Mortality review.
Robert Francis QC report on Mid-Staffs enquiry.
RCP and West African College of Physicians launch the Millennium Development Goal 6 Partnership for African Clinical Training (M-PACT) for treating HIV/AIDS, malaria and tuberculosis.

2014

RCP celebrates 50 years in Regent's Park.
NHS England publishes its *Five Year Forward View.*
Commonwealth Fund review of international healthcare systems: NHS is rated as the best system in terms of efficiency, effective care, safe care, coordinated care, patient-centred care and cost-related problems.

2015

RCP launches its inaugural annual conference entitled *Medicine 2015.*

2016

UK referendum vote to leave the European Union. Junior doctors' strike.

2017

Launch of RCP North Centre of Excellence.

2018

Royal College of Physicians' Quincentennial celebrations.

The College in 2018 is a very different organisation from that of 1948. It has become more outward-looking, welcoming thousands of visitors to exhibitions and with a public lecture series, open house days, garden tours and treasures evenings. It has an active, ambitious healthcare agenda to improve patient care and to lead public health and policy debates, deliver medical education, and provide support and facilities for its members and fellows. The College has expanded nationally and internationally, providing curricula across 29 medical disciplines, coordinating globally with its sister physician colleges in Edinburgh and Glasgow. Together they produce the most widely accepted postgraduate clinical examination in medicine, guidelines and reports across a range of public health, environmental and clinical topics. Nationally, regional offices have existed since the 1960s and 1970s and the opening of a 'RCP North' in Liverpool in 2017 is a signal of its national reach. Professionally, from a homogenous group of 767 fellows in 1948, it now has a diverse membership of 30,000 members and fellows across the globe, who continue to lead the RCP mission to obtain the best health and healthcare for all.

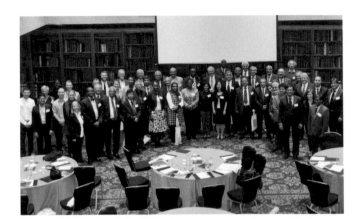

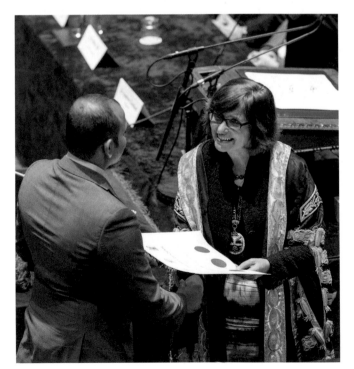

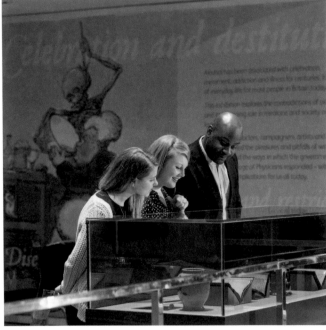

Above left: Annual meeting of the international advisors in the Dorchester Library.

Left: The current President Jane Dacre, in ceremonial robes, giving a membership certificate to a new member of the Royal College of Physicians.

Above: Visitors looking at historical exhibits at the *This bewitching poison* exhibition.

Right: Presidents of the Royal College of Physicians, 1941–2018.

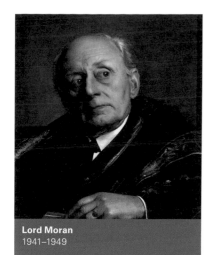

Lord Moran
1941–1949

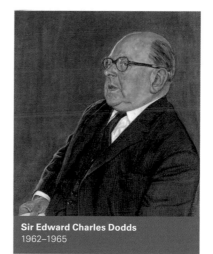

Sir Walter Russell Brain
1950–1956

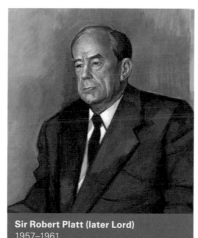

Sir Robert Platt (later Lord)
1957–1961

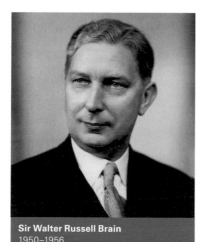

Sir Edward Charles Dodds
1962–1965

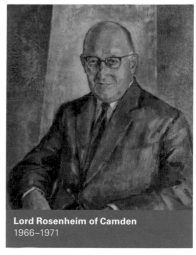

Lord Rosenheim of Camden
1966–1971

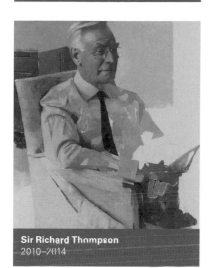

Sir Richard Thompson
2010–2014

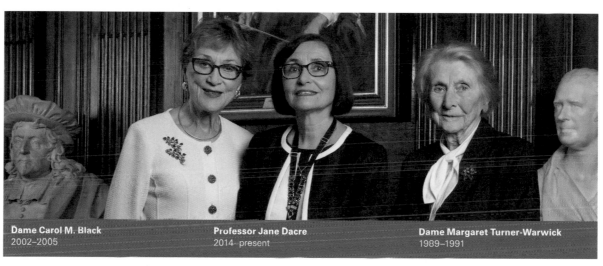

Dame Carol M. Black
2002–2005

Professor Jane Dacre
2014–present

Dame Margaret Turner-Warwick
1989–1991

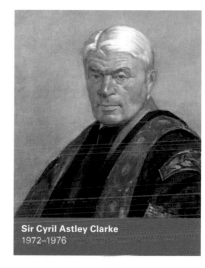

Sir Cyril Astley Clarke
1972–1976

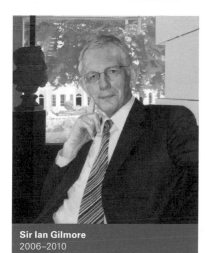

Sir Ian Gilmore
2006–2010

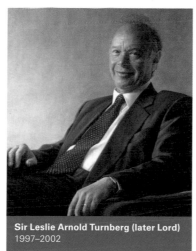

Sir Leslie Arnold Turnberg (later Lord)
1997–2002

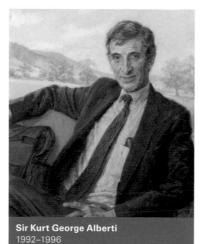

Sir Kurt George Alberti
1992–1996

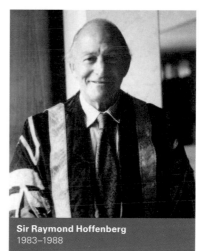

Sir Raymond Hoffenberg
1983–1988

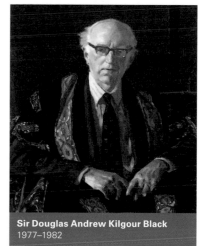

Sir Douglas Andrew Kilgour Black
1977–1982

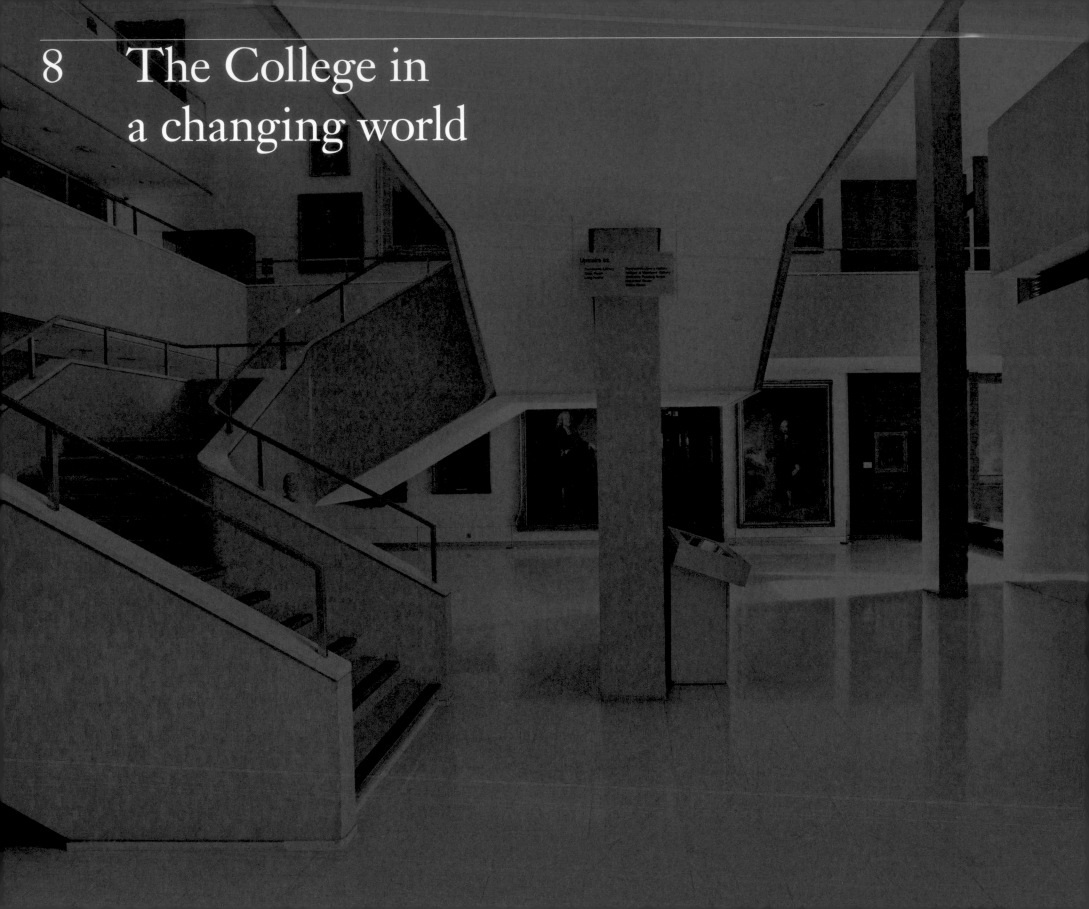

8   The College in
a changing world

When Linacre and colleagues received the royal charter from Henry VIII in 1518, and established the College of Physicians in Linacre's home near St Paul's Cathedral, they could not have imagined the 2018 College – with its headquarters in a Grade I-listed building in Regent's Park, honoured by the patronage of Queen Elizabeth II, and comprised of 34,000 fellows and members and 430 staff, with a new centre of excellence in Liverpool (RCP North).

The College has perpetuated its early objectives of admitting only physicians of the highest standard, who strive to improve clinical care. However, while retaining the established ceremonies, the College has also modernised to embrace a broader and international membership, now including medical students, physician associates and those who have retired, as well as leading physicians and clinical scientists from around the world.

The Council is the RCP's governing body for all professional and clinical matters, and is supported by a wide range of sub-committees and led by the President, who is elected annually by the Fellowship, for a maximum of four years. The College officers are Fellows, appointed in the case of the Treasurer and Registrar, but elected to the positions of academic, education and training and clinical vice-presidents, and all are re-elected by the Fellowship annually. Council meets bimonthly and is composed of the President, College officers, the Vice-President for Wales and ten to twelve elected councillors and is supported by regional advisors, representatives from specialist societies, faculties and College subcommittees. The Executive Leadership Team, who are members of staff, support and oversee the work of the College.

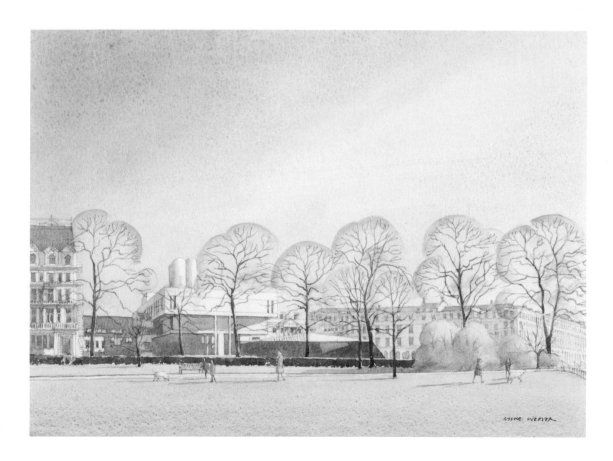

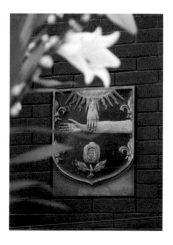

Far left: The Lasdun Hall with the presidential portraits in the RCP headquarters in Regent's Park, London.

Left: Watercolour painted in 1970 prior to the addition of the Council chamber and the Wolfson Theatre by Mike Weaver, an architect, impressed by the Lasdun building. Watercolours, depicting summer and winter scenes, were kindly donated to the College in 2014 and 2015, as part of the 2016 50th-anniversary celebrations of the move to Regent's Park.

Right: RCP coat of arms.

Right: An infographic demonstrating the core elements of the Board of Trustees, Council and the Executive Leadership Team and the five main work streams of the RCP: resources; education; policy; strategy and communications; membership support and care quality improvement, together with other key groups including federation; faculties; specialist societies and medical royal colleges.

Below: President's address at a membership ceremony.

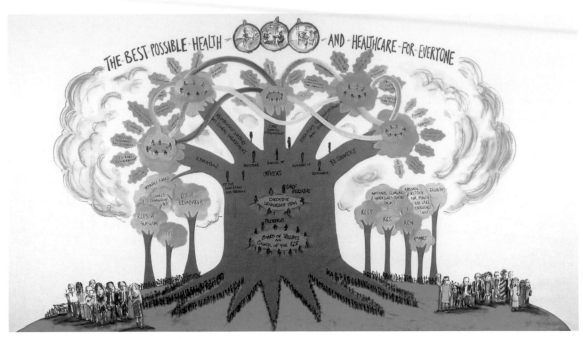

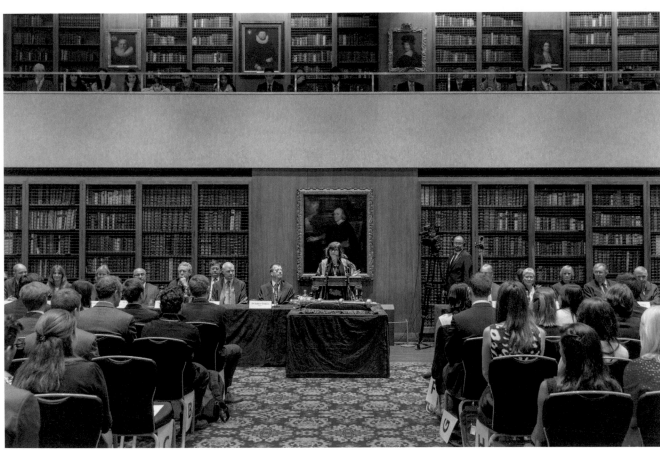

As a charity, the Board of Trustees (BoT) is the RCP's governing body and meets four times a year to provide direction with regard to risk, finance, the fulfilment of charitable responsibilities and the College's commitment to public benefit. The Trustees include the six senior officers of the RCP, four fellows nominated from Council and four lay members appointed by the BoT. It works closely and liaises with the Council but ultimately, all decisions (apart from changes to the bye-laws and regulations) are taken by, or on behalf of, the BoT, and reported to the fellows for agreement and ratification at the AGM.

The RCP vision is 'the best health and healthcare for all' and the 2015–20 strategy is, therefore, focused on five work strands: improving care for patients, developing physicians throughout their careers, leading and supporting members, shaping the future of health and healthcare and investing in our future, and building on our heritage. The College underpins this work by providing an independent view on medical professionalism, leadership and quality improvements in clinical practice. It communicates these values through stakeholder meetings, social media, the press, peer publications and a public engagement programme, which includes exhibitions, lectures and tours.

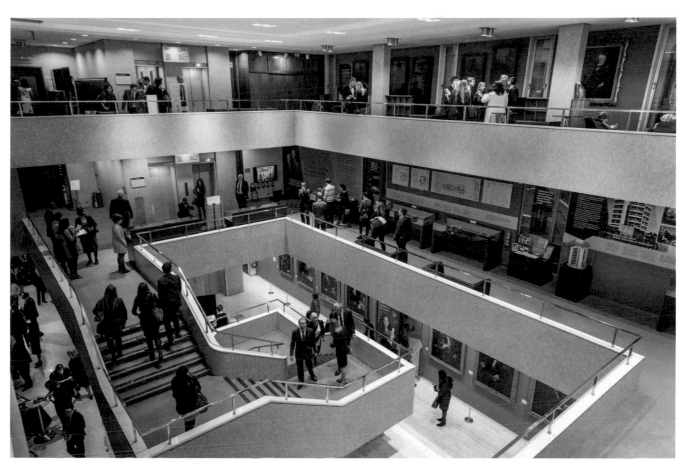

Above right: Lasdun's 'floating' staircase, at the centre of College life, in the Lasdun Hall at the Royal College of Physicians.

Right: Visitors examining exhibits at the Lasdun exhibition in 2014, celebrating 50 years of the opening of the RCP and Lasdun building in Regent's Park.

Far right: The public engagement programme began in 2014 and aims to provide the general public with information about the RCP and evidence- based information about health and medicine. Additionally, the public are invited to lectures, exhibitions and programmes related to the medicinal garden, heritage and to Quincentennial Society meetings.

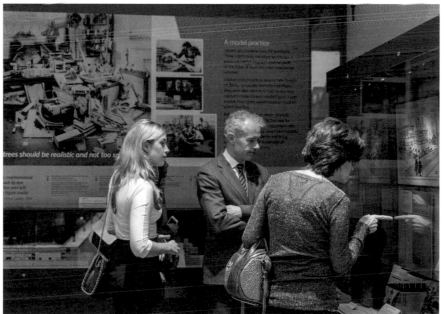

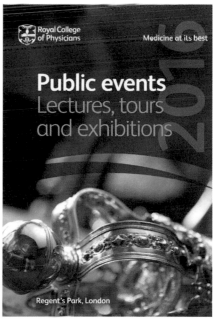

> '*The Future Hospital Commission… produced the most important statement about the future of British medicine for a generation.*'
>
> Richard Horton, editor of *The Lancet*

The College is focused on quality improvement in all aspects of patient care, with support from the patient and carers' network to ensure proposals and strategies are relevant. A broad range of initiatives have been brought together in the Quality Improvement Hub, including important developments to establish and disseminate good standards of core medical practice for the unique medical and social needs of adolescents and young adults and the specific healthcare needs of the homeless and excluded community.

The Clinical Effectiveness and Evaluation Unit has undertaken national clinical audits on chronic obstructive pulmonary disease; falls; end of life care; inflammatory bowel disease; stroke; and, most recently, lung cancer, which have enabled the identification of quality improvement initiatives. In addition, the RCP has introduced accreditation services for example in endoscopy and allergy, supporting departments to drive up their quality of care and influence national policy.

The National Guideline Centre, working with NICE, has a track record in developing high-quality clinical guidelines, which reduce variations in standards of care, address clinical uncertainties and improve the quality of life for patients.

The Future Hospital Programme aims to evaluate methods for raising the standards of care and to disseminate good practice. Innovative service approaches are being piloted and evaluated and eight development and training programmes have been set in place for effective clinical leadership.

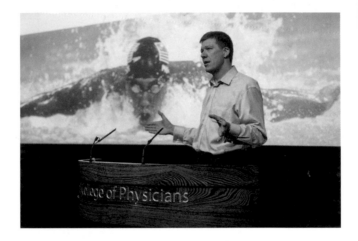

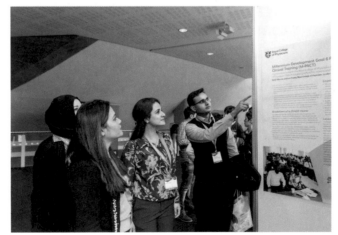

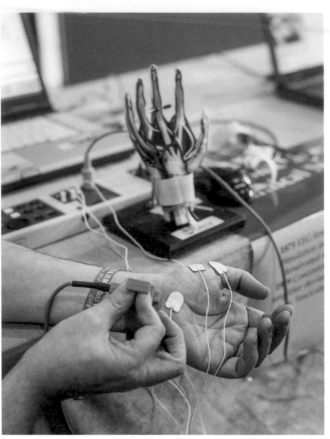

Above left: Richard Budgett FRCP, Medical and Scientific Director of the International Olympic Committee and Chief Medical Officer to the 2012 Summer Olympic Games, held in London, giving a lecture at the Royal College of Physicians in 2012.

Above right: Demonstration of the neurophysiological technique (electromyography) to assess the median nerve supply of the hand muscles at Careers Day.

Left: Junior doctor describing his research work to colleagues at the annual conference.

Below left: Professor Don Berwick, former Head of the US Centers for Medicare & Medicaid Services, delivering an inspirational talk at the RCP Medicine 2016 conference.

Below right: National Medical Director's Clinical Fellow working at the Royal College of Physicians and discussing career opportunities with a colleague.

Bottom right: The junior doctors took strike action in January 2016 over the imposition by the Health Secretary, Jeremy Hunt, of a new seven-day contract, which they considered would impact negatively on medical training, was unsafe for patient care and conflated two issues: the need for a seven-day service and junior doctors' working and training arrangements, without addressing the chronic understaffing and underfunding of the NHS.

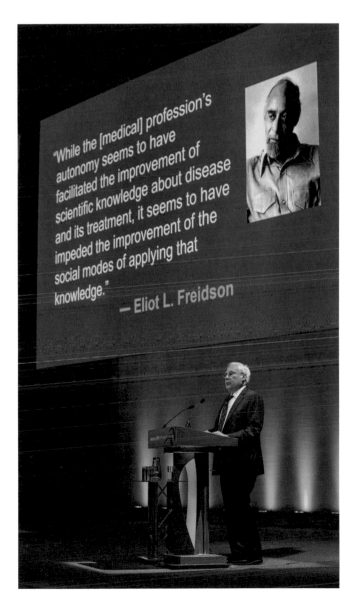

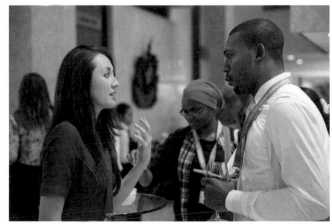

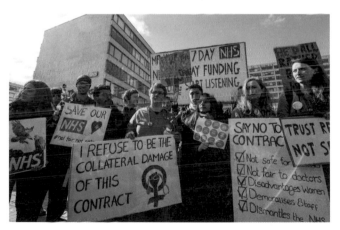

The fellows and members are the Royal College of Physicians, and their voice informs College activities through personal contract and via the College's advisors and tutors, membership research group surveys, elected representatives on Council and the international office and advisors. The number of RCP members increased by 50 per cent between 2006 and 2016, with current retention rates of 92–95 per cent, and with growth in all membership groups. Approximately 75 per cent of the UK membership is outside London and the South East and an objective of RCP North, opened at the end of 2017, is to facilitate access to College activities to a greater number of our members and fellows. The College continues to pursue a robust process to ensure that every consultant physician is considered for Fellowship, and strives to honour distinguished scientific and medical non-physician colleagues, who have made outstanding contributions to medicine, as honorary fellows.

The annual census of UK consultant physicians and trainees, *Focus on Physicians*, establishes data on physician demographics, working patterns, specialty uptake and job satisfaction. For example, the annual census has demonstrated an increased number of consultants (male and female) working flexibly and an increase in female consultants from 18 per cent in 2000 to 34 per cent in 2015. Through an understanding of the environment in which physicians work and the pressures in the NHS, the College can both provide appropriate education and professional training and advocate for physician-related issues to improve healthcare, both within hospital trusts and government.

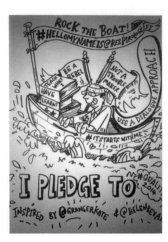

Above: One of a series of cartoons disseminated on social media, pledging to uphold and celebrate the NHS's standards of care. Dr Steve Smith established *Big Up the NHS* in 2013 to emphasise that while there are many problems in the NHS, it is the best healthcare system in the world and 'the casual unjustified swipe at the NHS in the media will cause real harm to real people'.

Right: RCP evening meeting.

Middle right: In 2015, the RCP launched the Faculty of Physician Associates, a new profession of healthcare workers, with the attitudes, skills and knowledge base to deliver holistic care and treatment within the general medical and/or general practice team, under defined levels of supervision. Shown here is one of its publications.

Far right: The College hosts four training faculties: the Faculty of Forensic and Legal Medicine (see crest); the Faculty for Pharmaceutical Medicine; the Faculty of Occupational Medicine (see logo); and the Faculty of Physician Associates.

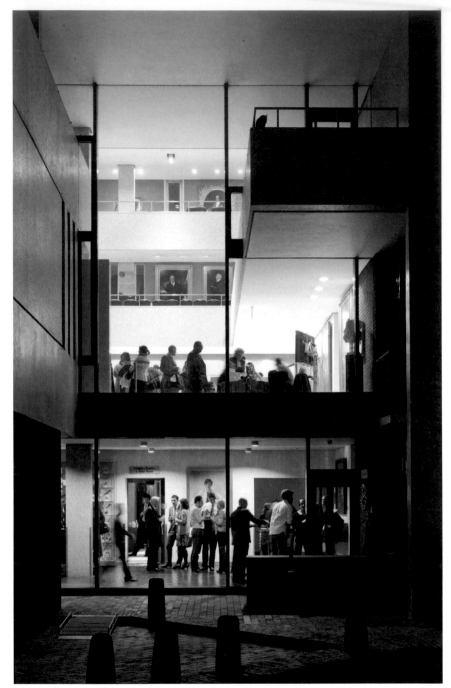

The RCP supports members across all specialties and grades – regionally, nationally and internationally – and engages with its members and fellows through a range of relevant professional platforms, including a recently established annual national conference.

The College network and local knowledge enables support through College advisors and tutors to trainees and, at consultant level, through advisory consultant physician appointments, clinical excellence awards and national honours committees. In cases of local professional difficulties, an RCP-invited service review and/or clinical record review can provide clarity and solutions and, if required, a supported programme of change.

New student and foundation doctor membership categories, with a virtual network, are expanding, supported for example by a careers' programme, financial support for student educational programmes and elective bursaries, which have been as diverse as driving to deliver an ambulance to Mongolia and training in cardiac genetics through work on zebrafish at Harvard. The RCP Trainees Committee provides valued junior representation on all RCP committees and many external bodies, encouraging physicians-in-training to develop active roles in shaping the future of medicine.

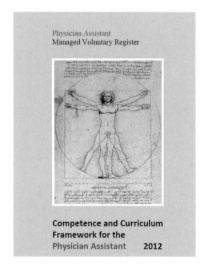

Physician Assistant
Managed Voluntary Register

Competence and Curriculum Framework for the Physician Assistant 2012

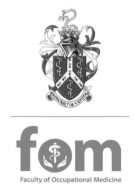

fom
Faculty of Occupational Medicine

'This increase in patient need is outpacing the resources we have to care for them safely… our hospitals are overfull, with too few qualified staff, and our primary, community and social care and public health services are struggling or failing to cope… Our NHS is underfunded, underdoctored and overstretched… People's lives are being put at risk or on hold…'

Extract from RCP Council letter to the Prime Minister, January 2017

Members' views are routinely sought via an online research group enabling problems, such as those detailed in *Hospitals on the Edge*, to be identified. This, in turn, enables early solutions, as exemplified in the RCP's response to the recommendations of the Francis Report and the establishment of the *Future Hospital Programme* to drive change.

The publication of *Underfunded, Underdoctored, Overstretched* and *Being a Junior Doctor* highlighted current issues in the National Health Service, and the series of 'Valuing Junior Doctors' discussions and the 'Keeping Medicine Brilliant' initiative aim to identify solutions to improve doctors' morale, retention and current professional concerns.

Retired colleagues are encouraged to engage in RCP activities and the Quincentennial Society provides a forum for regular meetings of like-minded retired physicians and widows and widowers of physicians on a range of non-medical topics.

Right: Medical student members driving an ambulance from the UK across Europe and Asia to deliver it to Mongolia, as part of their elective in Mongolia, as there was no ambulance in the district in which they were going to work.

Far right: RCP new members' ceremony in the Dorchester Library with the President.

Below: Cartoon illustrating the concerns undermining the NHS.

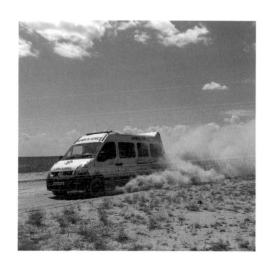

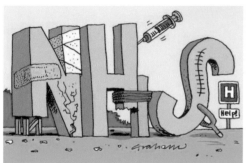

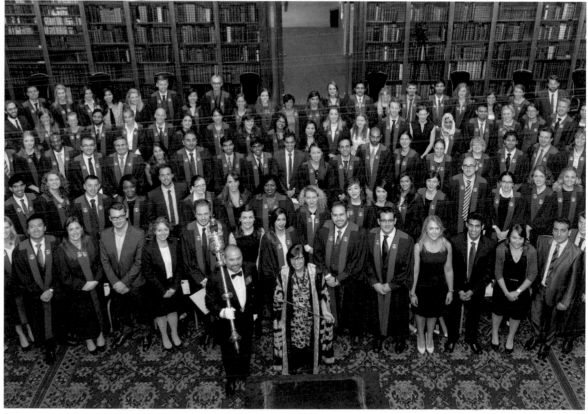

The international office, international fellows, who comprise 17 per cent of the membership based in 80 countries, and 53 international advisors work jointly to embed regionally relevant, physician-led improvements, including access to medical education, quality improvement programmes and organisational, capacity-building initiatives. The RCP is an internationally recognised organisation for training and examining physicians, and oversees the MRCP (UK) with its two Scottish sister colleges.

The RCP International Medical Training (IMT) programme has expanded rapidly, from 79 trainees in 2011 to 300 in 2017. It enables international medical graduates to work and train in medicine in the UK and consolidate their knowledge and skills through the new Diploma in UK Medical Practice, run jointly with the Liverpool School of Tropical Medicine.

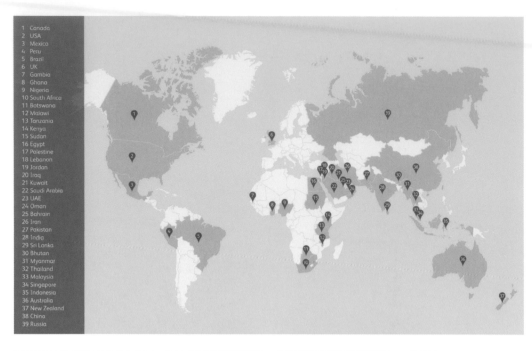

1 Canada
2 USA
3 Mexico
4 Peru
5 Brazil
6 UK
7 Gambia
8 Ghana
9 Nigeria
10 South Africa
11 Botswana
12 Malawi
13 Tanzania
14 Kenya
15 Sudan
16 Egypt
17 Palestine
18 Lebanon
19 Jordan
20 Iraq
21 Kuwait
22 Saudi Arabia
23 UAE
24 Oman
25 Bahrain
26 Iran
27 Pakistan
28 India
29 Sri Lanka
30 Bhutan
31 Myanmar
32 Thailand
33 Malaysia
34 Singapore
35 Indonesia
36 Australia
37 New Zealand
38 China
39 Russia

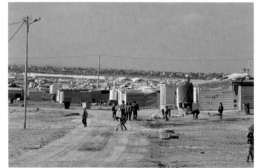

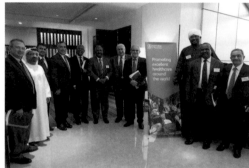

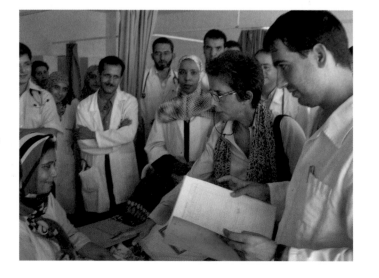

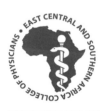

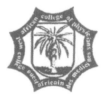

Top: Map illustrating the home countries of the 2017 cohort of current Medical Training Initiative colleagues recruited through RCP.

Middle left: The Zataari refugee camp, 10 kilometres east of Mafraq in Jordan, is gradually evolving into a permanent settlement. Opened in July 2012, it has a population of just under 80,000 (down from a peak of 150,000). The RCP programme aims to pre-empt future healthcare challenges and reduce the need for a medical emergency response.

Middle right: Regional international advisors' meeting.

Bottom left: Professor Dame Parveen Kumar, author with Dr Michael Clark of the internationally respected textbook, *Clinical Medicine*, teaching doctors in Libya.

Bottom right: Logos of the newly established East, Central and Southern Africa College of Physicians and the West African College of Physicians, established in 1976.

Medicine is advancing globally, and the RCP offers its experience and resources to organisations which are promoting good practice. Its international priorities focus on the Middle East, Asia and Africa. Examples include support for the West African College of Physicians, including the current M-PACT programme for infectious diseases training. In 2014, RCP was invited to the foundation meeting of the East, Central and Southern Africa College of Physicians (ECSACOP) with representatives of nine countries: Kenya, Lesotho, Malawi, Mauritius, Swaziland, Tanzania, Uganda, Zambia and Zimbabwe and has continued to support the development of this college. In Oman and India, centres of medical excellence are being established and, in partnership with the Jamaican Ministry of Health and the University of the West Indies, a multi-disciplinary programme of curriculum development and skills training is underway. In Iceland, continuing professional development and core medical training curricula development are in progress, while intensive clinical and communication skills courses are being undertaken in Myanmar.

Following the UK referendum vote of June 2016, in which it was decided the UK would leave the European Union (Brexit), the RCP is advocating to retain the 20 per cent of European doctors (and the many other healthcare workers) in the NHS, which relies on these professionals.

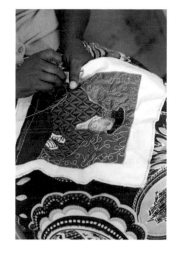

Above and right: Detail taken from the Keiskamma tapestry (see over) made in commemoration of 500 years of the Royal College of Physicians. The Keiskamma Art Project was established in 2000 in the tiny Eastern Cape coastal town of Hamburg. The project has transformed lives in this small community, employing more than 100 people, who have produced a magnificent tapestry to commemorate 500 years of the RCP.

Below left: RCP member and previous Chief Medical Officer's Clinical Fellow based at RCP providing medical support in the Haiti earthquake.

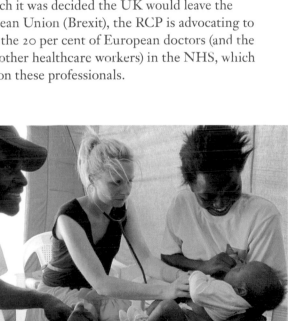

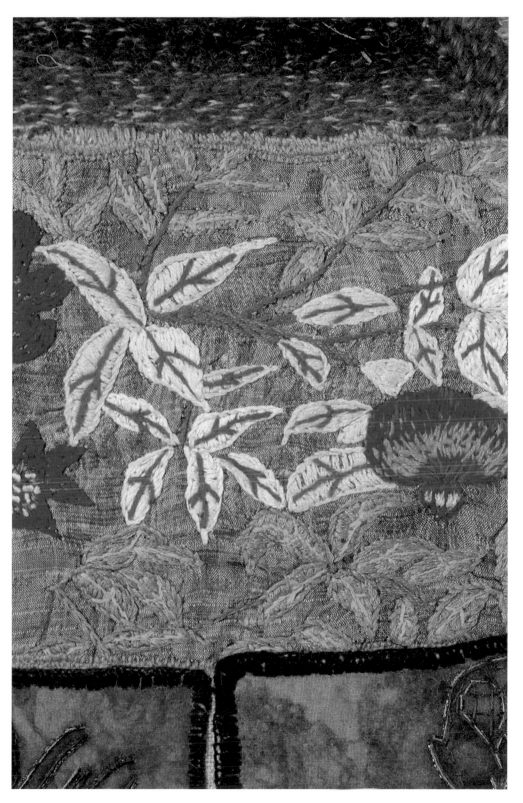

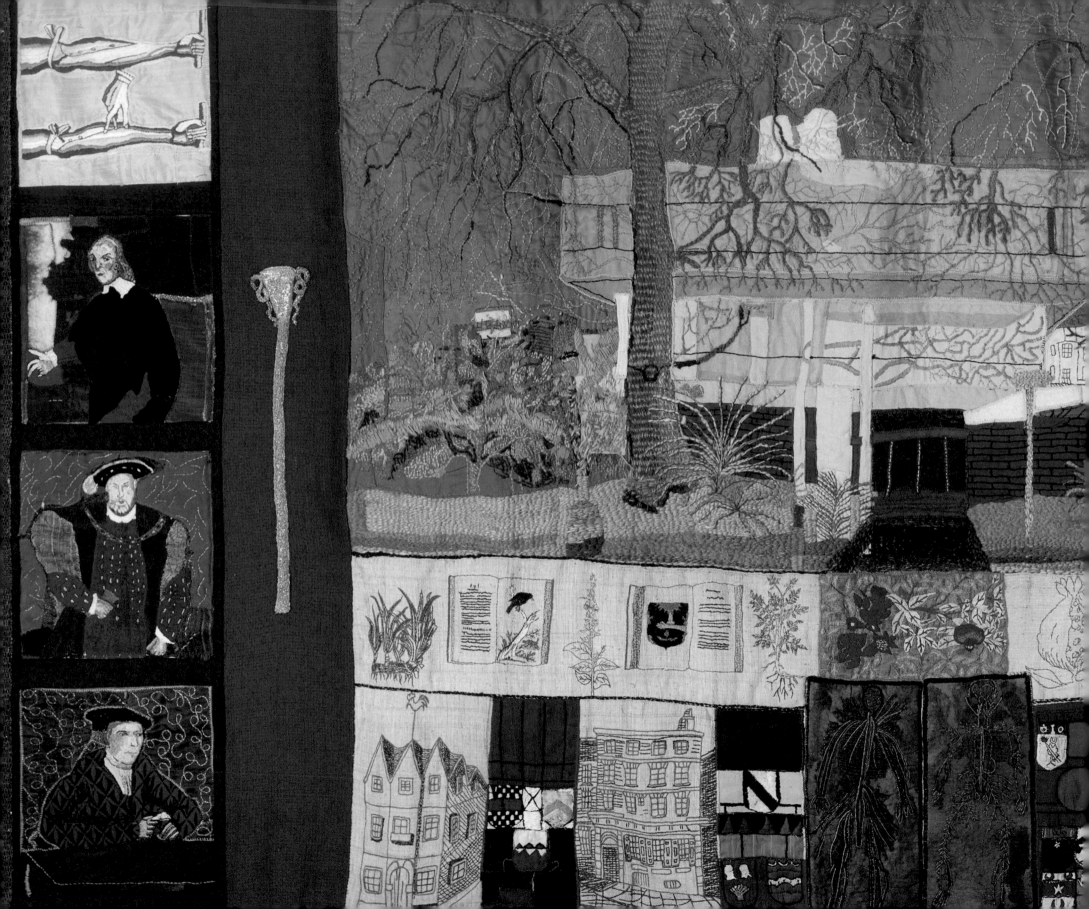

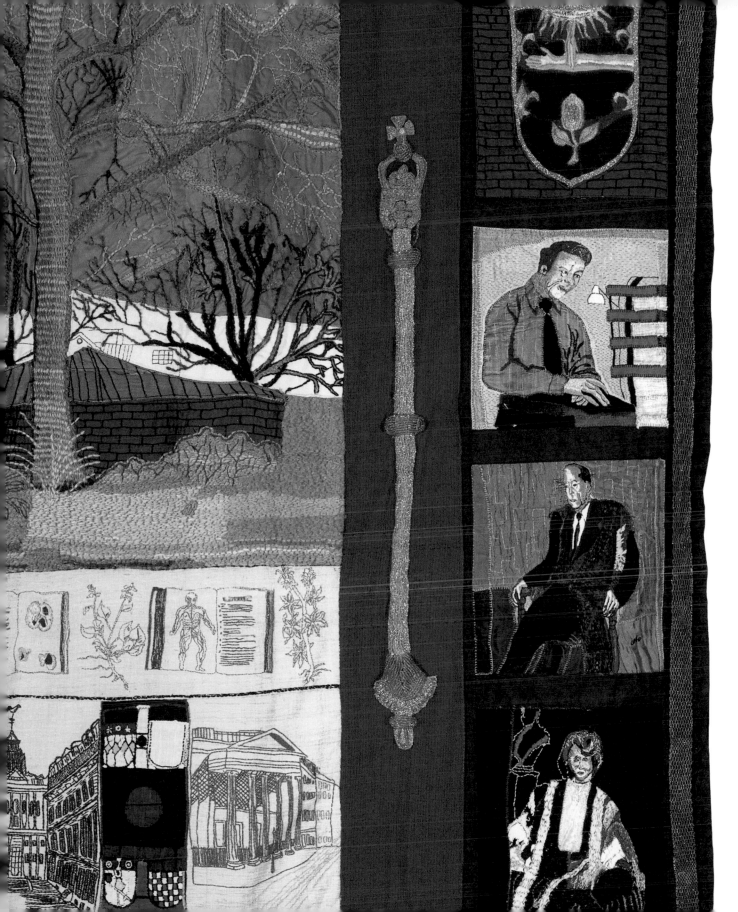

Left: The Keiskamma Commemoration Tapestry illustrating 500 years of the Royal College of Physicians. The tapestry includes images of treasures (caduceus, mace and rare books), the five homes of the College, medicinal plants, Henry VIII, Denys Lasdun, Presidents (Linacre, Platt and Turner-Warwick) and Harvey, with an illustration of his classical experiments.

> *'For public health, climate change is the defining issue for the 21st century.'*

Margaret Chan, former Director-General of the World Health Organization

Healthcare sustainability aims simultaneously to optimise the environmental, social and financial impacts (i.e. 'triple bottom line') of healthcare, without compromising the current and future health of patients and healthcare provision. There is irrefutable evidence that human and social systems are inextricably linked with climate change, which has been described by *The Lancet* 'as the most significant threat of the 21st century', undermining the fundamental determinants of good health globally. The burden and distribution of infectious diseases, poverty, health inequalities, and food and water security have all deteriorated. The health consequences of hurricanes, flooding, heatwaves and emergent infectious disease have all been clearly demonstrated in the last two years, throughout the world.

The College is now committed to the promotion of a programme of healthcare sustainability, not least as the NHS is one of the largest contributors to greenhouse gas emissions in the UK. Recent RCP publications *Every breath we take* and *Breaking the fever* have highlighted the direct effect of climate change and air pollution on increased mortality, morbidity and health service demand.

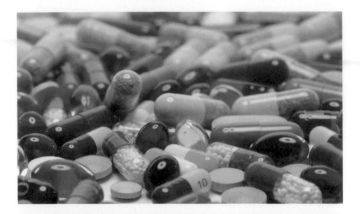

Left: Pharmaceuticals are responsible for the greatest part of the NHS procurement carbon footprint. Key initiatives include: reducing waste by review of every repeat prescription; introduction of a two-stage drug initiation system (where the first prescription is issued for one week, and then the longer course issued a week later, with no additional prescription charge); checking and ensuring drug compliance; minimising wastage and non-compliance with effective written details given to patients (and carers) on discharge.

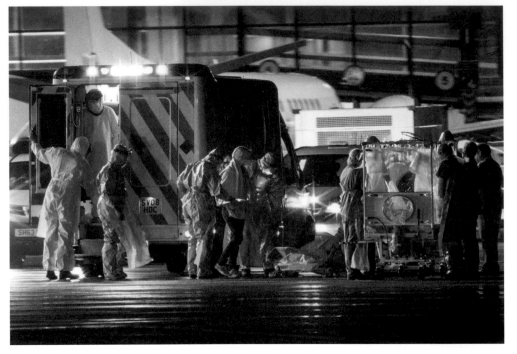

Left: Scottish healthcare worker, diagnosed with Ebola, being transferred in a quarantine transfer tent, from Glasgow Airport to the Infectious Diseases Unit at the Royal Free Hospital in London.

Right: *Anopheles minimus* mosquito, responsible for spreading the drug-resistant *P. falciparum* parasite in Thailand and Vietnam.

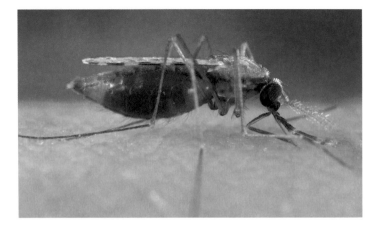

Training and lifelong education are fundamental requirements for physicians, and the Jerwood Education Centre provides national and international outreach programmes. The RCP engages with the General Medical Council, Health Education England, local education and training boards and patients to ensure that higher specialist training has appropriate standards and competencies in internal medicine and the 29 physician specialties. It also focuses on training in leadership and management, education methods (e.g. 'Doctors as educators' programme), research, communication, quality improvement, commissioning and medical professionalism.

The rapid changes in workforce and population demographics, patient needs, technology and healthcare provision, spanning health and social care, require new competencies and flexible curricula. The College initiatives, such as the establishment of RCP North and the Chief Registrar positions, are designed to ensure improved training and work environments for trainees. Electronic online resources include streamed lectures, podcasts, apps and e-learning modules, together with archives of filmed RCP events. To its portfolio of academic, research and clinical conferences, the RCP is now launching an annual educational conference, 'Medical Education: Supporting Learning in the Clinical Environment'.

RCP North will significantly enhance its ability to provide more medical training, examinations, quality improvement and research for doctors and healthcare professionals, in the UK and internationally.

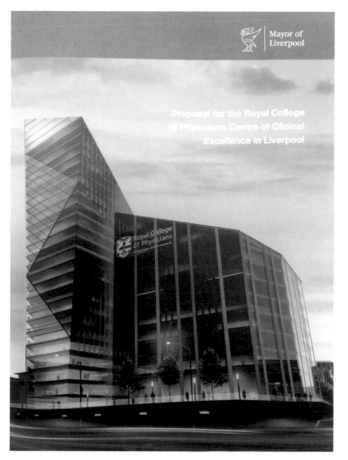

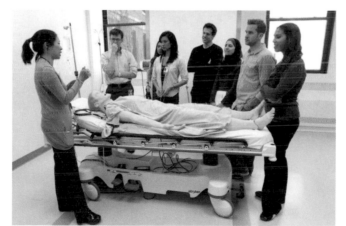

'[The RCP North initiative] animates our strategic commitment to be regionally present and relevant, demonstrating modernity to the membership and fellowship of the RCP, and changing the perception that the RCP is London-centric.'

Professor Jane Dacre, PRCP

Left: An artist's impression of the iconic RCP Centre of Excellence Phase 2 presented as part of Liverpool's bid to host the new RCP development.

Left below: Simulation-based education is a key element of medical training for the current generation. The RCP offers a programme of educating supervisors and is developing a simulation laboratory for future training in RCP North.

Below: Jerwood Medical Education Centre plaque: RCP medical education trains doctors as educators in the clinical environment. There is an MSc programme in medical education and plans to develop research capacity in this area, in addition to training in accreditation, quality improvement and leadership. Lectures, conferences, workshops and electronic resources provide education at all career stages and the RCP has supported educational development of the Faculty of Physician Associates.

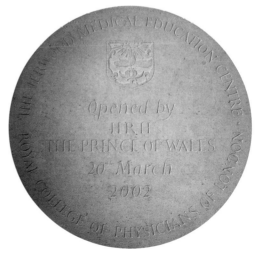

The UK is a world leader in research with 31 Nobel laureates in physiology or medicine and the highest impact factor/head of population (14 per cent most cited articles with 0.88 per cent world population). Embedding research into every physician's practice is a priority for RCP, with expertise in clinical trials, translational science, healthcare improvement, medical education and audit. The recent RCP *Research for all* survey identified that many more physicians would like to engage in research, but are limited by lack of time or funding, and, in response, the joint RCP NIHR *Research Engagement Toolkit* tackles the perceived barriers to research for the jobbing physician. RCP advocates that there should be research time in every physician's job plan, it promotes meetings for research-active trainees and physicians, and has awarded joint (Medical Research Council, Wellcome, Academy of Medical Sciences and National Institute for Health Research) and individual research funding of £526,000 between 2013 and 2014. The 2018 'Giving Health' fundraising appeal will further facilitate RCP's future commitment to research.

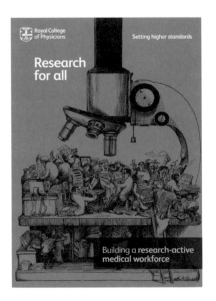

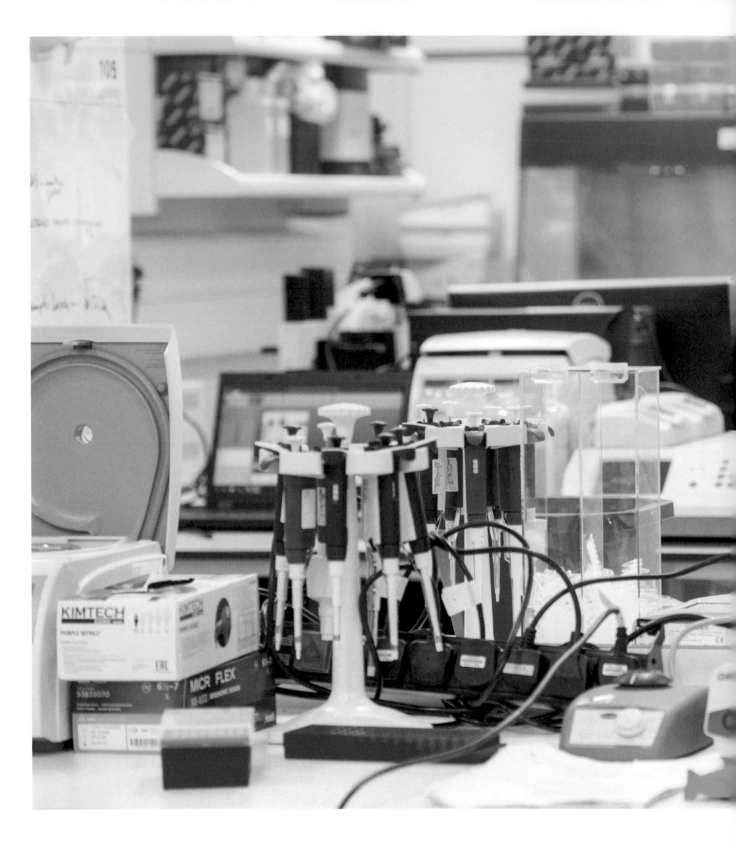

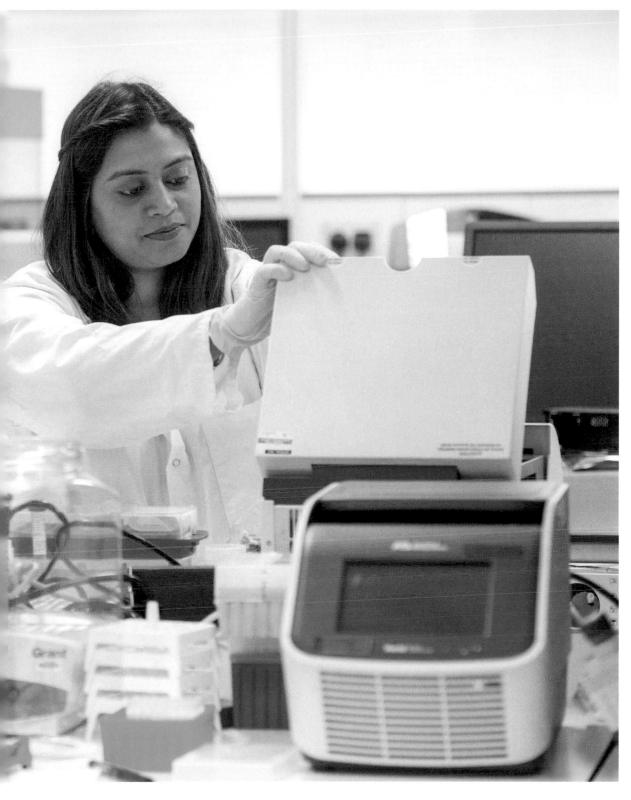

'*Research is to see what everybody else has seen, and to think what nobody else has thought.*'

Albert Szent-Györgyi, who was awarded the Nobel Prize in Physiology or Medicine in 1937.

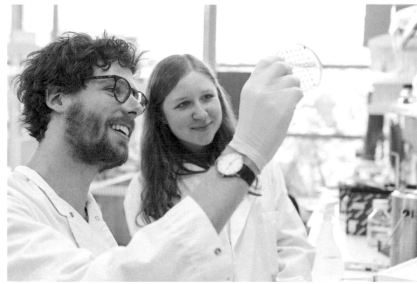

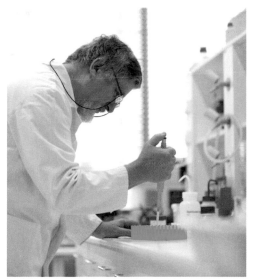

Far left: The UK is a world leader in research, but this is a challenging time for medicine. The RCP champions research for every physician and believes that the only way to continue to keep people well and provide the best treatment is by investing in research that results in better treatments and service solutions.

Left and above: Fellows and members of the Royal College of Physicians undertake research independently and in collaboration in hospitals, universities, scientific institutes, such as the newly opened Crick Institute, and research centres around the world.

The technological revolution is driving progress in biomedical science and healthcare. Nanotechnology, artificial intelligence, wireless technologies, genomics, pharmacogenetics, robotics, stem cell research, imaging advances and other diagnostic technologies, together with universal electronic patient health records, clinical prescribing and warning systems, telemedicine and the analysis of 'big data' are a few of the developments that are likely to transform the practice and sustainability of medicine. In the last few decades, major advances in public health policies, for example smoking campaigns, have led to significant improvements in health, as exemplified by longer life expectancy and a 45 per cent reduction in standardised mortality rates over the last 30 years, with the biggest improvements in the UK in heart disease and stroke.

As medicine continues to change at an accelerating pace, the training and role of physicians must adapt accordingly. Climate change, globalisation and health inequalities, unless countered, will significantly alter disease presentation. The demographics and health needs of the population are no longer focused on single disease pathology in mid-life, but are centred on multiple co-morbidities in the elderly. Added to these changes, the demographics, expectations and diversity of physicians are changing. Flexible and evolving patterns of work and an appropriate work/life balance are major considerations. Healthcare and social care organisational restructuring, as outlined by the RCP's Future Hospital Commission, help improve clinical care, and patient-centred and personalised medicine are becoming the norm. Medicine will become more focused on prevention and early detection of disease, not primarily diagnosis and treatment.

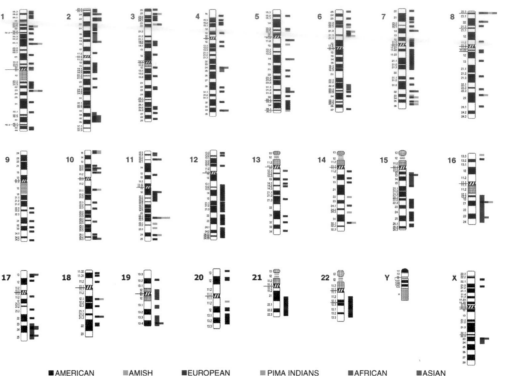

■AMERICAN   ■AMISH   ■EUROPEAN   ■PIMA INDIANS   ■AFRICAN   ■ASIAN

Left: Common obesity is polygenic and about 60 genomic regions are involved in the regulation, the distribution and the quantity of fat-mass, energetic expenditure and regulation of circulating insulin and leptin concentrations (satiety hormones). These regions vary between different populations, as exemplified by the colours listed in the key.

Below left: Deterministic cerebral tractography showing 60 per cent of the observable long-range white matter fibre tracts in a healthy male, captured using a 64-direction diffusion tensor imaging MRI sequence. Viewed sagittally, red, green and blue lines show those tracts which are mainly in the superior-inferior, mediolateral and anteroposterior axes respectively.

Right: New RCP 500 charter: In celebration of its 500-year anniversary in September 2018, the Royal College of Physicians devised a modern charter of its members' professional values.

Opposite right: Physicians of the future networking at the College.

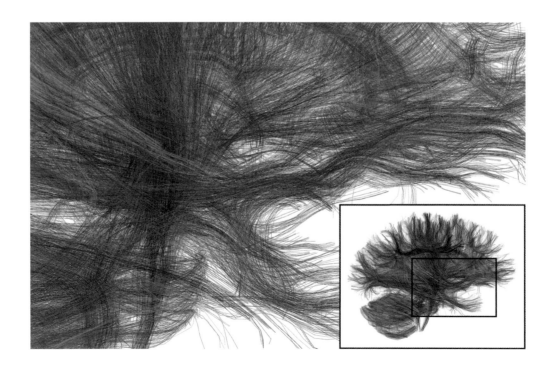

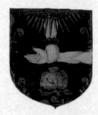

RCP500 Charter

On this, the five-hundredth anniversary of the Royal College of Physicians' 1518 royal charter, we the fellows and members make this profession to our Sovereign, our governments and ourselves, but above all, to our patients.

....

We promise to seek to provide the highest standards of patient care at all times, working with others to treat patients in the manner in which we would wish to be treated ourselves, and to involve patients, their families and carers in decisions about their care.

We promise to train, develop and support other doctors and healthcare professionals at all career stages, to champion research and innovation that improves the care we provide to patients and to commit to our own continuous professional development throughout our careers.

We promise to act as leaders to develop, influence and sustain high-quality healthcare both locally and more widely, to act in our patients' and society's interests over our own and to speak up when it is right and necessary to do so.

We promise to promote good health and prevention of ill health across society, to look after our own health so that we are best placed to look after others and to use our healthcare resources justly and wisely.

....

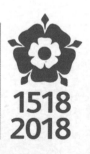

1518
2018

The Royal College of Physicians will remain centred on capturing, harnessing, evaluating and disseminating the rapidly increasing wealth of medical developments and changes to promote excellence in medicine and medical care. Equally importantly, as from its foundation, the RCP will remain a vibrant and welcoming centre for physicians and like-minded individuals to meet, discuss, learn, engage and formulate opinion in all aspects of their academic and professional lives.

'The best preparation for tomorrow is to do today's work superbly well.'

William Osler

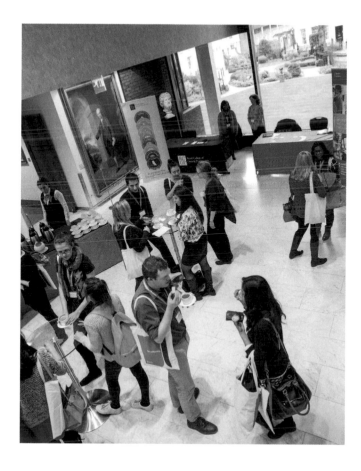

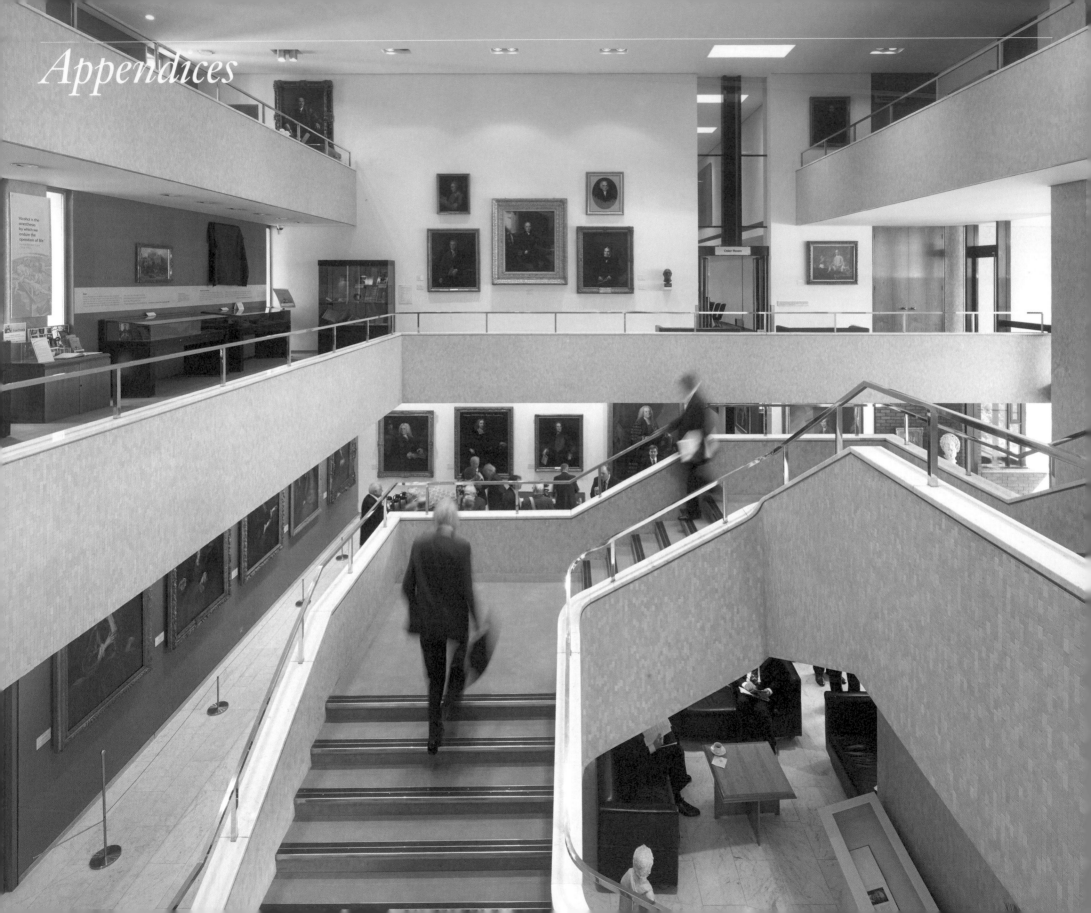

Index

List of subscribers

For consistency, names have been edited to remove titles and postnominals.

Dzifa Wosornu Abban
Sam Abraham
Bhavyang Rameshchandra Acharya
Peter Ackrill
Philip C. Adams
Peter Adnitt
Benjamin Afful
Rasheed Ahmad
Asim Ahmed
Makhzan Israr Ahmed
E. Akoto
Ali Al-Memar
Norildin Al-Refaie
K.G.M.M. Alberti
Mark Aldersley
Nicholas Alexander
Bob Allan
B. Roger Allen
Samuel H. Allen
Stephen Allen
Miles Allison
Qusay Alrahim
Mona Alrukhaimi
Almurtadha Raad Abdulkadhim Altae
Debie Alvares
Osama Shukir Muhammed Amin
Thomas Andrew Scott Amos
Samantha Kay Anandappa
Seetharam Anandram
John Anderton
William James Appleyard
Oscar Aquilina
Judy O.S. Archer
Mary Armitage
Rob Armstrong
Mansel Aylward
Michael Azad
Bijay Baburajan
Trevor Baglin
Alan Bailey
Dale Bailey
Daniel Bailey
Mark Baker
Robert Baldwin
Chitrabhanu Ballav
John Bamford
Andrew Bamji

Soma Banerjee
Ann Banister
David C. Banks
Nicholas Banner
Amerjeet Banning
Ankush Bansal
Peter C. Barnes
Harold Barry
Humayun Bashir
Naghman Bashir
Kolitha Basnayake
Margaret Bassendine
Lofty L. Basta
Anthony Batchelor
Robert Batey
Geoffrey Bayliss
Erol Baysal
Kristin Becker
Gareth Beevers
John Bell
Sam Benady
John Bennett
Stephen Bentley
Jeffrey D. Bernhard
Ranajoy Sankar Bhattacharya
Andrew J. Birnie
David Black
Paul Blake
Carol Blow
Robert Bluglass
Simon Peter Borg-Bartolo
Adetola Borisade
David Bossingham
Brian Bourke
Anthony Bowdler
Noel Gerard Boyle
Gail C. Bridgman
Verena Briner
Warwick Britton
Clement Brown
Ian Brown
Martin M. Brown
Aleck Brownjohn
Murray Brunt
Dudley Bruton
Lawrence Bryson
Jacqueline Bucknall
Ian Bullock
Peter Burdett-Smith
John Burn
Ekaterina Burova
James Burton
Richard Buxton
James Patrick Henry Byrne
Margaret Byron
Joseph Cacciottolo
Julius Cairn
Alexander James Campbell
Martin Carmalt
James Catania
Graeme Catto
Chin Pang Ian Chan
Johnny Ka-Ho Chan
Leslie Chau Nyen Chan
Tai-Kwong Chan
Vivian Nap-Yee Chan
Graham Chance

Joseph Chandy
Carolyn Charlesworth
Amitesh Kumar Chattopadhyay
Owais B. Chaudhri
Humayun Chaudhry
Hugh Chaun
Man Fung Cheng
Chi-Chi Cheung
Chew Chin Hin
Clarence Patrick Chikusu
Teresa Veronica Ching
Peter L. Chiodini
Siew Eng Choon
Theodoros Christophides
Felix Chua
Raymond Chynoweth
Roy B. Clague
Chris Clark
Jennifer Clark
Geoffrey Clarke
Rosemary Clarke
Davis Coakley
Stephanie S. Cobbold
Clive Cockram
Bernard Coleiro
Duncan Colin-Jones
Brian Colvin
C.K. Connolly
Clive Constable
Mehrengise Cooper
John Adrian Copplestone
Chris Corrigan
John Costello
David Cove
George Cowan
Matthew Cowan
Sean F. Cowley
Alan Craft
June Crown
Derek R. Cullen
Philip John Comyn Cummin
Shamaila Dar
Dipankar Datta
Brian Davies
Edward T.L. Davies
Simon W. Davies
Ursula M. Davies and
    Andrew S. Laurie
Josu de la Fuente
Jacob F. de Wolff
John Dean
John Deanfield
Doddabele S. Deepak
Mark Andrew Delicata
Dhanaraja Padubidri Devadiga
Vinod Devalia
Graeme Dewhurst
Ketan Dhatariya
Elissa Kaur Dhillon
John Dibble
M.J. Dillon
David Dingli
Gar-Ling Diong
Peter Disler
Shalin Diwanji
Philip Charles Doré
Huw Dorkins

Mark Dorreen
Thomas Downes
Adrian Draper
Jan Droste
Lewis Drusin
Chris Durkin
Deepak Dwarakanath
Hugh Dyson
Roland Ede
Felicity Edwards
Ruthraj Edwards
Mayen Egbe
Ruvan A.I. Ekanayaka
Jimmy Eric Elizabeth
David Elliman
Cyril Elliott
Michael Ellis
Jan Willem F. Elte
Peter Emerson
Allswell Eno
C.C. Evans
John Howell Evans
Nicholas Evans
Nigel Evans
Sara Evans
Timothy W. Evans
Caroline Everett
David Ewins
Lewis Farrow
John Feehally
David Fegan
Joerg Felber
Garrick Fiddler
Steve Field
J. David Fielding
Roger Finch
Jo-David Fine
Leon Fine
Andrew Y. Finlay
Mihai-Ionut Firescu
John Firth
Murray Fletcher
E. Jane Flint Bridgewater
David Flower
William Martyn Flowers
John Ford
Malcolm Forsythe
Clare J. Fowler
Tim Fowler
Ian M. Franklin
Anne Freeman
Kirk Freeman
Robert Freercks
Jacqueline (Jacky) Frisby
John Fysh
Simon Gabe
Tarek Gaber
Michael D. Gaitonde
Michael Galloway
David Galton
Helena Gardiner
Clifford Garratt
J. Michael Gaziano
Helen Gentles
George Ghaly
T. Michael Gibson
Edward Gilby

Paul Giles
Martin Gillings
William Peter Goddard
Michael Goggin
Ian Gooding
Moj Goonewardene
Mahendra V. Govani
Allison Graham
David Grant
Charles Greenfield
John W. Gregory
Robert Gregory
Bill Gunnyeon
Thea Haldane
John A.S. Hall
Michael Hall
Russell Hall
Henry L. Halliday
Garry Hambleton
Clare Hammond
J.F. Hare
John Gordon Harold
Malcolm Harrington
Kevin Harris
Rodney Harris
Brian Harrison
Peter and Verity Harrison
Lorraine Hart
Timothy Harvey
Stanley Hawkins
Kamila Hawthorne
Nicola Hay
Christopher J. Healey
Barbara Heffernan
Edward B. Henderson
Amy Heskett
Peter S. Hetzel
Geoffrey Hibbard
Caroline Higenbottam
Christopher Hillman
Rowan Hillson
Henry F. Hiscocks
A. Victor Hoffbrand
Barry Hoffbrand
King Holmes
Mary Holt
Gregory Hood
David Charles Domett Hope
Neil Hopkinson
S. Hoque
Richard Houlston
Oliver Howard
James Howe
Nicholas Hudd
Martin Hudson
Elizabeth Hughes
Paul J. Hughes
William Hunter
Nigel Hurst
Elmahdi Hussain
Sin Man Emily Ieng
Stephen Illingworth
Richard J.M. Ingram
Alan Ireland
Sten Iwarson
Michael James
John Casimir Janssen

Ali Jawad
Thilak Jayalath
Ruwanthi Jayasekara
Tilak Jayasuriya
B. Nihal M. Jayawardhana
Ian Jeffery
David Jefferys
Geraint H. Jenkins
Gillian Jenner
Suthipun Jitpimolmard
Howard Jones
Lydia Jones
Phil Jones
Roy Jones
Jith Mathew Joseph
Ajay Kakkar
Dheeraj Kalladka
Peter Kaufmann
Arvind Kaul
Ravindra Kumar Kedia
Mike Kelly
Ruth Kent-Rogers
Kayvan Khadjooi
Roeinton Khambatta
Nassir uddin Azam Khan
Chris Kibbler
Richard Kinder
Brian Kirby
Martin Knapp
Robin Knill-Jones
Thomas Gerrard Koczian
Calvin Koh
Dow-Rhoon Koh
Chin Yong Kok
Behabay Koroma
Christopher Krasucki
Channarayapatna Venkatachala Setty
    Krishna
S.A.M. Kularatne
Parveen Kumar
Bikas Kundu
Mahantesh Kuppasad
Harriet Kwarko
Nikolaos Kyriakakis
Salvador Labrador Y Descalzo
Evmorfia Ladoyanni
Mayur Keshavji Lakhani
Vincent Lamy
Peter Lance
John M. Land
Fernando Larach
A.J. Larner
Mark Lawden
Malcolm Lawson
John Lazarus
B.K. Lee
Thomas Lee
Yuk Tong Lee
David Neil Leitch
King Sun Leong
Richard Keith Levick
Lionel Lewis
Malcolm J. Lewis
Gerald Libby
Zhong Hong Liew
Wei Fong Lim
Robert Lisak

Bernard Lloyd
Howell Lloyd
Alan Lobo
Fiona Lofts
Kathleen Logan
Tuck-Kay Loke
Djamchid Lotfi
Ray Lowenthal
David Lubel
Sing-Leung Lui
John Ma
Graham Macdonald
Andrew F. Macleod
Anita Macnab
Yashwant Mahida
Laurence P. Maidon
Carmel Mallia
James Malpas
Reginah T. Manyeula
Christopher Marguerie
Richard Markham
Gianni Marone
Valerie Marrian
Philip Marriott
Phillip Marshall
David Martin
Raymond Massay
Faris Massoud
Alan Christopher Walter Matheson
Michael Lewis Mattison
Peter Mayer
Janet McGee
Ian McKinlay
Karen McKnight
Brendan Mclean
Chris McManus
Ben Mearns
Thomas Medveczky
Anthony Mee
Harry Mee
Bhasker Mehta
Leon Menezes
Louis Merton
F.R.I. Middleton
Alastair Miller
David Miller
Roger J. Mills
Yalda Savannah Mirzanejad
Andrew R.J. Mitchell
Peter Mohr
Kenneth Moles
Aoife Molloy
Pauline Monro
Anthony Morgan
Terence Morris
Robin Mortimer
John Mucklow
Siobhain Mulrennan
Iain Murray-Lyon
Yulius Mustafa
Chathuranganie Nanayakkara
Firoze Narielvala
Daniel Nelmes
Charles R.J.C. Newton
Chin-Teck Ng
Claire Nicholl
David Nicholl

Gary John Nicholls
Peter Nightingale
Chuka Nwokolo
Peadar O'Mórdha
John Stephen Obbo
Terence Ong
Kofi Oppong
Michael Orme
T. Peter Ormerod
Clive Ostler
Manish Pagaria
Arabinda Pal
Reema Pal
N.D. Pandita-Gunawardena
Peter Panegyres
Tanya Pankhurst
Niranjala Shanthimanoharie
    Paramothayan
Liakat Ali Parapia
David Parker
Robert Parker
William Parker
Michael H. Parkinson
Sonia Parmar
Michael Parr
Nicholas Parry-Jones
Nilima Parry-Jones
Martyn R. Partridge
Maggie Paterson
David Patient
David Patterson
Linda Patterson
James Pattison
Munro Peacock
Ben Pearson
Jeremy Pearson
Stanley Pearson
Richard Peatfield
Amanda Pegden
Ed Poile
Justin Penge
Mark Popys
Alan Perkins
Damian Perrin
Ana Phelps
Marcus Pittman
Anura Piyadigamage
Christopher Pokorny
Joyce Popoola
Madakashira D. Pranesh
Ronald Prineas
Peter Prouse
Robert Prowse and Dorothy Keefe
Charles Pusey
Mohammed Qayyum
Angus I. Rae
David Rainford
Vijayaraghavan Rajendran
Roby Rakhit and Natasha Kapur
V.S. Ramachandran
The Royal College of Surgeons
    of Edinburgh Library
Alan Rees
Paul Rees
Philip Reid
Spyros Retsas
Adrian Reuben

Lesley Elizabeth Rhodes
Michael Richardson
Geoff Ridgway
N.R. Clifford Roberton
Clive J.C. Roberts
Wing Roberts
David Rogers
Richard Rondel
Tony Roques
Alison Ross
Peter Rothwell
Neville Rowell
Derek Rowlands
John Rowley
Adrian Ruddle
Michael Rudolf
Francis Rugman
Louise Sadler
Shahideh Safavi
Harsha Samarajiwa
Sattianathan Sangeelee
Nikhil Sanyal
Amit Saraf
Martin Sarner
Jeremy Saunders
John Saunders
Michael Saunders
Elliott Savdie
Joanna Sawicka
Zuzanna Sawicka
Christopher Sawyer
Howard Scarffe
Stephen C. Schoenbaum
Victoria Scott-Lang
Thomas Sears
Giles Sechiari
Abbas Sedaghat
Jane Selwyn
Carrock Sewell
Kanagaratnam Shanmugaratnam
Pankaj Sharma
James Shawcross
Jeremy Shearman
William Shedden
Bav Shergill
Charles Sherrington
Jeremy Shindler
John Shneerson
Edward Shotter
Alison Shurz
Paul Siklos
Quintus Silva
John Silver
Fiona Sim
Marcus Simmgen
Paul Simmons
Chong Yoon Sin
Kim Yoon Siow
Veluppillai Sivasubramanian
Helen Skinner
Peter J. Sleight
Piotr Ślezak
Sarah Small
Rod Smallwood
Anthony Smith
Russell Smith
David G. Smithard

John and Sarah Smithson
    (née Slaney)
Noel Snell
Upendra Somasundram
Krishna Somers
Ruchit Sood
Illahi Bakhsh Soomro
Gehan Soosaipillai
Geoff Sparrow
Mark Spring
Ramalingam Srinivasan
Margaret Stark
Ian Starke
Andrew Steel
John Stein
Terence Stephenson
Jeremy Stern
John Stoker
Peter Stride
John A. Summerfield
Beatrice Summers
Philip Swales
Howard Swanton
Alan Sweatman
Gillian Swift
Wing-Kin Syn
Soad Tabaqchali
Denis Charles Talbot
P.K. Talukdar
Alfred Yat Cheung Tam
Endean Tan
Evelyn Tan
Francis S.K. Tan
Tilli Tansey
David Taylor-Robinson
I.K. Taylor
James F.N. Taylor
Rod Taylor
Leo-Suan Teh
Yee Sin Tey
Ashish Thakur
Binda Bihari Thakur
Isaac Thambar
Harold Thimbleby
Adrian M.K. Thomas
Gwynne Wilton Thomas
Mark Thomas
Julia Thompson
Graham Thorpe
Michael Tibbs
Fatharrahman Tijany
Sophie Tomlinson
Bing Chung Tong
Nadeem Toodayan
Zaheer Toodayan
Simon Travis
Michael Trimble
Yen Chow Tsao
John Tucker
W. Michael G. Tunbridge
David Turner
Graham Turner
John Turney
Martin Tweeddale
Ploutarchos Tzoulis
Shaughan Ude
Kiran Vadapalli

Allister Vale
Richard van der Star
Mangalakumar Veerasamy
Francisco Vega-Lopez
Athasit Vejjajiva
Sivapragasam Visvanathan
Klaus von Werder
Keith Waddell
Mahmood Wahed
David J. Walker
David Wall
Ian Wall
Ian Wallace
William Wallace
Katherine Walland
Anthony B. Ward
Simon Warren
Steven Warrington
Danie Watson
Roger Watt
Stephen Webster
Jadwiga Wedzicha
Anthony Weetman
Frank Wells
Terence West
Daniel Teo Kok Wey
Robert Whiting
Sheila Willatts
Alan John Williams
Jessica Williams
Meurig Williams
Paul Williams
Roger Williams
Audrey S. Willis
Ivor Wilson
Jean Wilson
Jeremy Wilson
Harith Wimalaratna
Gerrit Woltmann
Ernest Wong
Siew San Wong
Keith Wood
Philip Wood
David F. Woodings
Stephen Woolley
Catherine (Katie) Wright
David Wright
Kevan Wylie
David Yates
Siow Ing Yeo
Andrew Yeoman
Anthony Yip
David Young
Richard Yu
Michael Zatouroff
Ronald Zeegen

Picture credits

pp.6, 9L, 10L, 17, 26–7, 29, 30, 34, 35, 36, 37M & R, 40, 41, 43, 44, 45L, 46L, 47, 48, 49L, 52, 54L, 56, 57, 59, 60L, 62, 64, 66, 67, 69, 71R, 75, 76, 77, 79, 80R, 81L, 82R, 83, 84, 85, 86, 87, 92B, 97, 98L, 99, 105B, 106T & L, 108TL, BL & BM, 110L, 113, 115L, 117L, 130, 131T & R, 132BL, 136, 137BR, 138, 139R, 150, 153TL & TR, 155T, 156, 156–7, 158BL, 162, 163, 166, 167, 169R, 170T, 175TL, 175R, 176MR, 181BL, 182, 183B, 185 **RCP**; pp.8, 9R, 10R, 11BL, 13L, 15, 16L, 18BL & BR, 21T, 23, 25, 39, 42R, 70R, 71 ©**Henry Oakeley**; p.42L ©**Henry Oakeley with kind permission of RCP**; pp.11TL, 14R, 16R, 20L, 22–3, 31, 32, 33T & B, 37BL, 38, 54R, 60R, 61, 63, 68, 74–5, 78, 90, 93, 101, 102T & L, 103, 104L, 106R, 107R, 108TR, 110B, 111TR, 111BR, 112B, 112–13, 116L & T, 118R, 119R, 125L, 128L, 132TL & BR, 133, 134R, 139TL, 161B **Wellcome Collection**; pp.11R, 14L, 24, 45L, 155B, 161TL **RCP/ Mike Fear**; p.12 **DEA/G. Dagli Orti/ De Agostini/Getty Images**; p.13R **LuVo/iStock**; p.18T **Photo12/UIG via Getty Images**; p.19 **HAYKIRDI/ Getty Images**; p.20R **AtWag/ iStock**; p.20B **AlexSid/iStock**; p.28 ©**Courtesy of the Worshipful Company of Barbers/Bridgeman Images**; p.33L ©**Museum of London**; p.46R **The Provost and Fellows of Worcester College, University of Oxford**; p.49R **VCG Wilson/Corbis via Getty Images**; pp.50–51 **age fotostock/ Alamy**; pp.53, 151TL, 159BL & BR, 167 (Brain) ©**National Portrait Gallery, London**; pp.55, 100, 114 **Hulton Archive/Getty Images**;

pp.58–9 **Museum of Fine Arts (Szepmuveszeti) Budapest, Hungary/Bridgeman Images**; pp.62–3 **Look and Learn**; p.65 **Gallerie dell'Accademia, Venice, Italy/Bridgeman Images**; pp.72–3, 82L **Lordprice Collection/Alamy**; p.109TR **Guildhall Library & Art Gallery/Heritage Images/Getty Images**; pp.80L, 119L, 127R **Paul Fearn/Alamy**; p.81R **Emmanuel College, University of Cambridge**; p.88 **Leemage/Corbis via Getty Images**; p.89 **Royal Academy of Arts, London**; p.91 **ART Collection/ Alamy**; p.92L **Florilegius/SSPL/ Getty Images**; p.92T **John Hepner and James Lind Library**; pp.94–5, 96 **Private Collection/Bridgeman Images**; p.98R **Hulton Archive**; p.102R **Private Collection/©Look and Learn/Bernard Platman Antiquarian Collection/ Bridgeman Images**; pp.104R, 115R, 117R, 128R **Punch**; endpapers, pp.105T & R, 122 **Antiqua Print Gallery/Alamy**; p.107B **Time Life Pictures/Mansell/The LIFE Picture Collection/Getty Images**; p.107T **Florence Nightingale Museum, London, UK/Bridgeman Images**; p.108TM **Gordon Museum, King's College London**; p.109TL **Chronicle/Alamy**; p.109B **The Print Collector/Print Collector/ Getty Images**; p.111L **Académie de Médecine, Paris, France/ Archives Charmet/Bridgeman Images**; p.111MR ©**SCM/Science & Society Picture Library. All rights reserved**; p.112T **The New York Academy of Medicine**; p.116R **SSPL/Getty Images**; pp.120–21 **Science History Images/Alamy**; p.123 **The Queen Square Archives**; pp.124, 149TL, 149BL **Popperfoto/ Getty Images**; p.125R **World History Archive/Alamy**; p.126 **Peter Macdiarmid/Getty Images**; p.127L **Bettmann/Getty Images**; p.129 **Courtesy of Dr Andrew Bamji**; pp.130–31, 137L, 139L, 140–41, 145 ©**IWM**; p.132TR **Pictorial Press Ltd/ Alamy**; p.134L **Lebrecht Music and Arts Photo Library/Alamy**; p.135 **ullstein bild/ullstein bild via Getty Images**; p.137TR **British Medical Journal**; p.140 ©**Victoria Crowe/ National Portrait Gallery, London**; p.141TR **Instituto Cajal del Consejo Superior de Investigaciones Científicas, Madrid/CSIC**; p.141BR **Hospital Archives, The Hospital for Sick Children, Toronto, Canada**; pp.142–3 ©**Arcaid 2017**; p.144L ©**Evening Standard**; p.146 **Trafford Healthcare NHS/Press**

Association Images; p.147T **with kind permission of Guy's and St Thomas' NHS Foundation Trust and London Metropolitan Archive**; p.147B **Guy's and St Thomas' NHS Foundation Trust**; p.148L **Mark Kauffman/The LIFE Picture Collection/Getty Images**; p.149TR **gbimages/Alamy**; p.149BR **Heritage Image Partnership Ltd/ Alamy**; p.151TR **Lasdun Archive/ RIBA Collections**; p.151B **from Architectural Design: Ruminations on Architecture by Ken Allison, 2012**; pp.152, 168, 170B, 171, 172, 173L & T, 174TM & BM, 176BL, 186 **RCP/Jonathan Perugia**; p.153BL **James O. Davies/English Heritage**; p.153BR **RCP/Hélène Binet**; p.154 **RCP/Hufton + Crow**; p.158TL & R **St Christopher's Hospice**; p.159TL & TR ©**UPPA Commercial Photographers**; p.160 **Keystone Pictures USA/Alamy**; p.161TR **The Advertising Archives**; p.164 **The King's Fund**; p.165T & R **Imperial College Archives**; p.169L **RCP with kind permission of Michael Weaver**; p.173B **Chris Ratcliffe/ Getty Images**; p.174 **bigupthenhs. com with kind permission of Dr Steve Smith**; p.174TR **Faculty of Forensic and Legal Medicine**; p.174BR **Faculty of Occupational Medicine**; p.176T & ML **RCP/ Iain Fossey, International team**; p.176BR **East, Central and Southern Africa College of Physicians**; p.176BR **West African College of Physicians**; p.177L **Dr C.E.M. Coltart**; pp.177T & R, 178–9 **Keiskamma Trust**; p.180T **aabeele/Shutterstock**; p.180M **AFP/Getty Images**; p.180B **Media for Medical/Getty Images**; p.181T **RCP with kind permission of Liverpool NHS, Universities and City Council Consortium**; p.181R **RCP with kind permission of the Jerwood Foundation**; pp.182–3, 183T **with kind permission of the Francis Crick Institute**; p.184T **from 'Unraveling the Genetics of Human Obesity' by David M. Mutch and Karine Clément, published December 29, 2006 by PLOS Genetics**; p.184B **John McGonigle, Imperial College London**

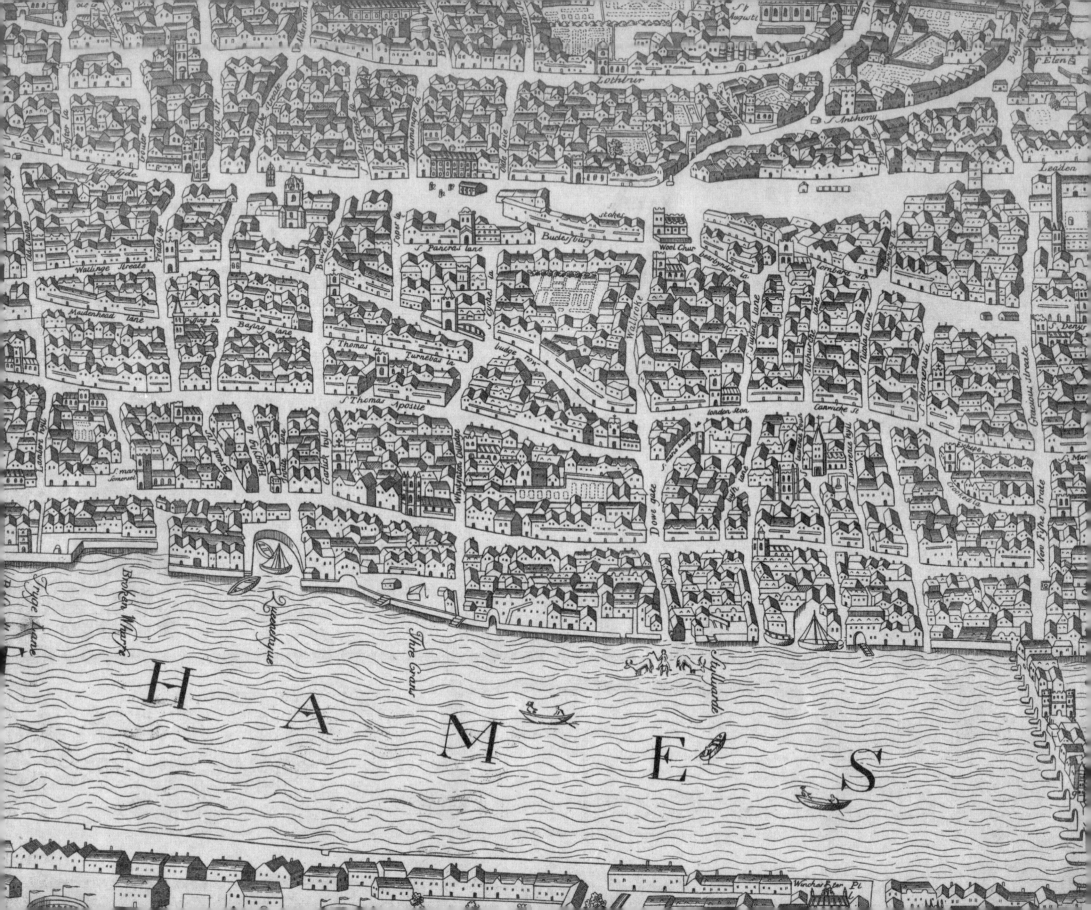